Immunological Insights and Emerging Therapeutics in Medical Mycology

Immunological Insights and Emerging Therapeutics in Medical Mycology

Edited by

Paschalis Vergidis
Section of Infectious Diseases, Department of Medicine, Mayo Clinic, Rochester, MN, United States

Dimitrios P. Kontoyiannis
Department of Infectious Diseases, Infection Control, and Employee Health, University of Texas MD Anderson Cancer Center, Houston, TX, United States

ELSEVIER

ACADEMIC PRESS
An imprint of Elsevier

Academic Press is an imprint of Elsevier
125 London Wall, London EC2Y 5AS, United Kingdom
50 Hampshire Street, 5th Floor, Cambridge, MA 02139, United States

For accessibility purposes, images in electronic versions of this book are accompanied by alt text descriptions independently provided by Elsevier, generated with the aid of AI. For more information, see https://www.elsevier.com/about/accessibility or Radarweg 29, 1043 NX Amsterdam, Netherlands.

Books and Journals published by Elsevier comply with applicable product safety requirements. For any product safety concerns or queries, please contact our authorised representative, Elsevier B.V., at productsafety@elsevier.com.

Publisher's note: Elsevier takes a neutral position with respect to territorial disputes or jurisdictional claims in its published content, including in maps and institutional affiliations.

Notices

Knowledge and best practice in this field are constantly changing. As new research and experience broaden our understanding, changes in research methods, professional practices, or medical treatment may become necessary.

Practitioners and researchers must always rely on their own experience and knowledge in evaluating and using any information, methods, compounds, or experiments described herein. In using such information or methods they should be mindful of their own safety and the safety of others, including parties for whom they have a professional responsibility.

To the fullest extent of the law, neither the Publisher nor the authors, contributors, or editors, assume any liability for any injury and/or damage to persons or property as a matter of products liability, negligence or otherwise, or from any use or operation of any methods, products, instructions, or ideas contained in the material herein.

ISBN: 978-0-443-23636-5

For Information on all Academic Press publications
visit our website at https://www.elsevier.com/books-and-journals

Publisher: Andre Wolff
Acquisitions Editor: Wendi Baker
Editorial Project Manager: Ashavari Bhattacharya
Production Project Manager: Punithavathy Govindaradjane
Cover Designer: Greg Harris

Typeset by MPS Limited, Chennai, India

Contents

List of contributors

Anna Apostolopoulou
Division of Infectious Diseases, Weill Cornell Medicine, New York, NY, United States

Stefano Colombo
Faculty of Biology, Medicine, and Health, Lydia Becker Institute of Immunology and Inflammation, University of Manchester, Manchester, United Kingdom

Oliver A. Cornely
University of Cologne, Faculty of Medicine and University Hospital Cologne, Department I of Internal Medicine, Excellence Centre for Medical Mycology (ECMM), Cologne, Germany; University of Cologne, Faculty of Medicine and University Hospital Cologne, Chair Translational Research, Cologne Excellence Cluster on Cellular Stress Responses in Aging-Associated Diseases (CECAD), Cologne, Germany; Faculty of Medicine and University Hospital Cologne, University of Cologne, Cologne, North Rhine-Westphalia, Germany

David B. Corry
Departments of Medicine and Pathology & Immunology, Dan L. Duncan Comprehensive Cancer Center, Michael E. DeBakey VA Center for Translational Research in Inflammatory Diseases, Baylor College of Medicine, Houston, TX, United States

Bradford Leonard Crowther
Department of Molecular and Cellular Biosciences, University of Cincinnati College of Medicine, Cincinnati, OH, United States; Division of Infectious Diseases, Department of Internal Medicine, University of Cincinnati College of Medicine, Cincinnati, OH, United States

Taiane Nascimento de Souza
Department of Microbiology and Immunology, Albert Einstein College of Medicine, Bronx, NY, United States

George Samuel Deepe
Division of Infectious Diseases, Department of Internal Medicine, University of Cincinnati College of Medicine, Cincinnati, OH, United States

Simon Feys
Department of Microbiology, Immunology and Transplantation, Leuven, Flemish Brabant, Belgium; Medical Intensive Care, University Hospitals Leuven, Leuven, Flemish Brabant, Belgium

Thomas S. Harrison
Institute for Infection and Immunity, City St George's University of London, London, United Kingdom; MRC Centre for Medical Mycology, University of Exeter, Exeter, United Kingdom

Amy P. Hsu
Laboratory of Clinical Immunology and Microbiology, National Institute of Allergy and Infectious Diseases, National Institutes of Health, Bethesda, MD, United States

Joseph N. Jarvis
Department of Clinical Research, Faculty of Infectious and Tropical Diseases, London School of Hygiene and Tropical Medicine, London, United Kingdom; Botswana Harvard Health Partnership, Gaborone, Botswana

Farrah Kheradmand
Departments of Medicine and Pathology & Immunology, Dan L. Duncan Comprehensive Cancer Center, Michael E. DeBakey VA Center for Translational Research in Inflammatory Diseases, Baylor College of Medicine, Houston, TX, United States

John M. Knight
Department of Pathology & Immunology, Baylor College of Medicine, Houston, TX, United States

Dimitrios P. Kontoyiannis
Department of Infectious Diseases, Infection Control, and Employee Health, University of Texas MD Anderson Cancer Center, Houston, TX, United States

Chris Kosmidis
National Aspergillosis Centre, Manchester University NHS Foundation Trust, Manchester, United Kingdom; Faculty of Biology, Medicine, and Health, Manchester Fungal Infection Group, University of Manchester, Manchester, United Kingdom

David S. Lawrence
Department of Clinical Research, Faculty of Infectious and Tropical Diseases, London School of Hygiene and Tropical Medicine, London, United Kingdom; Botswana Harvard Health Partnership, Gaborone, Botswana

Juergen Loeffler
Department of Internal Medicine II, University Hospital of Wuerzburg, Wuerzburg, Germany

Amber U. Luong
Department of Otorhinolaryngology–Head and Neck Surgery, McGovern Medical School, The University of Texas Health Science Center at Houston, Houston, TX, United States

Michael Karim Mansour
Division of Infectious Diseases, Massachusetts General Hospital, Boston, MA, United States

Sibylle C. Mellinghoff
University of Cologne, Faculty of Medicine and University Hospital Cologne, Department I of Internal Medicine, Excellence Centre for Medical Mycology (ECMM), Cologne, Germany; University of Cologne, Faculty of Medicine and University Hospital Cologne, Chair Translational Research, Cologne Excellence Cluster on Cellular Stress Responses in Aging-Associated Diseases (CECAD), Cologne, Germany

Nour Nassour
Division of Internal Medicine, University of Buffalo, Buffalo, NY, United States

Leonardo Nimrichter
Paulo de Góes Microbiology Institute, Federal University of Rio de Janeiro, UFRJ, Rio de Janeiro, RJ, Brazil

Joshua D. Nosanchuk
Departments of Medicine (Division of Infectious Diseases) and Microbiology and Immunology, Albert Einstein College of Medicine, Bronx, NY, United States

Clara Pralon
Paulo de Góes Microbiology Institute, Federal University of Rio de Janeiro, UFRJ, Rio de Janeiro, RJ, Brazil

Laura Seldeslachts
Department of Imaging & Pathology, KU Leuven, Leuven, Flemish Brabant, Belgium

Rosanne Sprute
University of Cologne, Faculty of Medicine and University Hospital Cologne, Department I of Internal Medicine, Excellence Centre for Medical Mycology (ECMM), Cologne, Germany; University of Cologne, Faculty of Medicine and University Hospital Cologne, Chair Translational Research, Cologne Excellence Cluster on Cellular Stress Responses in Aging-Associated Diseases (CECAD), Cologne, Germany

Hua Sun
Department of Otorhinolaryngology–Head and Neck Surgery, McGovern Medical School, The University of Texas Health Science Center at Houston, Houston, TX, United States

Beeke Tappe
Department of Internal Medicine II, University Hospital of Wuerzburg, Wuerzburg, Germany

Alessandro F. Valdez
Paulo de Góes Microbiology Institute, Federal University of Rio de Janeiro, UFRJ, Rio de Janeiro, RJ, Brazil

Greetje Vande Velde
Department of Imaging & Pathology, KU Leuven, Leuven, Flemish Brabant, Belgium

Paschalis Vergidis
Section of Infectious Diseases, Department of Medicine, Mayo Clinic, Rochester, MN, United States

Michael von Bergwelt-Baildon
Department of Medicine III, University Hospital, LMU Munich, Munich, Germany

Joost Wauters
Department of Microbiology, Immunology and Transplantation, Leuven, Flemish Brabant, Belgium; Medical Intensive Care, University Hospitals Leuven, Leuven, Flemish Brabant, Belgium

Sebastian Wurster
Department of Infectious Diseases, Infection Control and Employee Health, The University of Texas MD Anderson Cancer Center, Houston, TX, United States

Daniel Zamith-Miranda
Departments of Medicine (Division of Infectious Diseases) and Microbiology and Immunology, Albert Einstein College of Medicine, Bronx, NY, United States

Preface

Invasive fungal diseases (IFDs) are increasingly recognized as important causes of infectious mortality and clinical morbidity in millions of patients worldwide. The development of antifungal small molecules has been a major advance during the past five decades in the ongoing battle against IFDs; however, the increasing emergence of resistance to antifungal agents and severe immunosuppression limit the efficacy of these compounds. Instead, there is an ever-pressing demand to harness current knowledge of immunotherapeutics, as well as innate and adaptive host defenses, to combat these emerging IFDs.

The field of immunotherapeutics against IFDs is on the threshold of major new advances in detection, immune-based risk stratifications, and targeted intervention in patients with life-threatening mycoses. Following several decades of fundamental discoveries of innate and adaptive host defense mechanisms against invasive fungal pathogens, the field of medical mycology has reached the threshold of potentially transformational developments in immunotherapeutics for treatment and prevention of IFDs.

The ever-expanding heterogeneity of patients with IFDs warrants selective therapeutic approaches based upon the ontogeny and phenotype of their immune dysregulation. Utilizing increasingly available tools for genomics, proteomics, transcriptomics, and other host biomarkers from blood, bronchoalveolar fluid, and cerebrospinal fluid (CSF), where appropriate, can identify specific patterns of immune deficits, their severity, and the probability for development or progression of IFDs.

Accelerated recovery from profound neutropenia by filgrastim (granulocyte colony-stimulating factor [G-CSF]) and sargramostim (granulocyte-macrophage colony-stimulating factor [GM-CSF]) is one of the earliest and widely utilized immunotherapeutic modalities for prevention or treatment of IFDs. The use of interferon-gamma (INF-γ) for prevention and adjunctive treatment of invasive pulmonary aspergillosis in patients with chronic granulomatous disease was also an early landmark event of fungal immunotherapeutics. Among neutropenic and nonneutropenic patients with immune dysregulation, INF-γ, GM-CSF, INF-γ, PD-1 inhibitors, and antifungal monoclonal antibodies warrant further investigation in augmenting innate host responses against IFDs. Immunologic approaches of targeted reduction of deleterious inflammatory responses that injure infected tissue and release danger-associated molecular pattern molecules are also being studied.

Immunological Insights and Emerging Therapeutics in Medical Mycology delineates these advances and discoveries across a wide range of IFDs, immune mechanisms, and novel immunopharmacological strategies. The editors, Paschalis Vergidis, MD, MS, and Dimitrios P. Kontoyiannis, MD, ScD, PhD (hon), are highly distinguished physician-scientists in medical mycology who have carefully chosen internationally recognized experts as authors of the individual chapters. Paschalis Vergidis is as a professor of medicine, attending physician, and expert in medical mycology in infectious diseases at the Mayo Clinic in Rochester, MN, United States. Dimitrios P. Kontoyiannis is a professor and Robert C. Hickey Chair in Clinical Care at the University of Texas MD Anderson Cancer Center, Houston, TX, United States; president of the Mycoses Study Group Education and Research Consortium; and a founding board member of the International Immunotherapeutics Society for Fungal Diseases.

In parallel with their expertise, Professors Vergidis and Kontoyiannis have assembled a slate of world-class authors to address the host defenses, immune risk factors, and possible immunotherapeutic approaches to a wide range of IFDs, including candidiasis, cryptococcosis, aspergillosis, histoplasmosis, and coccidioidomycosis. The text is further enriched by authoritative reviews of immune checkpoint inhibitors and bioengineered T cells. In summary, this book is a timely and essential addition to our understanding of the rapidly evolving field of fungal host defense, immune risk stratification, and evolving immunotherapeutic strategies.

Thomas J. Walsh, MD, PhD (Hon)
Founding Director, Center for Innovative Therapeutics and Diagnostics
Henry Schueler Foundation Scholar in Mucormycosis
Adjunct Professor of Medicine and Microbiology & Immunology
University of Maryland School of Medicine

CHAPTER

1

The case for studying clinically relevant topics in fungal immunology

Paschalis Vergidis[1] and Dimitrios P. Kontoyiannis[2]

[1]*Section of Infectious Diseases, Department of Medicine, Mayo Clinic, Rochester, MN, United States,*

[2]*Department of Infectious Diseases, Infection Control, and Employee Health, University of Texas MD Anderson Cancer Center, Houston, TX, United States*

Despite advances in diagnosis and treatment, invasive fungal infections remain an important cause of morbidity and mortality, and their incidence and prevalence are on the rise due to an ever-expanding population of high-risk individuals with profound and persistent immunosuppression, frailty, and critical illness. Climate change is contributing to the geographic expansion of pathogenic fungi and a rising incidence of allergic airway disease. The rising trends in antifungal resistance due to extensive environmental and iatrogenic use of antifungals frequently devitalize our antifungal armamentarium. Our limited and incomplete understanding of antifungal host immunity, both in health and disease, hinders our efforts to devise effective therapeutic strategies against a variety of clinically important fungi. Furthermore, a better understanding of immune responses would provide the framework for developing novel immunotherapies for our vulnerable patients. This book seeks to address hot clinically relevant topics in Fungal Immunology and brings together contributions from leading experts, covering a broad spectrum of fungal infections. We envision it as a valuable resource for clinicians and researchers seeking a deeper understanding of the field.

Invasive candidiasis is the leading cause of fungal infection among hospitalized patients. There is a vast spectrum of clinical manifestations of invasive candidiasis, from candidemia to deep-seated candidiasis and disseminated infection. Key to the pathogenesis of invasive candidiasis is the transition of *Candida* sp. from a commensal organism on mucosal surfaces and skin to an opportunistic pathogen under conditions that disrupt mucosal barriers and decrease local and systemic host defenses. Neutrophils play a central role in this host defense against *Candida* spp. by employing multiple mechanisms, as reviewed by Anna Apostolopoulou et al. in Chapter 2. Besides phagocytosis, degranulation, and reactive oxygen species production, the authors discuss the formation of neutrophil extracellular traps. Our ability to assess neutrophil responses remains limited. As mentioned by the authors, the only commercially available test is dihydrorhodamine flow cytometry

Immunological Insights and Emerging Therapeutics in Medical Mycology. DOI: https://doi.org/10.1016/B978-0-443-23636-5.00004-6

used for the diagnosis of chronic granulomatous disease. Being able to comprehensively assess neutrophil effector capacity both quantitatively and qualitatively would refine clinical decisions by stratifying susceptible individuals and prognosticating patients with established candidiasis. While progress has been made, further development is required before a comprehensive functional assay can be adopted in clinical practice.

Cryptococcal meningitis is a severe opportunistic fungal infection of the central nervous system, and a major affliction in patients living with HIV. This infection is a leading cause of death and disability worldwide, especially in regions with limited access to antiretroviral therapy. Early fungicidal activity (EFA), which involves serial quantitative cerebrospinal fluid fungal cultures to determine *Cryptococcus* clearance rates in the first 2 weeks of antifungal treatment, has become an important tool in evaluating antifungal regimens for cryptococcal meningitis. EFA serves as both a prognostic indicator and a tool for evaluating the effectiveness of antifungal treatment regimens. In Chapter 3, Joe Jarvis et al. summarize the findings of clinical trials that informed the current guidelines for treating HIV-associated cryptococcal meningitis. The authors discuss the rationale for adding interferon-gamma (IFN-γ) adjunctively to antifungal therapy. A consortium has been formed to conduct an adaptive, open-label, randomized clinical trial using EFA as an important surrogate for response. Interestingly, one or two doses of subcutaneous IFN-γ have shown promise in pilot studies. The alarmingly high mortality rates of cryptococcal meningitis and the unpredictable occurrence of paradoxical and overzealous immune responses, driven by excessive inflammation following treatment, are also reviewed in the chapter and remind us that effective management requires both antifungal strategies and careful immune modulation.

Turning to Chapter 4, Chris Kosmidis and Stefano Colombo review the cytokine immunology and the role of adjunctive IFN-γ in invasive and chronic aspergillosis. For context, invasive aspergillosis typically occurs in severely immunocompromised patients and is characterized by rapid progression, often accompanied by vascular invasion by fungal hyphae. In contrast, chronic pulmonary aspergillosis develops in patients with underlying structural lung disease without severe immunocompromise and progresses slowly over several months or even years. Unfortunately, evidence regarding the impact of IFN-γ on the outcomes of invasive aspergillosis has been limited to case series. Designing a clinical trial presents the challenge of defining primary endpoints that can demonstrate a meaningful benefit of IFN-γ when combined with antifungal therapy. Subcutaneous IFN-γ may be difficult to tolerate, mainly due to constitutional "flu-like" symptoms and injection site reactions. In a study led by Chris Kosmidis, patients with chronic pulmonary aspergillosis who were able to tolerate IFN-γ had a significantly decreased rate of acute exacerbations and hospital admissions. Future clinical trials should be paired with immune profiling to better understand how adjunctive immunotherapy can shape effective immune responses in chronic aspergillosis syndromes.

In addition to the long-recognized risk for patients with hematologic malignancy and transplantation developing invasive aspergillosis, several new at-risk populations have been identified in recent years, such as critically ill patients with severe viral respiratory tract infection (influenza and COVID-19) requiring intensive care. Direct damage to the airway epithelium and virus-associated immune dysregulation, both systemically and locally at the mucosal level, underlie the pathogenesis of the disease. Furthermore, immunomodulatory interventions used in the treatment of SARS-CoV-2 pneumonia (glucocorticoids and interleukin-6 inhibitors) may further impair host immune responses. In Chapter 5, Simon Feys et al. provide a primer on severe postviral *Aspergillus* pneumonia and summarize recent findings on the multilevel disruption of antifungal immunity. Defective conidial phagocytosis, hampered killing of *Aspergillus* hyphae by neutrophils due to impaired NETosis, and reduced *Aspergillus* recognition are the main implicated mechanisms. Much remains to be explored in the field of viral-associated pulmonary aspergillosis, and the unique opportunity to study the disease on a large scale is unlikely to arise again now that the pandemic has passed.

As a medical and scientific community, we recognize substantial gaps in understanding, diagnosis, and management of allergic fungal rhinosinusitis and allergic bronchopulmonary mycoses. The clinical and immunopathological features of these disorders are heterogeneous and often overlap with asthma, leading to frequent underdiagnosis. Furthermore, it remains challenging to establish primary endpoints for clinical trials, as these entities are characterized by relapses and remissions, making it difficult to attribute changes in clinical status specifically to pharmacologic interventions rather than to background disease fluctuations. In Chapter 6, Amber Luong et al. summarize the evidence linking fungi to allergic airway disease and elucidate the immune mechanisms underlying airway mycosis-related allergic disease. They describe the role of immune defenses produced in response to fungal stimuli at the level of the airways. The authors emphasize that patients with allergic mycoses are often excluded from clinical trials of biologic agents, limiting our understanding of their role in fungal airway disease. Several antifungal medications are currently in the late stages of clinical development. Whether these medications can be explored as therapeutic options for airway mycoses remains to be determined.

Histoplasmosis is a fungal infection that can affect both immunocompetent and immunocompromised individuals, although disseminated infection is far more common in those with severely impaired T-cell immunity. Its geographic expansion beyond traditional endemic regions has been linked to global warming. The disease can have protean clinical manifestations, is underrecognized in world regions with limited diagnostic capacity, and is frequently misdiagnosed as tuberculosis. In Chapter 7, Alessandro Valdez et al. review host-pathogen interactions. *Histoplasma* is a thermally dimorphic fungus. Infection is acquired by inhalation of microconidia or mycelial fragments, which convert to yeast forms at body temperature in tissues. These yeasts proliferate within the phagolysosomes of macrophages using specific and sophisticated strategies for intracellular survival. As with other T-cell-associated bacterial, fungal, and mycobacterial pathogens, *Histoplasma* is typically contained within granulomas. Tumor necrosis factor-alpha (TNF-α) is a vital component of the host immune defense and plays a key role in maintaining granuloma integrity. In Chapter 8, Bradford Leonard Crowther III and George Samuel Deepe Jr review key aspects of histoplasmosis associated with TNF-α antagonists (e.g., infliximab and adalimumab), which are biologic agents widely used for the treatment of rheumatoid arthritis, inflammatory bowel disease, and other autoimmune conditions.

Coccidioidomycosis has several distinguishing features that set it apart from other fungal infections. The disease is endemic to arid regions of the southwestern United States and Mexico, and its geographic footprint has been expanding, in part because of climate change and natural events. In the environment, *Coccidioides* grows as mycelia that produce arthroconidia. Following inhalation, the arthroconidia transform within lung tissue into large spherules. Although it commonly presents as a self-limited respiratory illness, coccidioidomycosis can rarely disseminate, such as in patients with severely impaired cellular immunity. However, disseminated coccidioidomycosis can also occur in apparently immunocompetent hosts and in certain ethnic groups, such as Africans and Filipinos. Susceptibility to severe and/or disseminated coccidioidomycosis is likely multifactorial, involving complex genetic deficiencies in innate immune pathways. In Chapter 9, Amy P. Hsu reviews the early events following infection with an emphasis on immune responses triggered by spherule rupture that facilitate fungal recognition. The rarity of disseminated disease presents a significant challenge in establishing associations between genetic variants and risk of severe disease. Hsu et al. discovered a new pathway involved in fungal recognition and response: using whole-exome sequencing, they identified an overrepresentation of variants that impair beta-D-glucan sensing and H_2O_2 production by the pulmonary epithelial NADPH oxidase at the airway level. With advances in whole-genome sequencing, larger patient cohorts, and the application of artificial intelligence, significant progress can be anticipated in understanding the immunogenetics of "outliers" such as apparently immunocompetent patients with severe or disseminated fungal infections.

In recent years, immunomodulatory interventions have been explored as adjunctive therapies for infectious diseases. Among these, immune checkpoint inhibitors (ICIs) stand out, largely due to the extensive clinical experience with their tremendously successful use in cancer treatment. We believe there is merit in exploring immune checkpoint inhibition for infections that lack effective therapies. In Chapter 10, Sibylle Mellinghoff et al. outline the rationale behind immune checkpoint inhibition for the treatment of fungal infections, review preclinical animal studies, and discuss the anecdotal clinical data available. Most importantly, they provide valuable perspectives on strategies to advance ICI therapy toward clinical application. As with any clinical intervention, two key questions need to be addressed: (1) Are ICIs effective? Since these agents are expected to be used adjunctively to antifungal agents, clinical trials with clear endpoints should be carefully designed. The timing of administration is also important: Should ICIs be used early in the course of infection to prevent progression, or should they be reserved for cases refractory to antifungal agents? (2) Are ICIs safe? Potent immune activation in the lungs following reversal of immune exhaustion by ICIs could exacerbate lung inflammation caused by pulmonary fungal infection.

Building on the concept of immunomodulatory therapy, Beeke Tappe and Juergen Loeffler discuss in Chapter 11 another innovative approach to treating invasive aspergillosis: chimeric antigen receptor (CAR)-T-cell therapy. This form of adoptive cellular immunotherapy has revolutionized the treatment of certain malignancies (e.g., B-cell acute lymphoblastic leukemia (ALL), lymphomas and multiple myeloma) over the past decade. It involves the engineering of autologous T-lymphocytes to express synthetic receptors that recognize specific antigens on tumor cells, enabling targeted cytotoxicity. The process entails leukapheresis for the collection of T-cells, *ex vivo* genetic modification, expansion of the modified cells, and reinfusion of the cells into the patient. To date, no clinical studies have evaluated this strategy for the treatment of fungal infections. Implementing CAR-T-cell antifungal therapy presents even greater challenges than immune checkpoint inhibition. First, there are substantial logistical hurdles. The harvesting and modification of T-cells is a laborious and expensive process, which prohibits the use of autologous CAR-T cells in a timely manner. Cytokine release syndrome (CRS) is a well-recognized complication of CAR-T-cell therapy. The risk of severe CRS requiring immunosuppressive treatment may cause hesitancy in using CAR-T cell therapy for invasive fungal infections. Nonetheless, the potential for actively engaging the immune system at the site of infection makes CAR-T cell therapy an appealing direction for future exploration.

The rise in immunocompromised populations, the emergence of drug-resistant fungi, and climate-driven shifts in fungal epidemiology have brought mycoses into sharper clinical focus. Advances in immunology have shed light on the intricate balance between host defenses and fungal virulence, revealing that disease outcomes are often determined by host-pathogen interactions, where host damage is the key outcome influenced by both sides. These insights are catalyzing novel immunotherapeutic approaches that seek to recalibrate host immunity for optimal recovery. The convergence of basic science, translational research, and clinical practice promises a future where fungal infections are not merely managed but strategically intercepted through immunity-informed interventions and personalized approaches. We believe that this book will provide physicians and researchers in clinical microbiology, immunology, and infectious diseases with a deeper understanding of the advancements in Fungal Immunology, which are shaping the mycology field. It is our hope that readers will find the chapters as engaging and inspiring as we did while compiling them.

CHAPTER

2

The role of neutrophil responses in invasive candidiasis

Anna Apostolopoulou[1], Nour Nassour[2] and Michael Karim Mansour[3]

[1]Division of Infectious Diseases, Weill Cornell Medicine, New York, NY, United States,
[2]Division of Internal Medicine, University of Buffalo, Buffalo, NY, United States,
[3]Division of Infectious Diseases, Massachusetts General Hospital, Boston, MA, United States

Introduction

Neutrophils are the dominant cells of the innate immune system. They serve as the first line of defense against invasive fungal infections before a more specific acquired immune process is activated. Infectious and inflammatory processes in an infected tissue area trigger neutrophil recruitment and extravasation from the peripheral blood through the use of proinflammatory cytokines and chemokines. There, neutrophils will recognize and engage pathogens for the goal of elimination. *Candida* spp. are fungi that can be found ubiquitously in the environment. Several species, including *Candida albicans,* are commensals of the human skin and mucosal surfaces (Jarvis, 1995; Romo and Kumamoto, 2020), although in immunocompromised patients, they can cause significant disease ranging from mucocutaneous to invasive infections.

Fungal pathogen recognition

The first step in the neutrophil-pathogen interaction is pathogen recognition. Neutrophils express pathogen recognition receptors (PRRs), such as C-type lectin receptors including dectin-1 and dectin-2, toll-like receptors (TLRs), integrins (e.g., complement receptor 3 [CR3]), mannose receptor, nucleotide-binding oligomerization domain-like receptors, which bind to pathogen-associated molecular patterns (PAMPs). Some of the key PAMPs involved in fungal pathogen recognition include TLR2, TLR4, and Mincle, which bind to the fungal cell wall mannans; TLR9, which binds to fungal DNA; dectin-1, which recognizes fungal beta-glucan; and CR3, which recognizes both beta-glucans and mannans (Brown, 2011; Brown and Gordon, 2001; Netea et al., 2010; Sato et al., 2006; Taylor et al., 2007). The binding of PRRs to pathogen motifs through receptors, such as dectin-1, activates downstream signal transduction pathways involving immunoreceptor tyrosine-based

Immunological Insights and Emerging Therapeutics in Medical Mycology. DOI: https://doi.org/10.1016/B978-0-443-23636-5.00006-X

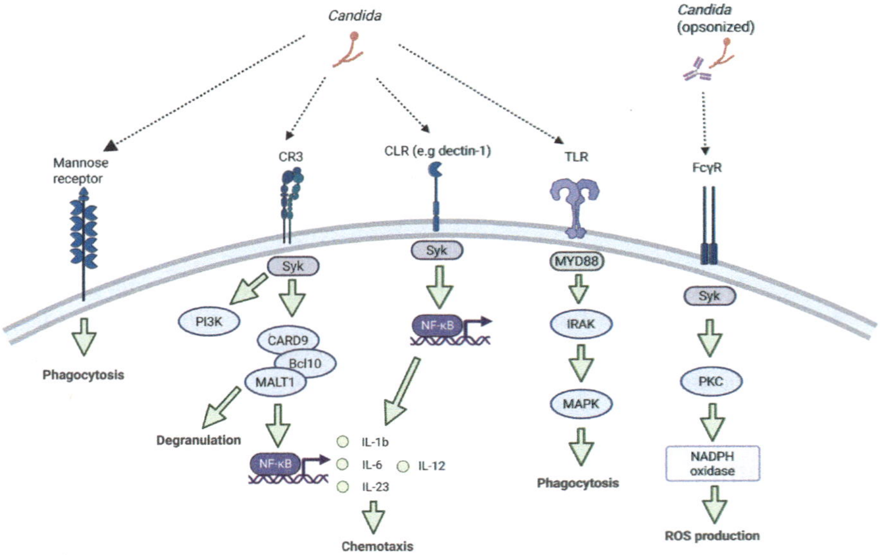

FIGURE 2.1 ***Candida*** recognition and signal transduction.

The schematic shows the process by which neutrophils recognize unopsonized (left) and opsonized (right) Candida and the downstream signal transduction leading to neutrophil activation. BCL10 = B-cell lymphoma/leukemia 10, CARD9 = caspase recruitment domain-containing protein 9, CLR = C-type lectin receptor, CR3 = complement receptor 3, IRAK = interleukin-1 receptor-associated kinase, MAPK = mitogen-activated protein kinase, PI3K = phosphoinositide 3-kinase, PKC = phospholipid-dependent protein kinase, TLR = toll-like receptor.

Created in BioRender. Apostolopoulou, A. (2025) https://BioRender.com/s947p4x.

activation motifs and activation of the spleen tyrosine kinase (SYK) directly. Intracellular signal activation results in the induction of several pathways, including the CARD9-Bcl10-MALT1 cytosolic complex, which leads to NF-κB translocation to the nucleus and expression of proinflammatory cytokines (IL-1β, IL-6, IL-23, and IL-12) as shown in Fig. 2.1. These cytokines promote the differentiation of T-lymphocytes into Th1 and Th17. The downstream effects of the Th1/Th17 response include the interferon (IFN)-γ-dependent activation of phagocytes, further neutrophil recruitment, and production of antimicrobial peptides at mucosal surfaces.

Neutrophil cytotoxicity

Neutrophils possess a multifaceted armamentarium for fungal pathogen killing and control of systemic fungal infections, as shown in Fig. 2.2. Phagocytosis, the

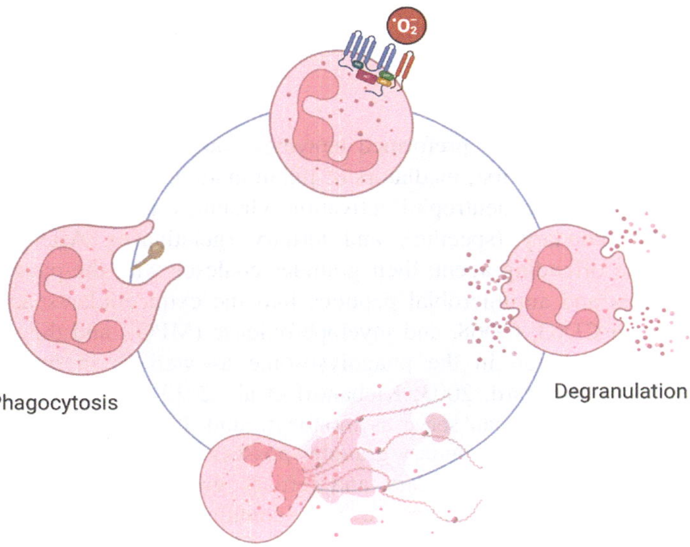

FIGURE 2.2 Key mechanisms of neutrophil cytotoxicity against invasive fungal infections.

The schematic shows the four cardinal mechanisms of neutrophil cytotoxicity against fungal infections: ROS production, degranulation, NET formation, and phagocytosis. NET: neutrophil extracellular traps, ROS: reactive oxygen species.

Source: *Created in BioRender. Apostolopoulou, A. (2025).*

formation of neutrophil extracellular traps (NETs), the generation of reactive oxygen species (ROS), and the release of cytotoxic granules (degranulation) are the key mechanisms of neutrophil cytotoxicity (Mortaz et al., 2018; Selders et al., 2017; Hellebrekers et al., 2018).

Phagocytosis

Phagocytosis is instrumental in pathogen elimination and resolution of inflammation. Human neutrophils have the ability to phagocytose both opsonized and unopsonized *Candida* yeast and hyphae for the purpose of elimination following phagolysosomal fusion. Opsonized yeast interacts with the Fcγ receptors, resulting in vigorous phagocytosis. Both opsonized and unopsonized yeast killing relies on the signaling proteins phosphatidylinositol-3-kinase and CARD9. Both pathways are activated by SYK, as shown in Fig. 2.1. However, these two pathways are independent of each other, as evidenced by the paradigm of chronic granulomatous disease (CGD). In patients with CGD, neutrophils are able to clear unopsonized *Candida*, but not opsonized *Candida* (Gazendam et al., 2014). On the other hand,

CARD9-deficient neutrophils are selectively susceptible to unopsonized *Candida* (Drewniak et al., 2013).

Degranulation

Neutrophil granules contain preformed enzymes, antimicrobial proteins, components of the respiratory burst, mediators of inflammation, and adhesion molecules, which are released upon neutrophil activation. Granules are divided into primary (azurophilic), secondary (specific), and tertiary (gelatinase). After neutrophils phagocytose the offending agent, their granules coalesce with the phagosome and release enzymes and antimicrobial peptides into the extracellular space. Primary granules contain CD63, CD68, and myeloperoxidase (MPO), and they participate in microbial degradation in the phagolysosome as well as in oxidative burst (Faurschou and Borregaard, 2003; Klebanoff et al., 2013). Primary granules also contain defensins, which can serve as monocyte and T-lymphocyte chemoattractants (Yang et al., 2000). Secondary granules possess CD66b and contain multiple enzymes and lactoferrin. Secondary and tertiary granules share lysozyme and CD11b/CD18 markers. Secretory vesicles contain plasma proteins, alkaline phosphatase, and membrane receptors including CD13, CD14, CD18, and CD45. Neutrophil degranulation is a crucial mechanism of killing large *Candida* hyphae that can escape phagocytosis. The importance of neutrophil degranulation in containing invasive candidiasis is highlighted in a mutant murine model with an intrinsic degranulation defect. In this model, systemic *C. albicans* infection led to decreased survival and increased growth of the fungal burden in the kidneys compared to wild-type mice (Swamydas et al., 2016).

Reactive oxygen species production

The NADPH oxidase system is an enzyme system that comprises four cytosolic proteins (p47phox, p67phox, p40phox, and Rac2) and two transmembrane proteins (p22phox and gp91phox). The activation of the NADPH oxidase system has multipotent cytotoxic effects. At an intracellular level, the NADPH oxidase potentiates the transfer of electrons into the phagosome that reduces O_2 to superoxide anion and H_2O_2, which pair with chloride anions to form HOCl (bleach). The production of ROS directly leads to fungal cell killing by oxidative burst and apoptosis. It also activates autophagy, induces NET formation, and leads to inflammasome activation. At an extracellular level, ROS may serve as a regulator for chemotaxis for phagocytes (Hattori et al., 2010; Nauseef, 2019; Röhm et al., 2014).

Neutrophil extracellular traps formation

Neutrophils are also capable of pathogen elimination through the formation of NETs. NETs are web-like structures composed of DNA, histones, and antimicrobial proteins (e.g., neutrophil elastase [NE], MPO) that were first discovered in the early 2000s. The formation and expulsion of NETs are important in the control of pathogen dissemination, especially for large-sized pathogens that are challenging to internalize. This is particularly relevant for fungi, such as *Candida* sp. that form long filaments (hyphae), leading to more effective proliferation and tissue invasion. Both *Candida* hyphae and yeast-form cells induce NET formation and release, followed by entrapment and extracellular killing of the yeast (Urban et al., 2006). NETs are crucial for killing of unopsonized *C. albicans* (Wu et al., 2019). Proteomic analysis of NETs in a mouse model showed that calprotectin contained in the NETs is crucial to the antifungal response against *C. albicans* systemic infections (Urban et al., 2009).

Epidemiology of invasive candidiasis in patients with neutrophil defects

Individuals with congenital or acquired neutrophil defects are at increased risk of invasive fungal infection, including invasive candidiasis (Mortaz et al., 2018). According to the Centers for Disease Control and Prevention (CDC) 2012–16 surveillance data (N = 3492), the crude incidence of candidemia in the United States is 8.7 per 100,000 people, and candidemia accounts for all-cause mortality of up to 30% (Toda et al., 2019). Neutropenia associated with cancer or cancer therapies is the most common cause of acquired neutropenia. Four percent of patients in this cohort had underlying neutropenia (Toda et al., 2019), although in non-US cohorts, reported rates of underlying neutropenia are higher (15%–30%) (Ye et al., 2022; Kim et al., 2021).

Invasive candidiasis can also affect individuals with chronic medical conditions that are not associated with neutropenia, such as diabetes mellitus (DM), solid malignancy, chronic liver and kidney disease, and those who are iatrogenically immunosuppressed, such as solid organ transplant recipients. Patients with DM appear to have a 1.38-fold increased risk of mycoses compared to the general population (Trof et al., 2007). According to the same CDC population-based surveillance study, patients with DM accounted for 33% of candidemia cases, whereas 17% had liver disease, 17% had solid malignancy, and 16% had chronic renal disease, of whom 12% had received hemodialysis during the 90 days preceding the diagnosis of candidemia. Lastly, patients with acquired immunodeficiency syndrome (AIDS) accounted for 3% of candidemia cases, and patients with solid organ or stem cell transplant collectively accounted for 2% of cases in this cohort (Toda et al., 2019).

It is important to note that there are several well-described forms of congenital neutrophil dysfunction that render individuals at an increased risk of invasive candidiasis. These syndromes are relatively rare and not captured well in population-based surveillance studies. Some of these disorders are listed below:

CGD: CGD is a rare congenital disorder of the innate immune system with an incidence of 1 in 250,000 persons that causes individuals to have defective phagocyte NADPH oxidase (Noack et al., 2001; Roos, 2016). Individuals with the disorder experience diminished superoxide production levels, which leaves them more vulnerable to bacterial and fungal infections (Noack et al., 2001). The majority of people experience symptoms in early childhood, and in addition to infections with catalase-positive bacterial and fungal species, patients experience dermatitis, gastrointestinal complications, and even failure to thrive (Lent-Schochet and Jialal, 2024). Amongst these patients, invasive fungal infections, such as those caused by *Aspergillus* sp., and *Candida* spp. amongst others, pose one of the highest risks of mortality (Marciano et al., 2015).

MPO deficiency: The most common disorder of neutrophil phagocytosis is MPO deficiency. The incidence of complete MPO deficiency is 1 in 4000 individuals. Even though MPO deficiency leads to defective in vitro fungicidal activity of *C. albicans*, patients are usually asymptomatic (Klebanoff et al., 2013).

Chediak–Higashi syndrome: Chediak–Higashi syndrome (CHS) is an autosomal recessive disorder that causes decreased phagocytosis and usually manifests as easy bruising, oculocutaneous albinism, and recurrent pyogenic infections (Ajitkumar et al., 2024). It is a rare disorder, with an estimated incidence of <1 in 1,000,000 (Kaplan et al., 2008). CHS typically manifests in early childhood, and the dysregulation it causes in leukocytes renders individuals at risk of both bacterial and fungal infections such as *Candida* (Elin et al., 1974).

Leukocyte adhesion deficiency (LAD): LAD is an immunodeficiency disorder characterized by impaired leukocyte migration and adhesion. It is inherited in an autosomal recessive way, and hundreds of cases have been identified, with an incidence of 1 in 1 million people globally (Dinauer, 2020). Classically, LAD presents with recurrent bacterial and/or fungal infections, neutrophil adhesion defects, and delayed umbilical cord separation at birth (Etzioni, 2007).

CARD9 deficiency: CARD9 deficiency is a rare autosomal recessive condition that renders individuals susceptible to chronic mucocutaneous candidiasis, systemic candidiasis, and invasive aspergillosis (CARD9 Deficiency and Other Syndromes of Susceptibility to Candidiasis, 2019; Rieber et al., 2021; Corvilain et al., 2018). A review study published in 2018 that examined all reported cases of fungal infection in these patients identified fewer than a hundred cases reported worldwide in the literature. The most common fungal infection in these cases was invasive candidiasis, where 15% of cases had central nervous system infections, 8.1% had osteomyelitis and endophthalmitis, and 2.7% had colitis (Vaezi et al., 2018). Individuals with CARD9 deficiency appear to be more vulnerable to *Candida* meningitis compared to individuals with an intact CARD9 signaling pathway (Drewniak et al., 2013; Drummond et al., 2015; Gavino et al., 2014).

Diagnostics

Chemotaxis

Neutrophils follow chemoattractant concentration gradients, such as CXC-type chemokines. Quantitative measurement of neutrophil chemotaxis is usually performed using the transwell migration "Boyden" assay, or similar modified assays (Boyden, 1962; Dinauer, 2020; Zigmond, 1977). These assays utilize a Millipore filter system between two chambers with a gradient across the filter. Chemotactic agents (e.g., N-formyl methionyl-leucyl-phenylalanine [fMLP], keratinocyte chemoattractant) are added to stimulate the neutrophils and their migration, and locomotion is visualized and measured. New experimental data involve the use of microfluidic platforms loaded with a chemoattractant priming solution and time-lapse imaging (Tsai et al., 2019; Ellett et al., 2022).

Phagocytosis

There are two main methods for the assessment of neutrophil phagocytosis. The most commonly used assay is based on flow cytometry and the use of fluorescent targets, for instance, pathogen strains expressing fluorescent proteins. Upon the phagocytosis of these fluorescent targets, neutrophils' fluorescence intensity increases (Lehmann et al., 2000). The second method is microscopy for direct visualization of ingested pathogens, especially electron microscopy, which provides high resolution (Hampton and Winterbourn, 1999). Flow cytometry is less laborious than electron microscopy, and it has the advantage of processing numerous samples in a shorter amount of time. One potential challenge of flow-cytometric assessment of neutrophil phagocytosis is distinguishing between engulfed pathogens and those attached to the neutrophil cell wall. To overcome this potential overlap, a phagocytosis inhibitor, such as cytochalasin D, an actin polymerization inhibitor, can be used as a negative control (Viens et al., 2022).

Reactive oxygen species production

The generation of ROS by stimulated neutrophils has been studied using a variety of methods, including assays of oxygen consumption (Kalyanaraman et al., 2012; Nauseef, 2014), the production of oxygen derivatives (e.g., hydrogen peroxide, superoxide) (Hashiguchi et al., 2005; Yamamoto et al., 1993), chemiluminescence (Hopke et al., 2020; Dinauer, 2020), and the formation of products of redox reactions (e.g., nitroblue tetrazolium reduction) (Gordon et al., 1973). Some of these methods are limited by a lack of specificity or an inability to quantify the production of ROS. Flow cytometry has effectively become the standard diagnostic approach for the measurement of ROS generation. At present, the only commercially available test able to assess neutrophil function in vitro is the dihydrorhodamine (DHR) flow cytometry test. The test specifically evaluates the activity of neutrophil NADPH oxidase by incubating neutrophils with DHR 123, which is oxidized to rhodamine 123, a fluorescent substance detected by flow cytometry (Vowells et al., 1995; Yu et al., 2018). It is a quick, inexpensive, and easy way to evaluate NADPH oxidase activity, and it has superseded the nitroblue tetrazolium test as the gold standard diagnostic tool for CGD (Richardson et al., 1998).

Degranulation

Neutrophil degranulation can be assessed by measuring the expression or enzymatic activity of specific granule markers. Some research protocols use sodium dodecyl-sulfate polyacrylamide gel electrophoresis and Western blot to measure the activity of MPO in neutrophil supernatants after cell lysis (Bedouhène et al., 2020). Others measure the expression of CD markers found in neutrophil granules that move to the cell membrane by flow cytometry. Such markers include CD63 for primary granules, CD15 and CD66b for secondary granules, and CD11b for tertiary granules. Secretory vesicles can be identified by staining for CD13, CD14, CD18, and CD45 (Hashiguchi et al., 2005; Naegelen et al., 2015).

Multiparametric assays

As previously mentioned, flow cytometry-based assays are a promising method to assess neutrophil function and neutrophil–pathogen interaction (Fig. 2.3). Flow cytometry enables simultaneous assessment of several neutrophil functions such as phagocytosis, ROS production, and degranulation (Gupta-Wright et al., 2017; Hesselink et al., 2020; Reiné et al., 2020; Timmer et al., 2023). Such high-throughput assays allow for an efficient assessment of several different neutrophil functions simultaneously. These approaches additionally permit the correlation of specific functions assigned to individual cells, revealing potential subgroups within phagocyte populations.

Swarming assays

First described in 2008 using seminal intravital imaging, researchers have discovered an additional mechanism by which neutrophils eliminate large pathogen molecules such as fungi: a process called "swarming" in which clusters of neutrophils coordinate an attack against a relatively larger target (Chtanova et al., 2008;

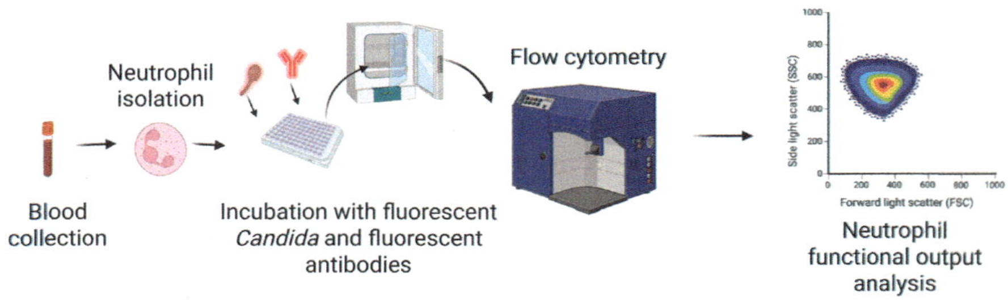

FIGURE 2.3 Workflow of cytometry-based assay for neutrophil functional output analysis.

The schematic shows the laboratory process from neutrophil isolation from whole blood, incubation with fluorescent *Candida* and antibodies, followed by flow cytometry for neutrophil functional output analysis.

Created in BioRender. Apostolopoulou, A. (2025) https://BioRender.com/dmi3rap.

Kienle and Lämmermann, 2016; Peters et al., 2008). The mechanism of swarming has been assessed using several methods in both mouse and human models. While important, mouse models present several limitations that restrict their usefulness, including low throughput, poor molecular signal assessment, and difficulty in translating such protocols in human studies (Hopke and Irimia, 2020).

The use of microscale and microfluid technologies has been instrumental in the understanding of human neutrophil swarming. These technologies enable the concurrent evaluation of the signaling molecules coordinating the process and their interactions with other immune and nonimmune cells (Hopke and Irimia, 2020). In ex vivo experiments, pathogens are organized in arrays, separated inside individual wells in a 16-cell arrangement (Hopke et al., 2020). Commercially available multiwell attachments are used to create the individual wells above microarrays of poly-l-lysine/ZETAG printed onto glass slides, which allow for simultaneous testing processes under different conditions (different microbial targets, neutrophil sources, and treatment conditions) (Hopke and Irimia, 2020). When added to the wells, neutrophils undergo a coordinated swarming response depending on the size of the pathogen clusters (Reátegui et al., 2017). Mediators such as leukotriene B4, a dihydroxy fatty acid, have been demonstrated to play a critical role in mediating the neutrophil swarming process (Hopke et al., 2022; Lämmermann et al., 2013). Swarming responses are directly visualized by time-lapse microscopy, and the area of the swarm can be outlined and quantified (Fig. 2.4).

Assessment of neutrophil extracellular NET-osis

For assessment of NET formation, fluorescence microscopy or spectrophotometry can be used to detect the expulsion of neutrophil DNA into the extracellular space can be used (Urban et al., 2006). This can be achieved by using fluorescent probes (e.g., SYTOX Green) or pathogen strains expressing fluorescent proteins (e.g., *C. albicans* expressing red fluorescent protein) to measure the neutrophil fluorescence intensity (Dinauer, 2020). Other researchers have developed a modified sandwich enzyme-linked immunosorbent assay (ELISA) to measure NETs in human plasma using antiMPO and antiNE monoclonal antibodies as well as a specific antiDNA antibody to detect circulating MPO- or NE-DNA immunoconjugates (Kano et al., 2017). Lastly, Wu et al. have studied neutrophil killing by neutrophil extracellular NET-osis using micrococcal nuclease (MNase), an enzyme that digests neutrophil DNA. By coincubating mouse neutrophils with *C. albicans* and either MNase or heat-inactivated MNase, they observed the difference between NET-independent and NET-mediated killing of *Candida* (Wu and Wu-Hsieh, 2020).

Neutrophil profiling

A comprehensive assessment of neutrophil function includes the assessment of cytokine, growth factor, chemokine, and signaling protein expression. Traditionally,

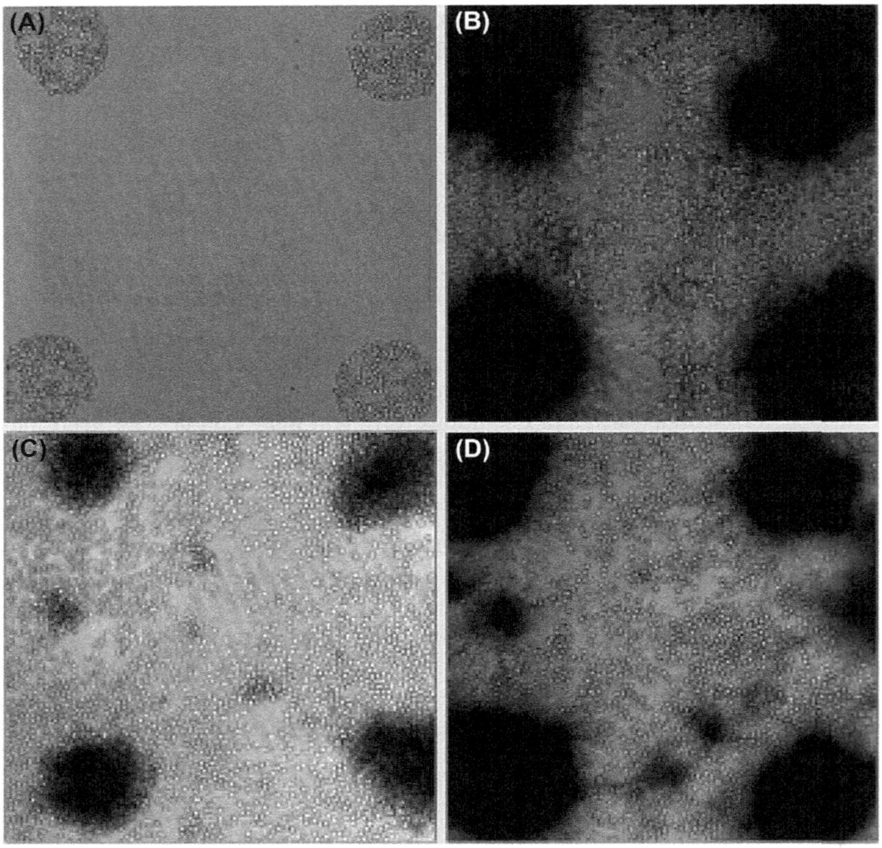

FIGURE 2.4 Neutrophil swarming responses visualized by time-lapse microscopy.

Micrograph images from glass slides spotted with live *Candida albicans* at four corners, then submerged in media at 37°C to allow for growth. Panels represent *C. albicans* alone on the spots at rest, time = 0 (Panel A), *C. albicans* alone after full germination for 24 hours (Panel B), *C. albicans* cocultured with healthy control neutrophils (Panel C), and a matched sample from a patient with neutrophil dysfunction (Panel D). When examined visually, healthy neutrophils restrict control of *Candida* (smaller biomass) to a greater degree than neutrophils from the patient.

ELISA and Western blot have been used to measure the expression of these proteins; however, a composite cytometric bead assay is also available for this purpose. The latter includes fluorescent beads and binding antibodies that can simultaneously detect up to 30 proteins at very low concentrations (<1 pg/mL), allowing for high sensitivity (Naegelen et al., 2015).

Neutrophil killing of *Candida*

In general, there are two methods to assess neutrophil killing of a pathogen: one involving direct enumeration of colony-forming units (CFU) and the other using colorimetric assays of pathogen metabolic activity. Direct enumeration of CFU relies on the ability of the yeast to form colonies on agar after incubation of neutrophils with *Candida*. By comparing this with the corresponding inoculum on a control nutrient agar plate, the reduction in fungal growth can be determined. Manual CFU counting is simple but labor-intensive and relies on the ability of the individual performing it. Challenges exist in the enumeration of hyphae-forming pathogens like *C. albicans* or *Aspergillus* sp., as they may clump, thus limiting the reproducibility and accuracy of the assay. As such, a different methodology, which relies on the reduction of XTT (2,3-bis [2-methoxy-4-nitro-5-sulfophenyl]-5-[(phenylamino) carbonyl]-2H-tetrazolium hydroxide) (a tetrazolium dye) by the fungal NADPH oxidase, was developed to assess fungal cell metabolic activity as a proxy for their viability (Kuhn et al., 2003; Levitz and Diamond, 1985; Meshulam et al., 1995). Reduction of tetrazolium salts or resazurin-based solutions produces colored formazan products, which can be quantified by absorbance or fluorescence.

Therapeutics

Restoring neutrophil count

Iatrogenic neutropenia, typically caused by myeloablative chemotherapy, is usually mitigated by using recombinant human granulocyte colony-stimulating factor (G-CSF), which acts to increase neutrophil generation and release from the bone marrow (Basu et al., 2002). In a multicenter prospective study of patients with hematologic malignancies who received myeloablative chemotherapy prior to autologous stem cell transplant, the magnitude of the leukocyte peak after G-CSF administration was independently associated with a lower incidence of infections (Straka et al., 2011).

A different approach to neutrophil count restoration involves the use of chemokine receptor CXCR4 antagonists for warts, hypogammaglobulinemia, infections, and myelokathexis (WHIM) syndrome, a rare congenital cause of neutropenia. The CXCR4 antagonist works by mobilizing leukocytes from the bone marrow to the peripheral circulation. In a recently published Phase III randomized clinical trial, the CXCR4 antagonist mavorixafor led to a significant increase in time above the absolute neutrophil count (ANC) threshold $\geq 500/\mu L$ and a decrease in the incidence and severity of infections compared to placebo (Badolato et al., 2024).

Neutrophil function augmentation in preclinical models

Priming neutrophils with growth factors and cytokines such as G-CSF, granulocyte-macrophage colony-stimulating factor (GM-CSF), and IFN-γ has been investigated as a neutrophil augmentation strategy against bacterial and fungal infections in both healthy and immunocompromised hosts. These investigations stemmed from the principle that these factors not only induce neutrophil proliferation, but also modulate neutrophil function. In neutrophils stimulated by the chemotactic factor fMLP, both G-CSF and GM-CSF significantly induced ROS production in healthy individuals and a small subset of patients with cyclic neutropenia in vitro (Balazovich et al., 1991).

However, the experimental use of growth factors and cytokines in models of systemic *Candida* infection has yielded variable results. In several in vitro studies of healthy donor neutrophils, pretreatment of mature neutrophils with G-CSF did not result in an increase in phagocytosis, ROS production, chemotaxis, or neutrophil killing of *C. albicans* (Gaviria et al., 1999; Roilides et al., 1991; Shimono et al., 1994), whereas in other studies G-CSF increased the antifungal activity of neutrophils against *C. albicans* and *Candida tropicalis* (Roilides et al., 1995; Roilides et al., 1992). Several studies of in vitro pretreatment of neutrophils with IFN-γ, IL-2, and GM-CSF demonstrated that pretreatment of neutrophils with these cytokines led to a significant increase in neutrophil killing of *C. albicans* (Djeu et al., 1993; Gaviria et al., 1999; Roilides et al., 1995; Yamamoto et al., 1993, 1992). In a recent in vitro study of neutrophils obtained from solid organ (N = 21) and stem cell transplant recipients (N = 19), priming neutrophils with G-CSF and GM-CSF enhanced their swarming and fungicidal activity against *C. albicans* (Barros et al., 2021). In immunocompromised hosts with systemic fungal infection, augmentation may be a promising approach, but larger prospective studies are needed to further investigate this hypothesis.

A different approach has been to leverage the programmed cell death-1 (PD-1)/programmed cell death ligand-1 (PD-L1) pathway as adjunct therapy for fungal infections. In mouse models of invasive fungal infection, blockade of the PD-1 pathway in infected mice is associated with increased survival compared to infected controls. In fact, in a mouse model of *C. albicans* sepsis in immunocompetent mice that received anti-PD-1, anti-PD-L1, or anti-CTLA-4 antibodies, a twofold improvement in survival was reported (Chang et al., 2013). Nevertheless, the effect of immune checkpoint blockade on neutrophils remains unclear, and the proposed mechanism of action of these agents lies in the reversal of the T-cell exhaustion occurring in the context of invasive candidiasis (Mellinghoff et al., 2022).

Neutrophil function augmentation in in vivo studies and case series

Early studies of in vivo administration of G-CSF to healthy individuals resulted in circulating neutrophils with increased MPO activity, opsonin receptor expression, and neutrophil recruitment to the site of infection in one study (Allen et al., 1997) and increased neutrophil degranulation and CD11b and CD66b production in another study (de Haas et al., 1994). On the other hand, an in vivo study of G-CSF administration to healthy donors did not show evidence of increased neutrophil killing of *C. albicans*, while neutrophil killing of *Aspergillus* and *Rhizopus* was significantly augmented (Liles et al., 1997). However, one study group found increased fungicidal activity by neutrophils after prolonged G-CSF pretreatment time (15 hours) (Yamamoto et al., 1993). The use of adjunctive G-CSF and GM-CSF has been associated with complete remission of *Candida* meningitis in two patients with congenital CARD9 deficiency (Du et al., 2020; Gavino et al., 2014). Similarly, in a patient with chronic mucocutaneous candidiasis, the disease was controlled with continuous G-CSF treatment, and recurred upon treatment discontinuation (Shahar et al., 2013). Lastly, we have published our experience of using chronic G-CSF therapy in a young female patient with recurrent infections and a dysfunctional neutrophil response to *C. albicans* as assessed by swarming and killing assays. Although the patient's underlying defect remained elusive after extensive evaluation for immunodeficiencies, her neutrophil response to *C. albicans* improved with in vitro cytokine augmentation, and her frequency and severity of infections decreased significantly (Alexander et al., 2021).

At present, the only practice-changing clinical study of growth factor augmentation in patients with neutrophil dysfunction was the Phase III randomized, double-blind, placebo-controlled trial of prophylactic use of subcutaneous IFN-γ in patients with CGD (International Chronic Granulomatous Disease Cooperative Study Group, 1991). This trial showed both relative risk reduction and delay in the incidence of primary serious infections in the treatment arm and led to the approval of subcutaneous IFN-γ by the Food and Drug Administration in 1990. A subsequent open-label study of long-term IFN-γ therapy in 67 patients with CGD reported very low rates of serious fungal infections and no life-threatening adverse events at the 9-year follow-up (Marciano et al., 2004). Lastly, a recent single-blinded trial randomized critically ill patients ($N = 37$) with reduced neutrophil phagocytosis to either subcutaneous GM-CSF or placebo. Neutrophil phagocytosis was determined as the proportion of neutrophils phagocytosing serum-opsonized zymosan particles as visualized by light microscopy, and <50% was the criterion for study inclusion. The study failed to show a significant difference in the primary endpoint, which was neutrophil phagocytosis at 48 hours after the first dose of the study drug (Pinder et al., 2018). The study was not powered to evaluate for infectious attack rate or mortality, and was unbalanced in terms of baseline neutrophil phagocytosis between the two arms, limiting extrapolation of its results.

Granulocyte and granulocyte-progenitor transfusions

Granulocyte transfusions have been investigated as another promising adjunct to antifungal therapy, albeit with mixed results. Granulocyte transfusions involve blood donation and leukapheresis after priming donors with G-CSF (Dignani et al., 1997). In a retrospective case-control study of neutropenic patients with candidemia, granulocyte transfusions in addition to antifungal therapy were associated with improved survival compared to antifungal therapy alone (Safdar et al., 2004).

Nevertheless, in clinical trials, granulocyte concentrate transfusions have not proven to be more effective than targeted antimicrobial therapy alone in improving survival or infection clearance in severely neutropenic patients with bacteremia or disseminated fungal infection (Fortuny et al., 1975; Price et al., 2015; Winston et al., 1982). This lack of efficacy may be attributed at least in part to the short lifespan of mature neutrophils.

To overcome this limitation of mature neutrophils, researchers focused on the development of granulocyte progenitor transfusions. In a preclinical murine model, ex vivo engineered granulocyte-macrophage progenitors (GMPs) were transfused into neutropenic mice and differentiated in vivo to mature neutrophils in the bone marrow and spleen. The GMPs successfully migrated to inflammatory foci in response to invasive candidiasis and improved the survival of the affected mice (Sykes et al., 2022). In a recent Phase II randomized multicenter double-blind clinical trial, patients with acute myeloid leukemia receiving induction chemotherapy were randomized to the allogeneic myeloid progenitor cell product CLT-008 (Romyelocel-L) in addition to G-CSF versus G-CSF alone. The investigators reported a statistically significant but clinically modest difference in the number of days with febrile episodes from day 15 to day 28 after induction. The median time to ANC recovery was identical in both arms (Desai et al., 2021).

Conclusions

Despite the quintessential role of neutrophils in eliminating invasive candidiasis, our ability to test neutrophil function in clinical practice remains limited. In nonneutropenic patients with chronic medical conditions (diabetes, chronic liver disease), congenital or acquired immunodeficiencies, or those who have undergone stem cell or solid organ transplantation, neutrophil functional assessment would aid in understanding their lifetime risk for fungal infections. Another cohort of interest would include critically ill patients in the intensive care unit, as evidence of neutrophil dysfunction has previously been reported in these groups (Wenisch et al., 2001). We envision that a comprehensive neutrophil functional assessment would help risk-stratify patients into higher- and lower-baseline risks for invasive mycoses and advise antifungal prophylaxis practices. It would also help with the prognostication of therapeutic response in patients who develop such infections.

At present, there is a variety of platforms and assays evaluating specific neutrophil functions, but most are not validated for clinical practice and are only used as part of experimental protocols. Multiparametric assays and protocols that can concurrently examine multiple neutrophil functions and allow for rapid data analysis would be an important area for future research. For restoration of neutrophil count in patients with severe neutropenia, G-CSF is the standard of care. Once identified, the potential use of chronic treatments for neutrophil augmentation, such as IFN-γ or colony-stimulating factors, may provide a safe and effective therapeutic intervention for susceptible patients, although large clinical studies are needed to establish its efficacy.

References

Ajitkumar, A., Yarrarapu, S.N.S., Ramphul, K., Ajitkumar, A., Yarrarapu, S.N.S., Ramphul, K., 2024. Chediak-Higashi Syndrome. StatPearls. StatPearls Publishing, Treasure Island (FL) 2024.

Alexander, N.J., Bozym, D.J., Farmer, J.R., Parris, P., Viens, A., Atallah, N., et al., 2021. Neutrophil functional profiling and cytokine augmentation for patients with multiple recurrent infections: a case study. Journal of Allergy and Clinical Immunology: In Practice 9 (2), 986–988. Available at https://doi.org/10.1016/j.jaip.2020.08.024, http://www.elsevier.com/journals/the-journal-of-allergy-and-clinical-immunology-in-practice/2213-2198.

Allen, R.C., Stevens, P.R., Price, T.H., Chatta, G.S., Dale, D.C., 1997. In vivo effects of recombinant human granulocyte colony-stimulating factor on neutrophil oxidative functions in normal human volunteers. Journal of Infectious Diseases 175 (5), 1184–1192. Available at https://doi.org/10.1086/595866, http://jid.oxfordjournals.org/content/current.

Badolato, R., Alsina, L., Azar, A., Bertrand, Y., Bolyard, A.A., Dale, D., et al., 2024. A phase 3 randomized trial of mavorixafor, a CXCR4 antagonist, for WHIM syndrome. Blood 144 (1), 35–45. Available at https://doi.org/10.1182/blood.2023022658, https://www.sciencedirect.com/science/journal/00064971.

Balazovich, K.J., Almeida, H.I., Boxer, L.A., 1991. Recombinant human G-CSF and GM-CSF prime human neutrophils for superoxide production through different signal transduction mechanisms. The Journal of Laboratory and Clinical Medicine 118 (6), 576–584.

Barros, N., Alexander, N., Viens, A., Timmer, K., Atallah, N., Knooihuizen, S.A.I., et al., 2021. Cytokine augmentation reverses transplant recipient neutrophil dysfunction against the human fungal pathogen Candida albicans. Journal of Infectious Diseases 224 (5), 894–902. Available at https://doi.org/10.1093/infdis/jiab009, http://jid.oxfordjournals.org/content/current.

Basu, S., Hodgson, G., Katz, M., Dunn, A.R., 2002. Evaluation of role of G-CSF in the production, survival, and release of neutrophils from bone marrow into circulation. Blood 100 (3), 854–861. Available at https://doi.org/10.1182/blood.V100.3.854, https://www.journals.elsevier.com/blood.

Bedouhène, S., Dang, P.M.C., Hurtado-Nedelec, M., El-Benna, J., 2020. Neutrophil degranulation of azurophil and specific granules. Methods in Molecular Biology 2087, 215–222. Available at https://doi.org/10.1007/978-1-0716-0154-9_16, http://www.springer.com/series/7651.

Boyden, S., 1962. The chemotactic effect of mixtures of antibody and antigen on polymorphonuclear leucocytes. The Journal of Experimental Medicine 115 (3), 453–466. Available at https://doi.org/10.1084/jem.115.3.453.

Brown, G.D., 2011. Innate antifungal immunity: the key role of phagocytes. Annual Review of Immunology 29, 1–21. Available at https://doi.org/10.1146/annurev-immunol-030409-101229.

Brown, G.D., Gordon, S., 2001. A new receptor for β-glucans. Nature 413 (6851), 36–37. Available at https://doi.org/10.1038/35092620, http://www.nature.com/nature/index.html.

CARD9 Deficiency and Other Syndromes of Susceptibility to Candidiasis I NIAID: National Institute of Allergy and Infectious Diseases. WWW Document, WWW Document, (2019).

Chang, K.C., Burnham, C.A., Compton, S.M., Rasche, D.P., Mazuski, R.J., SMcDonough, J., et al., 2013. Blockade ofthe negative co-stimulatory molecules PD-1 and CTLA-4 improves survival in primary and secondary fungal sepsis. Critical Care 17 (3). Available at https://doi.org/10.1186/cc12711, http://ccforum.com/content/17/3/R85.

Chtanova, T., Schaeffer, M., Han, S.J., van Dooren, G.G., Nollmann, M., Herzmark, P., et al., 2008. Dynamics of neutrophil migration in lymph nodes during infection. Immunity 29 (3), 487–496. Available at https://doi.org/10.1016/j.immuni.2008.07.012, www.immunity.com.

Corvilain, E., Casanova, J.L., Puel, A., 2018. Inherited CARD9 deficiency: invasive disease caused by ascomycete fungi in previously healthy children and adults. Journal of Clinical Immunology 38 (6), 656–693. Available at https://doi.org/10.1007/s10875-018-0539-2, http://www.wkap.nl/journalhome.htm/0271-9142.

Desai, P.M., Brown, J., Gill, S., Solh, M.M., Akard, L.P., Hsu, J.W., et al., 2021. Open-label phase II prospective, randomized, controlled study of romyelocel-l myeloid progenitor cells to reduce infection during induction chemotherapy for acute myeloid leukemia. Journal of Clinical Oncology 39 (29), 3261–3272. Available at https://doi.org/10.1200/JCO.20.01739, https://ascopubs.org/doi/pdf/10.1200/JCO.20.01739.

Dignani, M.C., Anaissie, E.J., Hester, J.P., O'Brien, S., Vartivarian, S.E., Rex, J.H., et al., 1997. Treatment of neutropenia-related fungal infections with granulocyte colony-stimulating factor-elicited white blood cell transfusions: a pilot study. Leukemia : Official Journal of the Leukemia Society of America, Leukemia Research Fund, U.K 11 (10), 1621–1630. Available at https://doi.org/10.1038/sj.leu.2400811, http://www.nature.com/leu/index.html.

Dinauer, M.C., 2020. Neutrophil defects and diagnosis disorders of neutrophil function: an overview. Methods in Molecular Biology 2087, 11–29. Available at https://doi.org/10.1007/978-1-0716-0154-9_2, http://www.springer.com/series/7651.

Djeu, J.Y., Liu, J.H., Wei, S., Rui, H., Pearson, C.A., Leonard, W.J., et al., 1993. Function associated with IL-2 receptor-beta on human neutrophils. Mechanism of activation of antifungal activity against Candida albicans by IL-2. The Journal of Immunology 150 (3), 960–970. Available at https://doi.org/10.4049/jimmunol.150.3.960.

Drewniak, A., Gazendam, R.P., Tool, A.T.J., Van Houdt, M., Jansen, M.H., Van Hamme, J.L., et al., 2013. Invasive fungal infection and impaired neutrophil killing in human CARD9 deficiency. Blood 121 (13), 2385–2392. Available at https://doi.org/10.1182/blood-2012-08-450551, http://www.bloodjournal.org/content/121/13/2385.full.pdf.

Drummond, R.A., Collar, A.L., Swamydas, M., Rodriguez, C.A., Lim, J.K., Mendez, L.M., et al., 2015. CARD9-dependent neutrophil recruitment protects against fungal invasion of the central nervous system. PLoS Pathogens 11 (12). Available at https://doi.org/10.1371/journal.ppat.1005293, http://pathogens.plosjournals.org/.

Du, B., Shen, N., Hu, J., Tao, Y., Mo, X., Cao, Q., 2020. Complete clinical remission of invasive Candida infection with CARD9 deficiency after G-CSF treatment. Comparative Immunology, Microbiology and Infectious Diseases 70, 101417. Available at https://doi.org/10.1016/j.cimid.2020.101417.

Elin, R.J., Edelin, J.B., Wolff, S.M., 1974. Infection and immunoglobulin concentrations in Chediak Higashi mice. Infection and Immunity 10 (1), 88–91. Available at https://doi.org/10.1128/iai.10.1.88-91.1974.

Ellett, F., Marand, A.L., Irimia, D., 2022. Multifactorial assessment of neutrophil chemotaxis efficiency from a drop of blood. Journal of Leukocyte Biology 111 (6), 1175–1184. Available at https://doi.org/10.1002/JLB.3MA0122-378RR, http://jlb.onlinelibrary.wiley.com/hub/journal/10.1002/(ISSN)1938-3673/.

Etzioni, A., 2007. Leukocyte Adhesion Deficiencies: Molecular Basis, Clinical Findings, and Therapeutic Options. Springer Science and Business Media LLC, pp. 51–60. Available at https://doi.org/10.1007/978-0-387-72005-0_5 160.

Faurschou, M., Borregaard, N., 2003. Neutrophil granules and secretory vesicles in inflammation. Microbes and Infection 5 (14), 1317–1327. Available at https://doi.org/10.1016/j.micinf.2003.09.008.

Fortuny, I.E., Bloomfield, C.D., Hadlock, D.C., Goldman, A., Kennedy, B.J., McCullough, J.J., 1975. Granulocyte transfusion: a controlled study in patients with acute nonlymphocytic leukemia. Transfusion 15 (6), 548–558. Available at https://doi.org/10.1046/j.1537-2995.1975.15676082229.x.

Gavino, C., Cotter, A., Lichtenstein, D., Lejtenyi, D., Fortin, C., Legault, C., et al., 2014. CARD9 deficiency and spontaneous central nervous system candidiasis: complete clinical remission with GM-CSF therapy. Clinical Infectious Diseases 59 (1), 81–84. Available at https://doi.org/10.1093/cid/ciu215.

Gaviria, J.M., Van Burik, J.A.H., Dale, D.C., Root, R.K., Liles, W.C., 1999. Comparison of interferon-γ, granulocyte colony-stimulating factor, and granulocyte-macrophage colony-stimulating factor for priming leukocyte- mediated hyphal damage of opportunistic fungal pathogens. Journal of Infectious Diseases 179 (4), 1038–1041. Available at https://doi.org/10.1086/314679.

Gazendam, R.P., Van Hamme, J.L., Tool, A.T.J., Van Houdt, M., Verkuijlen, P.J.J.H., Herbst, M., et al., 2014. Two independent killing mechanisms of Candida albicans by human neutrophils: evidence from innate immunity defects. Blood 124 (4), 590–597. Available at https://doi.org/10.1182/blood-2014-01-551473, http://www.bloodjournal.org/content/124/4/590.full-text.pdf+html.

Gordon, A.M., Rowan, R.M., Brown, T., Carson, H.G., 1973. Routine application of the nitroblue tetrazolium test in the clinical laboratory. Journal of Clinical Pathology 26 (1), 52–56. Available at https://doi.org/10.1136/jcp.26.1.52.

Gupta-Wright, A., Tembo, D., Jambo, K.C., Chimbayo, E., Mvaya, L., Caldwell, S., et al., 2017. Functional analysis of phagocyte activity in whole blood from HIV/tuberculosis-infected individuals using a novel flow cytometry-based assay. Frontiers in Immunology 8. Available at https://doi.org/10.3389/fimmu.2017.01222, https://www.frontiersin.org/articles/10.3389/fimmu.2017.01222/full.

de Haas, M., Kerst, J.M., van der Schoot, C.E., Calafat, J., Hack, C.E., Nuijens, J.H., et al., 1994. Granulocyte colony-stimulating factor administration to healthy volunteers: analysis of the immediate activating effects on circulating neutrophils. Blood 84 (11), 3885–3894. Available at https://doi.org/10.1182/blood.v84.11.3885.bloodjournal84113885.

Hampton, M.B., Winterbourn, C.C., 1999. Methods for quantifying phagocytosis and bacterial killing by human neutrophils. Journal of Immunological Methods 232 (1-2), 15–22. Available at https://doi.org/10.1016/S0022-1759(99)00147-7, www.elsevier.com/locate/jim.

Hashiguchi, N., Chen, Y., Rusu, C., Hoyt, D.B., Junger, W.G., 2005. Whole-blood assay to measure oxidative burst and degranulation of neutrophils for monitoring trauma patients.

European Journal of Trauma 31 (4), 379–388. Available at https://doi.org/10.1007/s00068-005-1025-0.

Hattori, H., Subramanian, K.K., Sakai, J., Jia, Y., Li, Y., Porter, T.F., et al., 2010. Small-molecule screen identifies reactive oxygen species as key regulators of neutrophil chemotaxis. Proceedings of the National Academy of Sciences of the United States of America 107 (8), 3546–3551. Available at https://doi.org/10.1073/pnas.0914351107, http://www.pnas.org/content/107/8/3546.full.pdf.

Hellebrekers, P., Vrisekoop, N., Koenderman, L., 2018. Neutrophil phenotypes in health and disease. European Journal of Clinical Investigation 48 (S2). Available at https://doi.org/10.1111/eci.12943.

Hesselink, L., Spijkerman, R., de Fraiture, E., Bongers, S., Van Wessem, K.J.P., Vrisekoop, N., et al., 2020. New automated analysis to monitor neutrophil function point-of-care in the intensive care unit after trauma. Intensive Care Medicine Experimental 8 (1). Available at https://doi.org/10.1186/s40635-020-0299-1, icm-experimental.springeropen.com/articles.

Hopke, A., Irimia, D., 2020. Ex vivo human neutrophil swarming against live microbial targets. Methods in Molecular Biology 2087, 107–116. Available at https://doi.org/10.1007/978-1-0716-0154-9_8, http://www.springer.com/series/7651.

Hopke, A., Scherer, A., Kreuzburg, S., Abers, M.S., Zerbe, C.S., Dinauer, M.C., et al., 2020. Neutrophil swarming delays the growth of clusters of pathogenic fungi. Nature Communications 11 (1). Available at https://doi.org/10.1038/s41467-020-15834-4.

Hopke, A., Lin, T., Scherer, A.K., Shay, A.E., Timmer, K.D., Wilson-Mifsud, B., et al., 2022. Transcellular biosynthesis of leukotriene B4 orchestrates neutrophil swarming to fungi. iScience 25 (10). Available at https://doi.org/10.1016/j.isci.2022.105226, www.cell.com/iscience.

International Chronic Granulomatous Disease Cooperative Study Group, 1991. A controlled trial of interferon gamma to prevent infection in chronic granulomatous disease. N. Engl. J. Med. New England Journal of Medicine 324 (8), 509–516. Available at https://doi.org/10.1056/nejm199102213240801.

Jarvis, W.R., 1995. Epidemiology of nosocomial fungal infections, with emphasis on candida species. Clinical Infectious Diseases 20 (6), 1526–1530. Available at https://doi.org/10.1093/clinids/20.6.1526.

Kalyanaraman, B., Darley-Usmar, V., Davies, K.J.A., Dennery, P.A., Forman, H.J., Grisham, M.B., et al., 2012. Measuring reactive oxygen and nitrogen species with fluorescent probes: challenges and limitations. Free Radical Biology and Medicine 52 (1), 1–6. Available at https://doi.org/10.1016/j.freeradbiomed.2011.09.030, www.elsevier.com/locate/freeradbiomed.

Kano, H., Aminul Huq, M., Tsuda, M., Noguchi, H., Takeyama, N., 2017. Sandwich ELISA for circulating myeloperoxidase- and neutrophil elastase-DNA complexes released from neutrophil extracellular traps. Advanced Techniques in Biology & Medicine 05 (01). Available at https://doi.org/10.4172/2379-1764.1000196.

Kaplan, J., De Domenico, I., Ward, D.M.V., 2008. Chediak-Higashi syndrome. Current Opinion in Hematology 15 (1), 22–29. Available at https://doi.org/10.1097/MOH.0b013e3282f2bcce.

Kienle, K., Lämmermann, T., 2016. Neutrophil swarming: an essential process of the neutrophil tissue response. Immunological Reviews 273 (1), 76–93. Available at https://doi.org/10.1111/imr.12458.

Kim, J.H., Suh, J.W., Kim, M.J., 2021. Epidemiological trends of candidemia and the impact of adherence to the candidemia guideline: six-year single-center experience.

Journal of Fungi 7 (4). Available at https://doi.org/10.3390/jof7040275, https://www.mdpi.com/2309-608X/7/4/275/pdf.

Klebanoff, S.J., Kettle, A.J., Rosen, H., Winterbourn, C.C., Nauseef, W.M., 2013. Myeloperoxidase: a front-line defender against phagocytosed microorganisms. Journal of Leukocyte Biology 93 (2), 185–198. Available at https://doi.org/10.1189/jlb.0712349, http://www.jleukbio.org/content/93/2/185.full.pdf+html.

Kuhn, D.M., Balkis, M., Chandra, J., Mukherjee, P.K., Ghannoum, M.A., 2003. Uses and limitations of the XTT assay in studies of Candida growth and metabolism. Journal of Clinical Microbiology 41 (1), 506–508. Available at https://doi.org/10.1128/jcm.41.1.506-508.2003.

Lämmermann, T., Afonso, P.V., Angermann, B.R., Wang, J.M., Kastenmüller, W., Parent, C.A., et al., 2013. Neutrophil swarms require LTB4 and integrins at sites of cell death in vivo. Nature 498 (7454), 371–375. Available at https://doi.org/10.1038/nature12175.

Lehmann, A.K., Sørnes, S., Halstensen, A., 2000. Phagocytosis: measurement by flow cytometry. Journal of Immunological Methods 243 (1-2), 229–242. Available at https://doi.org/10.1016/S0022-1759(00)00237-4.

Lent-Schochet, D., Jialal, I., 2024. Chronic Granulomatous Disease. StatPearls. StatPearls Publishing.

Levitz, S.M., Diamond, R.D., 1985. A rapid colorimetric assay of fungal viability with the tetrazolium salt MTT. Journal of Infectious Diseases 152 (5), 938–945. Available at https://doi.org/10.1093/infdis/152.5.938.

Liles, W.C., Huang, J.E., Van Burik, J.A.H., Bowden, R.A., Dale, D.C., 1997. Granulocyte colony-stimulating factor administered in vivo augments neutrophil-mediated activity against opportunistic fungal pathogens. Journal of Infectious Diseases 175 (4), 1012–1015. Available at https://doi.org/10.1086/513961, http://jid.oxfordjournals.org/content/current.

Marciano, B.E., Wesley, R., De Carlo, E.S., Anderson, V.L., Barnhart, L.A., Darnell, D., et al., 2004. Long-term interferon- therapy for patients with chronic granulomatous disease. Clinical Infectious Diseases 39 (5), 692–699. Available at https://doi.org/10.1086/422993.

Marciano, B.E., Spalding, C., Fitzgerald, A., Mann, D., Brown, T., Osgood, S., et al., 2015. Common severe infections in chronic granulomatous disease. Clinical Infectious Diseases 60 (8), 1176–1183. Available at https://doi.org/10.1093/cid/ciu1154, http://cid.oxfordjournals.org/content/by/year.

Mellinghoff, S.C., Thelen, M., Bruns, C., Garcia-Marquez, M., Hartmann, P., Lammertz, T., et al., 2022. T-cells of invasive candidiasis patients show patterns of T-cell-exhaustion suggesting checkpoint blockade as treatment option. Journal of Infection 84 (2), 237–247. Available at https://doi.org/10.1016/j.jinf.2021.12.009, http://www.elsevier.com/inca/publications/store/6/2/3/0/5/4/index.htt.

Meshulam, T., Levitz, S.M., Christin, L., Diamond, R.D., 1995. A simplified new assay for assessment of fungal cell damage with the tetrazolium dye, (2,3)-bis-(2-methoxy-4-nitro-5-sulphenyl)-(2H)-tetrazolium-5-carboxanilide (XTT). Journal of Infectious Diseases 172 (4), 1153–1156. Available at https://doi.org/10.1093/infdis/172.4.1153.

Mortaz, E., Alipoor, S.D., Adcock, I.M., Mumby, S., Koenderman, L., 2018. Update on neutrophil function in severe inflammation. Frontiers in Immunology 9. Available at https://doi.org/10.3389/fimmu.2018.02171, www.frontiersin.org/Immunology.

Naegelen, I., Beaume, N., Plançon, S., Schenten, V., Tschirhart, E.J., Bréchard, S., 2015. Regulation of neutrophil degranulation and cytokine secretion: a novel model approach based on linear fitting. Journal of Immunology Research 2015. Available at https://doi.org/10.1155/2015/817038, http://www.hindawi.com/journals/jir/.

Nauseef, W.M., 2014. Detection of superoxide anion and hydrogen peroxide production by cellular NADPH oxidases. Biochimica et Biophysica Acta - General Subjects 1840 (2), 757–767. Available at https://doi.org/10.1016/j.bbagen.2013.04.040.

Nauseef, W.M., 2019. The phagocyte NOX2 NADPH oxidase in microbial killing and cell signaling. Current Opinion in Immunology 60, 130–140. Available at https://doi.org/10.1016/j.coi.2019.05.006, http://www.journals.elsevier.com/current-opinion-in-immunology/.

Netea, M.G., Gow, N.A.R., Joosten, L.A.B., Verschueren, I., Van Der Meer, J.W.M., Kullberg, B.J., 2010. Variable recognition of Candida albicans strains by TLR4 and lectin recognition receptors. Medical Mycology 48 (7), 897–903. Available at https://doi.org/10.3109/13693781003621575.

Noack, D., Rae, J., Cross, A.R., Ellis, B.A., Newburger, P.E., Curnutte, J.T., et al., 2001. Autosomal recessive chronic granulomatous disease caused by defects in NCF-1, the gene encoding the phagocyte p47-phox: mutations not arising in the NCF-1 pseudogenes. Blood 97 (1), 305–311. Available at https://doi.org/10.1182/blood.V97.1.305, https://www.journals.elsevier.com/blood.

Peters, N.C., Egen, J.G., Secundino, N., Debrabant, A., Kimblin, N., Kamhawi, S., et al., 2008. In vivo imaging reveals an essential role for neutrophils in leishmaniasis transmitted by sand flies. Science (New York, N.Y.) 321 (5891), 970–974. Available at https://doi.org/10.1126/science.1159194.

Pinder, E.M., Rostron, A.J., Hellyer, T.P., Ruchaud-Sparagano, M.H., Scott, J., MacFarlane, J.G., et al., 2018. Randomised controlled trial of GM-CSF in critically ill patients with impaired neutrophil phagocytosis. Thorax 73 (10), 918–925. Available at https://doi.org/10.1136/thoraxjnl-2017-211323, http://thorax.bmj.com/.

Price, T.H., Boeckh, M., Harrison, R.W., McCullough, J., Ness, P.M., Strauss, R.G., et al., 2015. Efficacy of transfusion with granulocytes from G-CSF/dexamethasone-treated donors in neutropenic patients with infection. Blood 126 (18), 2153–2161. Available at https://doi.org/10.1182/blood-2015-05-645986.

Reátegui, E., Jalali, F., Khankhel, A.H., Wong, E., Cho, H., Lee, J., et al., 2017. Microscale arrays for the profiling of start and stop signals coordinating human-neutrophil swarming. Nature Biomedical Engineering 1 (7). Available at https://doi.org/10.1038/s41551-017-0094, www.nature.com/natbiomedeng/.

Reiné, J., Rylance, J., Ferreira, D.M., Pennington, S.H., Welters, I.D., Parker, R., et al., 2020. The whole blood phagocytosis assay: a clinically relevant test of neutrophil function and dysfunction in community-acquired pneumonia. BMC Research Notes 13 (1). Available at https://doi.org/10.1186/s13104-020-05034-0.

Richardson, M.P., Ayliffe, M.J., Helbert, M., Davies, E.G., 1998. A simple flow cytometry assay using dihydrorhodamine for the measurement of the neutrophil respiratory burst in whole blood: comparison with the quantitative nitrobluetetrazolium test. Journal of Immunological Methods 219 (1-2), 187–193. Available at https://doi.org/10.1016/s0022-1759(98)00136-7.

Rieber, N., Gazendam, R.P., Freeman, A.F., Hsu, A.P., Collar, A.L., Sugui, J.A., et al., 2021. Extrapulmonary *Aspergillus* infection in patients with CARD9 deficiency. JCI Insight 1 (17). Available at https://doi.org/10.1172/jci.insight.89890, https://insight.jci.org/articles/view/89890/pdf.

Röhm, M., Grimm, M.J., D'Auria, A.C., Almyroudis, N.G., Segal, B.H., Urban, C.F., et al., 2014. NADPH Oxidase promotes neutrophil extracellular trap formation in pulmonary aspergillosis. Infection and Immunity 82 (5), 1766–1777. Available at https://doi.org/10.1128/iai.00096-14.

Roilides, E., Walsh, T.J., Pizzo, P.A., Rubin, M., 1991. Granulocyte colony-stimulating factor enhances the phagocytic and bactericidal activity of normal and defective human neutrophils. Journal of Infectious Diseases 163 (3), 579–583. Available at https://doi.org/10.1093/infdis/163.3.579.

Roilides, E., Holmes, A., Blake, C., Pizzo, P.A., Walsh, T.J., 1995. Effects of granulocyte colony-stimulating factor and interferon-γ on antifungal activity of human polymorphonuclear neutrophils against pseudohyphae of different medically important Candida species. Journal of Leukocyte Biology 57 (4), 651–656. Available at https://doi.org/10.1002/jlb.57.4.651, http://jlb.onlinelibrary.wiley.com/hub/journal/10.1002/(ISSN)1938-3673/.

Roilides, E., Uhlig, K., Venzon, D., Pizzo, P.A., Walsh, T.J., 1992. Neutrophil oxidative burst in response to blastoconidia and pseudohyphae of *Candida albicans*: augmentation by granulocyte colony-stimulating factor and interferon. Journal of Infectious Diseases 166 (3), 668–673. Available at https://doi.org/10.1093/infdis/166.3.668.

Romo, J.A., Kumamoto, C.A., 2020. On commensalism of candida. Journal of Fungi 6 (1). Available at https://doi.org/10.3390/jof6010016, https://www.mdpi.com/2309-608X/6/1/16/pdf.

Roos, D., 2016. Chronic granulomatous disease. British Medical Bulletin 118 (1), 50–63. Available at https://doi.org/10.1093/bmb/ldw009.

Safdar, A., Hanna, H.A., Boktour, M., Kontoyiannis, D.P., Hachem, R., Lichtiger, B., et al., 2004. Impact of high-dose granulocyte transfusions in patients with cancer with candidemia: retrospective case-control analysis of 491 episodes of candida species bloodstream infections. Cancer 101 (12), 2859–2865. Available at https://doi.org/10.1002/cncr.20710.

Sato, K., Yang, X.L., Yudate, T., Chung, J.S., Wu, J., Luby-Phelps, K., et al., 2006. Dectin-2 is a pattern recognition receptor for fungi that couples with the Fc receptor γ chain to induce innate immune responses. Journal of Biological Chemistry 281 (50), 38854–38866. Available at https://doi.org/10.1074/jbc.M606542200, http://www.jbc.org/cgi/reprint/281/50/38854.

Selders, G.S., Fetz, A.E., Radic, M.Z., Bowlin, G.L., 2017. An overview of the role of neutrophils in innate immunity, inflammation and host-biomaterial integration. Regenerative Biomaterials 4 (1), 55–68. Available at https://doi.org/10.1093/rb/rbw041, https://academic.oup.com/rb.

Shahar, E., Wildbaum, G., Katz, R., Karin, N., Etzioni, A., Pollack, S., 2013. Continuous G-CSF Ttreatment induces complete clinical remission and restoration of IL-17 secretion in autosomal dominant chronic mucocutaneous candidiasis. Journal of Allergy and Clinical Immunology 131 (2), AB231. Available at https://doi.org/10.1016/j.jaci.2012.12.1489.

Shimono, N., Okada, K., Takeda, D., Eguchi, K., Misumi, H., Sawae, Y., et al., 1994. Granulocyte colony-stimulating factor does not enhance phagocytosis or microbicidal activity of human mature polymorphonuclear neutrophils in vitro. Clinical Diagnostic Laboratory Immunology 1 (5), 556–562. Available at https://doi.org/10.1128/cdli.1.5.556-562.1994.

Straka, C., Sandherr, M., Salwender, H., Wandt, H., Metzner, B., Hübel, K., et al., 2011. Testing G-CSF responsiveness predicts the individual susceptibility to infection and consecutive treatment in recipients of high-dose chemotherapy. Blood 117 (7), 2121–2128. Available at https://doi.org/10.1182/blood-2010-06-290080.

Swamydas, M., Gao, J.L., Break, T.J., Johnson, M.D., Jaeger, M., Rodriguez, C.A., et al., 2016. CXCR1-mediated neutrophil degranulation and fungal killing promote Candida clearance and host survival. Science Translational Medicine 8 (322). Available at https://doi.org/10.1126/scitranslmed.aac7718, http://stm.sciencemag.org/content/scitransmed/8/322/322ra10.full.pdf.

Sykes, D.B., Martinelli, M.M., Negoro, P., Xu, S., Maxcy, K., Timmer, K., et al., 2022. Transfusable neutrophil progenitors as cellular therapy for the prevention of invasive fungal infections. Journal of Leukocyte Biology 111 (6), 1133–1145. Available at https://doi.org/10.1002/JLB.4HI1221-722R, http://jlb.onlinelibrary.wiley.com/hub/journal/10.1002/(ISSN)1938-3673/.

Taylor, P.R., Tsoni, S.V., Willment, J.A., Dennehy, K.M., Rosas, M., Findon, H., et al., 2007. Dectin-1 is required for β-glucan recognition and control of fungal infection. Nature Immunology 8 (1), 31–38. Available at https://doi.org/10.1038/ni1408.

Timmer, K.D., Floyd, D.J., Scherer, A.K., Crossen, A.J., Atallah, J., Viens, A.L., et al., 2023. Multiparametric profiling of neutrophil function via a high-throughput flow cytometry-based assay. Cells 12 (5). Available at https://doi.org/10.3390/cells12050743, https://www.mdpi.com/journal/cells.

Toda, M., Williams, S.R., Berkow, E.L., Farley, M.M., Harrison, L.H., Bonner, L., et al., 2019. Population-based active surveillance for culture-confirmed candidemia — four sites, United States, 2012–2016. MMWR. Surveillance Summaries. 68 (8), 1–15. Available at https://doi.org/10.15585/mmwr.ss6808a1.

Trof, R.J., Beishuizen, A., Debets-Ossenkopp, Y.J., Girbes, A.R.J., Groeneveld, A.B.J., 2007. Management of invasive pulmonary aspergillosis in non-neutropenic critically ill patients. Intensive Care Medicine 33 (10), 1694–1703. Available at https://doi.org/10.1007/s00134-007-0791-z.

Tsai, T.Y.C., Collins, S.R., Chan, C.K., Hadjitheodorou, A., Lam, P.Y., Lou, S.S., et al., 2019. Efficient front-rear coupling in neutrophil chemotaxis by dynamic myosin II localization. Developmental Cell 49 (2), 189. Available at https://doi.org/10.1016/j.devcel.2019.03.025.

Urban, C.F., Reichard, U., Brinkmann, V., Zychlinsky, A., 2006. Neutrophil extracellular traps capture and kill *Candida albicans* and hyphal forms. Cellular Microbiology 8 (4), 668–676. Available at https://doi.org/10.1111/j.1462-5822.2005.00659.x.

Urban, C.F., Ermert, D., Schmid, M., Abu-Abed, U., Goosmann, C., Nacken, W., et al., 2009. Neutrophil extracellular traps contain calprotectin, a cytosolic protein complex involved in host defense against *Candida albicans*. PLoS Pathogens 5 (10), e1000639. Available at https://doi.org/10.1371/journal.ppat.1000639.

Vaezi, A., Fakhim, H., Abtahian, Z., Khodavaisy, S., Geramishoar, M., Alizadeh, A., et al., 2018. Frequency and geographic distribution of CARD9 mutations in patients with severe fungal infections. Frontiers in Microbiology 9. Available at https://doi.org/10.3389/fmicb.2018.02434, https://www.frontiersin.org/journals/microbiology#.

Viens, A.L., Timmer, K.D., Alexander, N.J., Barghout, R., Milosevic, J., Hopke, A., et al., 2022. TLR signaling rescues fungicidal activity in syk-deficient neutrophils. Journal of Immunology 208 (7), 1664–1674. Available at https://doi.org/10.4049/jimmunol.2100599, https://www.jimmunol.org/content/jimmunol/208/7/1664.full.pdf.

Vowells, S.J., Sekhsaria, S., Malech, H.L., Shalit, M., Fleisher, T.A., 1995. Flow cytometric analysis of the granulocyte respiratory burst: a comparison study of fluorescent probes. Journal of Immunological Methods 178 (1), 89–97. Available at https://doi.org/10.1016/0022-1759(94)00247-t.

Wenisch, C., Fladerer, P., Patruta, S., Krause, R., Hörl, W., 2001. Assessment of neutrophil function in patients with septic shock: comparison of methods. Clinical Diagnostic Laboratory Immunology 8 (1), 178–180. Available at https://doi.org/10.1128/cdli.8.1.178-180.2001.

Winston, D.J., Ho, W.G., Gale, R.P., 1982. Therapeutic granulocyte transfusions for documented infections. A controlled trial in ninety-five infectious granulocytopenic episodes. Annals of Internal Medicine 97 (4), 509–515. Available at https://doi.org/10.7326/0003-4819-97-4-509.

Wu, S.Y., Wu-Hsieh, B.A., 2020. Neutrophil extracellular trap killing assay of *Candida albicans*. Bio-protocol 10 (16). Available at https://doi.org/10.21769/BioProtoc.3716, https://bio-protocol.org/en/archive?vol=10&issid=1246.

Wu, S.Y., Weng, C.L., Jheng, M.J., Kan, H.W., Hsieh, S.T., Liu, F.T., et al., 2019. *Candida albicans* triggers NADPH oxidase independent neutrophil extracellular traps through dectin-2. PLoS Pathogens 15 (11). Available at https://doi.org/10.1371/journal.ppat.1008096, https://journals.plos.org/plospathogens/article/file?id=10.1371/journal.ppat.1008096&type=printable.

Yamamoto, Y., Klein, T.W., Friedman, H., Kimura, S., Yamaguchi, H., 1993. Granulocyte colony-stimulating factor potentiates anti- *Candida albicans* growth inhibitory activity of polymorphonuclear cells. FEMS Immunology & Medical Microbiology 7 (1), 15–22. Available at https://doi.org/10.1111/j.1574-695x.1993.tb00376.x.

Yang, D., Chen, Q., Chertov, O., Oppenheim, J.J., 2000. Human neutrophil defensins selectively chemoattract naive T and immature dendritic cells. Journal of Leukocyte Biology 68 (1), 9–14. Available at https://doi.org/10.1189/jlb.68.1.9.

Ye, N., Liu, Z., Tang, W., Li, X., Chu, W., Zhou, Q., 2022. Systematic characterization of epidemiology, antifungal susceptibility, risk factors and outcomes of candidaemia: a six-year Chinese study. Infection and Drug Resistance 15, 4887–4898. Available at https://doi.org/10.2147/IDR.S378629, https://www.dovepress.com/getfile.php?fileID=83358.

Yu, J.E., Azar, A.E., Chong, H.J., Jongco, A.M., Prince, B.T., 2018. Considerations in the diagnosis of chronic granulomatous disease. Journal of the Pediatric Infectious Diseases Society 7, S6. Available at https://doi.org/10.1093/jpids/piy007, http://jpids.oxfordjournals.org/.

Zigmond, S.H., 1977. Ability of polymorphonuclear leukocytes to orient in gradients of chemotactic factors. Journal of Cell Biology 75 (2), 606–616. Available at https://doi.org/10.1083/jcb.75.2.606.

CHAPTER

3 Approaches to immunotherapy for cryptococcal meningitis

Joseph N. Jarvis[1,2], David S. Lawrence[1,2] and Thomas S. Harrison[3,4]

[1]*Department of Clinical Research, Faculty of Infectious and Tropical Diseases, London School of Hygiene and Tropical Medicine, London, United Kingdom,*
[2]*Botswana Harvard Health Partnership, Gaborone, Botswana,*
[3]*Institute for Infection and Immunity, City St George's University of London, London, United Kingdom,*
[4]*MRC Centre for Medical Mycology, University of Exeter, Exeter, United Kingdom*

Introduction

Much remains to be learnt about the frequency and circumstances of human exposure to *Cryptococcus species*, but evidence suggests such exposure, through inhalation of desiccated yeasts or basidiospores, is very common, commencing in early life (Goldman et al., 2001). However, in common with other, predominantly opportunistic fungal pathogens, exposure rarely leads to disease in immunocompetent hosts. Globally, advanced HIV disease is by some way the most important predisposing condition for reactivation of latent infection and progression to disease (Rajasingham et al., 2022), usually in the form of meningoencephalitis. In addition, a wide range of inherited and acquired immunodeficiency states have also been associated with cryptococcosis and cryptococcal meningitis (Meya and Williamson, 2024), and ongoing investigation of apparently immunocompetent patients with cryptococcal meningitis has revealed that many in fact do have specific immunological deficits or dysfunctions (Yan et al., 2021; Rosen et al., 2013). This epidemiology, on top of the challenges of and high mortality despite antifungal therapy, provides a strong rationale for exploration of adjunctive immunotherapeutic approaches.

Immunotherapy needs to be targeted to the particular immunological deficit or dysfunction of specific patient groups, and, ideally, individualized, based on patient-level immunodiagnostic tests. This is particularly clear, considering interventions in HIV-versus non-HIV-associated cryptococcal meningitis. The pathology of HIV-associated cryptococcal meningitis is driven by pathogen replication and high organism loads unchecked by inadequate T-cell–mediated immunity, while diverse immunopathologies predominate in non-HIV cryptococcal meningitis, and may challenge successful management. While this dichotomy is an

Immunological Insights and Emerging Therapeutics in Medical Mycology. DOI: https://doi.org/10.1016/B978-0-443-23636-5.00008-3

oversimplification, with disease in most patients reflecting a mix of pathogen and host-driven pathology, that may vary over time, it is perhaps not surprising that the U-shaped damage-response framework of microbial pathogenesis was developed by Casadevall and Pirofski while working on cryptococcal disease (Casadevall and Pirofski, 2003) (Fig. 3.1).

In this chapter, we review approaches to immunotherapy in HIV- and non-HIV-associated cryptococcal meningitis, with an emphasis on those that have reached, or are closest to, clinical evaluation, and put such approaches in the context of current best patient management, including that which directly affects host immunity, such as use of antiretrovirals and immunosuppressants for underlying conditions.

HIV-associated cryptococcal meningitis

Ongoing disease burden and need

Cryptococcal meningitis is the commonest form of adult meningitis in Sub-Saharan Africa (SSA) and is a key driver of global HIV mortality, resulting in >100,000 deaths/year with over 75% in SSA, and accounting for 15%–20% of all HIV-related deaths (Rajasingham et al., 2022). About one-third of HIV-infected individuals still

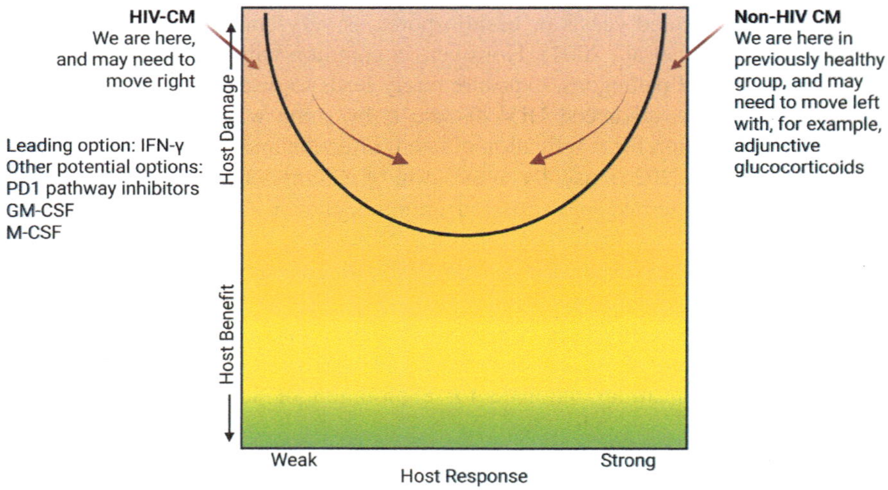

FIGURE 3.1

Parabolic curve of damage-response framework, as relates to cryptococcal meningitis in HIV and non-HIV hosts. *CM*, Cryptococcal meningitis; *GM-CSF*, granulocyte-macrophage colony-stimulating factor; *IFN-γ*, interferon-gamma; *PD-1*, programmed cell death protein-1; *M-CSF*, macrophage colony-stimulating factor.

Adapted from Casadevall and Pirofski. Nature Reviews Microbiology 2003 Oct; 1(1):17–24.

present for care with very low CD4 counts, despite access to antiretroviral therapy (ART). Furthermore, each year, a proportion of patients drop out of HIV care, later re-presenting with advanced HIV disease and complications such as cryptococcal meningitis. Consequently, cryptococcal meningitis rates are not decreasing in most of Africa (Tenforde et al., 2017), and targeting cryptococcal disease and other complications of advanced HIV disease is now widely recognized by WHO and all major stakeholders as an urgent and neglected priority in order to reduce persistently high HIV-related mortality (Ford et al., 2024).

Through a series of phase 2 and phase 3 trials across sites in SSA, the doses, combinations and schedules of amphotericin B (deoxycholate and AmBisome formulations), fluconazole, and flucytosine, have been optimized to maximize antifungal efficacy and minimize toxicity, in regimens that are also practical and cost-effective to implement globally (Molloy et al., 2018; Jarvis et al., 2022). A new phase 2 trial endpoint, early fungicidal activity (EFA), was developed (Brouwer et al., 2004) in order to rapidly assess the rate of clearance of infection from the cerebrospinal fluid (CSF) with a particular dose or combination, and to select the most promising regimens for testing in two large phase 3 trials, ACTA and AMBITION (Molloy et al., 2018; Jarvis et al., 2022). The AMBITION (single 10 mg/kg dose liposomal amphotericin B on day 1, plus fluconazole 1200 mg/d plus flucytosine for 2 weeks) and ACTA (amphotericin B deoxycholate plus flucytosine, for 1 week) trial antifungal regimens have been rapidly adopted by WHO and national guidelines as the preferred and second-line induction treatments, respectively (WHO, 2022), and have driven access to generic flucytosine, and to AmBisome. Implementation studies have confirmed a large reduction in mortality in routine care with the new treatments (Mashau et al., 2022).

Use of available drugs has been optimized, but nevertheless, 10-week mortality remains 25% or more (Jarvis et al., 2022), and further progress depends on novel drugs or approaches, with immunotherapy being one of the most promising. Such a host-directed approach would complement any future antifungal developments and would be unaffected by pathogen resistance, providing the potential for long-lasting utility.

Background and rationale for adjunctive interferon-gamma

Efficacy

In HIV-associated cryptococcal meningitis, there is compelling and consistent evidence that increased CSF interferon-gamma (IFN-γ) and pro-inflammatory cytokines (IL-6, IL-8, TNF-α) at baseline are associated with more rapid clearance of infection and survival. The data were based on a series of phase 2 trials in which both the rate of clearance of infection (EFA) and CSF cytokine profiles were measured, originally in Thailand (Siddiqui et al., 2005), and then in South Africa (Jarvis et al., 2015), and across sites in SSA (Jarvis et al., 2014).

Similarly, specific systemic immune responses were studied using baseline PBMC samples from patients with HIV-associated cryptococcal meningitis stimulated ex vivo with cryptococcal mannoprotein. Patients who survived had many more cryptococcal-specific memory CD4 T-cells making IFN-γ and TNF-α and polyfunctional cells making both cytokines, than patients who died, whose responses are dominated by T-cells making only the chemokine macrophage inflammatory protein (MIP)-1α (Jarvis et al., 2013).

Based on these data, in a small phase II clinical study, we demonstrated that exogenous IFN-γ significantly increased the rate of clearance of infection, and just two subcutaneous doses of 100 μg on days 1 and 3 had the same effect as six doses over the first 2 weeks (Jarvis et al., 2012). Of note, in patients with no baseline cryptococcal-specific memory CD4 T-cell IFN-γ or TNF-α response, the increase in EFA was very sizeable at 0.25 log CFU/ml CSF per day (Jarvis et al., 2013), certainly an increase that would be expected to translate into clinical benefit. For comparison, the addition of flucytosine to fluconazole, which reduces 10-week mortality by 35% (Shiri et al., 2020), was associated with an EFA increase of 0.17 log CFU/ml CSF per day (Nussbaum et al., 2010).

Furthermore, having no baseline IFN-γ or TNF-α response was strongly associated with a low CSF white cell count (Jarvis et al., 2013), a parameter available from routine laboratories, which could be used to target IFN-γ therapy. The fact that just two doses were effective is consistent with our earlier observation that although important for clearance and survival, the endogenous IFN-γ response is very short-lived, with CSF IFN-γ levels peaking at day 3 and resolving by day 14 (Siddiqui et al., 2005).

These efficacy results were consistent with an earlier study based on CSF culture conversion (Pappas et al., 2004). Seventy-five patients were randomized to placebo, IFN-γ 100 μg, or IFN-γ 200 μg, three times per week for 10 weeks. In the combined IFN-γ therapy groups, CSF fungal cultures were negative at 2 weeks for 16 (34%) of 47 patients compared with 3 (13%) of 23 placebo recipients (P=.064).

In addition, the results of the opposite immunotherapeutic approach in this patient group have been demonstrated by the CryptoDex study, which was stopped early on recommendation of the data and safety monitoring committee (Beardsley et al., 2016). Adjunctive dexamethasone was associated with numerically higher mortality, disability, and adverse events. The rate of clearance of infection was significantly reduced (from -0.31 to -0.21 log CFU/ml CSF per day, P<.001), emphasizing the significant role played by host immunity in clearing infection, even in the context of this highly immunosuppressed population, and of fungicidal drugs.

Finally, we have recently confirmed the strong association of baseline CSF IFN-γ with mortality in analyses of our larger AMBITION trial: geometric mean IFN-γ concentration was 16.5 pg/mL (95% confidence interval [CI] 12.8–21.1) in those surviving to 2 weeks versus 6.5 pg/mL (95% CI 2.2–6.7, P<.0001) in those who died. The odds of death fell by approximately 50% with each $\log_{10}$ increase in baseline IFN-γ concentration (OR 0.52; 95% CI 0.38–0.72, P<.0001) (authors' unpublished data).

Safety

Side effects of IFN-γ include flu-like symptoms of fever and chills, headache, nausea, vomiting, hypersensitivity reactions, and injection site tenderness. Of note, these data are based on prolonged three times per week use (Interferon-gamma prescribing information, 2015). In cryptococcal meningitis, IFN-γ was well-tolerated dosed three times per week at 100 mg for 10 weeks, with no adverse effects on HIV viral load or CD4 cell count (Pappas et al., 2004). The risks to patients from just one or two doses of IFN-γ are likely extremely low. No IFN-γ-specific side effects were identified in our prior phase II study of 2 or 6 doses in cryptococcal meningitis (Jarvis et al., 2012). There was no significant increase in immune reconstitution inflammatory syndrome (IRIS) events, and with exogenous IFN-γ, pro-inflammatory cytokine levels in CSF declined faster from baseline to day 14, suggesting more rapid clearance of infection led to more rapid resolution of inflammation.

The trial

Based on the above data, we have formed a consortium to carry out an adaptive phase 2B/3 open-label, randomized controlled clinical trial of newly diagnosed patients presenting to the hospital with symptomatic HIV-associated cryptococcal meningitis. We will use a two-step adaptive approach. Given the large implementation and cost advantages of one versus two doses of IFN-γ, if one dose was as effective, we would first test one and two doses of IFN-γ compared with the standard of care (AMBITION- trial antifungal regimen with no IFN-γ), based on EFA; and then continue with optimal dosing vs control. We will exclude patients recently started on ART (Rhein et al., 2018) and with evidence of an unmasking IRIS presentation, in whom IFN-γ is less likely to be beneficial.

Based on our prior data, it may be that the trial will provide compelling efficacy data in patients with a low CSF white cell count. As an alternative to using CSF white cell count, we will also build on ongoing work using nonlinear methods to model factors associated with outcome in the combined ACTA and AMBITION-CM datasets (Samuels et al., 2025), to examine the effect of adjunctive IFN-γ in subgroups of patients (readily identified in routine care at presentation) across the risk spectrum as an alternative approach to targeting IFN-γ immune therapy. The trial will provide vital evidence in order to optimize any targeting strategy.

Feasibility and sustainability

An ultra-short course of adjunctive IFN-γ immunotherapy could be both practical to deliver in resource-limited settings and also cost-effective. We will incorporate formal health economic and acceptability analyses, as for the ACTA and AMBITION trials (Chen et al., 2019; Lawrence et al., 2022). Of note, even at current NHS indicative pricing, a dose of IFN-γ is £155, and administration incurs negligible additional care costs. Even at this price, this additional drug cost is less than 10% of total hospital care costs and less than the additional drug costs associated with the AMBITION trial regimen, which nevertheless was shown to be highly cost-effective (Lawrence et al., 2022). Additionally, however, high-quality data demonstrating benefits can drive increased access and reduced costs to providers (Jarvis et al., 2023). Of note, IFN-γ is off patent, and there are already several manufacturers, which could enable cost reductions with increasing demand.

Alternative approaches in HIV-associated cryptococcal meningitis

The case for IFN-γ is compelling and ready for testing in phase IIB/III trials. Other potential immune-enhancing approaches for HIV-associated cryptococcal meningitis are at a much earlier stage but deserve further exploration. These include GM-CSF and M-CSF, given evidence of their importance in both HIV-associated and non-HIV-associated cryptococcal infection (Yang et al., 2021; Rosen et al., 2013; Kannambath et al., 2020; Jiang et al., 2024; Arango-Franco et al., 2024), and limited in vitro and animal model data (Tascini et al., 1999; Hansakon et al., 2024; Nassar, Brummer and Stevens, 1994, 1995), and PD-1 checkpoint inhibitors (Roussey et al., 2017; Che et al., 2018). Within the AMBITION trial cohort, PD-1 and PD-L1 expression on monocytes and PD-1 expression on T-cells were significantly higher in those who died from cryptococcal meningitis compared to survivors (unpublished data).

An extensive body of in vitro and animal model work has demonstrated the potential benefit of selected monoclonal antibodies (mAbs) against cryptococcal glucuronoxylomannan (GXM), glucosylceramides, melanin, and β-glucan [reviewed in (Antachopoulos and Walsh, 2012)]. The anti-GXM mAb 18B7 reached a phase 1 dose-escalating trial in HIV-associated cryptococcal meningitis patients successfully treated with antifungal drugs. Doses of up to 1 mg/kg were well tolerated, with a modest reduction in cryptococcal antigen titer seen with this dose (Larsen et al., 2005). Subsequently, radiolabelled mAb 18B7 was shown to be highly effective in a murine model of cryptococcal infection (Bryan et al., 2010).

Management of antiretroviral therapy in HIV-associated cryptococcal meningitis

Based in large part on the results of the COAT study (Boulware et al., 2014), current guidance suggests delaying the start or re-start of antiretroviral therapy in patients presenting with HIV-associated cryptococcal meningitis until 4–6 weeks after the start of antifungal therapy, in order to avoid or reduce immune reconstitution reactions. More recently, increased mortality has been noted in several studies among patients started on ART within 14 days prior to presentation with cryptococcal meningitis, compared with those ART-naïve or on ART for longer durations prior to cryptococcal meningitis presentation (Moyo et al., 2025; Rhein et al., 2018; Kalata et al., 2021). This led to the suggestion (Alufandika et al., 2020), adopted as guidance within the AMBITION-CM trial, that ART should be withheld in this specific group and restarted at 4–6 weeks, as for ART-naive patients. In an analysis of the AMBITION trial data for those started on ART within the 14 days prior to presentation, 2-week mortality was lower, 14% (7/49), in those in whom ART was withheld compared with 35% (8/23) in those in whom ART was continued (P=.06) (Moyo et al., 2025). Although it should be stressed that this was an uncontrolled analysis, it does support the practice of withholding ART in this group.

Non-HIV-associated cryptococcal meningitis

Non-HIV-associated cryptococcal meningitis occurs in patients with a range of types and severity of immunosuppression, most usually affecting T-cell-mediated immunity, and also in those apparently immunocompetent and previously healthy (Meya and Williamson, 2024). In this latter group in particular, cryptococcal organism load is low, and in patients refractory to antifungal treatment, the issue is most often related to excessive and/or dysfunctional immune responses, rather than achieving sterilization of cryptococcal infection.

In this context, in patients with iatrogenic immunosuppression, care must be taken with management and any reduction, if this is clinically feasible, of immunosuppressive medications. While a reduction in immunosuppression may help initial sterilization of cryptococcal infection, it may also predispose to immune reconstitution reactions, and organ rejection in transplant patients, and exacerbate underlying autoimmune diseases. Discontinuation of calcineurin inhibitors, in particular, predisposes to reconstitution reactions in transplant patients (Sun et al., 2015). In those on long-term steroids, modest initial reductions in dose may be safer. Management of immunosuppressive medications needs to be individualized based on the underlying disease and its activity, and the severity and form of cryptococcal infection.

In previously healthy patients with cryptococcal meningitis, Williamson and colleagues have described in detail the immunopathology of a subset of patients who develop a postinfectious inflammatory response syndrome (PIIRS), with deteriorating clinical condition, enhancing CNS mass lesions, and often elevated CSF pressures, despite sterilization of infection with antifungal drugs (Panackal et al., 2015). In a cohort of 17 such patients, they demonstrated intact Th1-type responses in the CNS, with activated $CD4^+$ and $CD8^+$ T-cells and dendritic cells identified in the CSF. Levels of, for example, IFN-γ and IL-6 in the CSF were greater than in healthy controls or patients with pulmonary cryptococcal infection (who had agreed to have a lumbar puncture for research purposes), and IFN-γ levels were comparable to those seen in HIV-associated cryptococcal meningitis survivors (Siddiqui et al., 2005). Further, both CSF $CD4^+$ and $CD8^+$ T-cells from these cryptococcal meningitis patients made significant amounts of IFN-γ when cocultured with autologous mature dendritic cells pulsed with cryptococcal cell homogenate or cryptococcal mannoprotein. Rather than a T-cell defect, there was evidence of ineffective monocyte-macrophage activation. Brain biopsies from 2 patients in the cohort and examination of prior autopsy tissue from similar cases showed T-cell and monocyte/macrophage infiltration, but nonprotective M2-type macrophage activation and poor colocalization and uptake of fungal cells (Panackal et al., 2015). Subsequently, $CXCR3^+$ $CD4^+$ T-cells, in particular, recruited to the CNS through high levels of the chemokine and CXCR3 ligand, CXCL10, secreted mainly by astrocytes, have been implicated in central nervous system pathology in a murine cryptococcal meningitis model that may be reflective of non-HIV-assocciated cryptococcal meningitis patients with PIIRS (Xu et al., 2020). Consistent data, showing significant IFN-γ and pro-inflammatory cytokine levels in CSF of a cohort of patients with non-HIV cryptococcal meningitis, have been reported from China (Jiang et al., 2022).

Given this immunopathology, Williamson and colleagues have developed a pulse- taper protocol of methylprednisolone for non-HIV cryptococcal meningitis patients with post infectious inflammatory response syndrome: methylprednisolone 1 g parenteral daily for 7 days followed by 1 mg/kg/day prednisone for 1 month and then tapered by 5 mg every month, based on clinical response and magnetic resonance brain imaging (Anjum et al., 2021). They reported marked and sustained clinical improvements: all 15 patients showed significant improvement in cognitive and performance scores, which were accompanied by a rapid reduction in markers of CSF inflammation (CSF: total white cell and $CD4^+$ and $CD8^+$ T-cell counts, protein, IL-6), and improvement in brain imaging with reductions in parenchymal and meningeal enhancement. Visual fields and hearing tests also improved. All patients were culture negative at initiation of corticosteroids for PIIRS, at a median of 6 weeks after starting antifungal therapy, and remained so for the 22-month median duration of the taper (Jiang et al., 2022), their practice being to keep patients on maintenance fluconazole for the duration of the taper, as well as prophylactic dose cotrimoxazole and valacyclovir.

The group published very useful practical clinical guidance on this immunomodulatory approach for patients with PIIRS in 2022, including diagnostic considerations and monitoring (Ssebambulidde et al., 2022). Amongst approximately 60 patients treated by that time, they reported best responses when steroids were started within 8 weeks of the start of antifungal therapy, and the need, not infrequently, to temporarily increase the oral prednisolone dose to treat recurrence of symptoms due to immunological flares.

Many questions remain. In particular, whether treating all or a broader range of non-HIV cryptococcal meningitis patients with adjunctive steroids earlier in the course of infection, could prevent or reduce the frequency and severity of PIIRS and obviate the need, in some patients, for higher and longer doses of corticosteroids later; could corticosteroids be more clearly targeted based on immunodiagnostic markers, such as CSF IL-6 and sCD25, currently used at NIH as supportive of PIIRS (Ssebambulidde et al., 2022), or markers of the CXCL10/CXCR3 axis (Xu et al., 2020), and if so, could such tests be made more widely available; and is there a role for steroid sparing agents or more specific immunomodulation in different patient groups, for example, the significant subset with anti-GM-CSF autoantibodies. To address the first question and collect data pertinent to the second, a randomized trial of steroid therapy in non-HIV cryptococcal meningitis has been proposed.

Conclusion

We have learnt a great deal about host immune responses to cryptococcal infection, both protective and those contributing to pathogenesis. Much remains to be done, and controlled trials are urgently needed to translate this knowledge into effective adjunctive immunotherapies targeted to individual patients' immune status and stage of infection. Host-directed therapies have the potential to make a sustained step-change improvement in patient outcomes in cryptococcal meningitis, as in other systemic fungal infections, complementing any advances in antifungal therapy and irrespective of rising antifungal resistance.

References

Alufandika, M., Lawrence, D.S., Boyer-Chammard, T., Kanyama, C., Ndhlovu, C.E., Mosepele, M., et al., 2020. A pragmatic approach to managing antiretroviral therapy-experienced patients diagnosed with HIV-associated cryptococcal meningitis: impact of antiretroviral therapy adherence and duration. AIDS (London, England) 34 (9), 1425–1428. Available at https://doi.org/10.1097/QAD.0000000000002556.

Anjum, S., Dean, O., Kosa, P., Magone, M.T., King, K.A., Fitzgibbon, E., et al., 2021. Outcomes in previously healthy cryptococcal meningoencephalitis patients treated with pulse taper corticosteroids for post-infectious inflammatory syndrome. Clinical Infectious Diseases 73 (9), e2789. Available at https://doi.org/10.1093/cid/ciaa1901.

Antachopoulos, C., Walsh, T.J., 2012. Immunotherapy of *Cryptococcus* infections. Clinical Microbiology and Infection 18 (2), 126–133. Available at https://doi.org/10.1111/j.1469-0691.2011.03741.x.

Arango-Franco, C.A., Rojas, J., Firacative, C., Migaud, M., Agudelo, C.I., Franco, J.L., et al., 2024. Autoantibodies neutralizing GM-CSF in HIV-negative colombian patients infected with *Cryptococcus gattii* and *C. neoformans*. Journal of Clinical Immunology 44 (7). Available at https://doi.org/10.1007/s10875-024-01757-y.

Beardsley, J., Wolbers, M., Kibengo, F.M., Ggayi, A.-B.M., Kamali, A., Cuc, N.T.K., et al., 2016. Adjunctive dexamethasone in HIV-associated cryptococcal meningitis. New England Journal of Medicine 374 (6), 542–554. Available at https://doi.org/10.1056/nejmoa1509024.

Boulware, D.R., Meya, D.B., Muzoora, C., Rolfes, M.A., Hullsiek, K.H., Musubire, A., et al., 2014. Timing of antiretroviral therapy after diagnosis of cryptococcal meningitis. New England Journal of Medicine 370 (26), 2487–2498. Available at https://doi.org/10.1056/NEJMoa1312884, http://www.nejm.org/doi/pdf/10.1056/NEJMoa1312884.

Brouwer, A.E., Rajanuwong, A., Chierakul, W., Griffin, G.E., Larsen, R.A., White, N.J., et al., 2004. Combination antifungal therapies for HIV-associated cryptococcal meningitis: a randomised trial. Lancet 363 (9423), 1764–1767. Available at https://doi.org/10.1016/S0140-6736(04)16301-0, http://www.journals.elsevier.com/the-lancet/.

Bryan, R.A., Jiang, Z., Howell, R.C., Morgenstern, A., Bruchertseifer, F., Casadeval, A., et al., 2010. Radioimmunotherapy is more effective than antifungal treatment in experimental Cryptococcal infection. Journal of Infectious Diseases 202 (4), 633–637. Available at https://doi.org/10.1086/654813.

Casadevall, A., Pirofski, L.A., 2003. The damage-response framework of microbial pathogenesis. Nature Reviews. Microbiology 1 (1), 17–24. Available at https://doi.org/10.1038/nrmicro732.

Che, Y.M., Zhang, Y., Li, M., Li, X.P., Zhang, L.L., 2018. In vitro and in vivo effect of PD-1/PD-L1 blockade on microglia/macrophage activation and T cell subset balance in cryptococcal meningitis. Journal of Cellular Biochemistry 119 (4), 3044–3057. Available at https://doi.org/10.1002/jcb.26432, http://onlinelibrary.wiley.com/journal/10.1002/(ISSN)1097-4644.

Chen, T., Mwenge, L., Lakhi, S., Chanda, D., Mwaba, P., Molloy, S.F., et al., 2019. Healthcare costs and life-years gained from treatments within the advancing cryptococcal meningitis treatment for Africa (ACTA) trial on cryptococcal meningitis: a comparison of antifungal induction strategies in sub-Saharan Africa. Clinical Infectious Diseases 69 (4), 588–595. Available at https://doi.org/10.1093/cid/ciy971.

Ford, N., Ehrenkranz, P., Jarvis, J., 2024. Advanced HIV as a neglected disease. New England Journal of Medicine 390 (6), 487–489. Available at https://doi.org/10.1056/NEJMp2313777, http://www.nejm.org/medical-index.

Goldman, D.L., Khine, H., Abadi, J., Lindenberg, D.J., Pirofski, L.-anne, Niang, R., et al., 2001. Serologic evidence for *Cryptococcus* neoformans infection in early childhood. Pediatrics 107 (5), e66. Available at https://doi.org/10.1542/peds.107.5.e66.

Hansakon, A., Khampoongern, R., Schiller, L., Jeerawattanawart, S., Angkasekwinai, P., 2024. Effect of intranasal administration of granulocyte-macrophage colony-stimulating factor on pulmonary *Cryptococcus gattii* infection. International Immunopharmacology 142 (Pt B), 113259. Available at https://doi.org/10.1016/j.intimp.2024.113259.

Interferon-gamma prescribing information. 2015 https://www.accessdata.fda.gov/drugsatfda_docs/label/2015/103836s5182lbl.pdf.

Jarvis, J.N., Meintjes, G., Rebe, K., Williams, G.N., Bicanic, T., Williams, A., et al., 2012. Adjunctive interferon-γ immunotherapy for the treatment of HIV-associated cryptococcal meningitis: a randomized controlled trial. AIDS (London, England) 26 (9), 1105–1113. Available at https://doi.org/10.1097/QAD.0b013e3283536a93.

Jarvis, J.N., Bicanic, T., Loyse, A., Namarika, D., Jackson, A., Nussbaum, J.C., et al., 2014. Determinants of mortality in a combined cohort of 501 patients with HIV-associated

cryptococcal meningitis: implications for improving outcomes. Clinical Infectious Diseases 58 (5), 736–745. Available at https://doi.org/10.1093/cid/cit794.
Jarvis, J.N., Lawrence, D.S., Meya, D.B., Kagimu, E., Kasibante, J., Mpoza, E., et al., 2022. Single-dose liposomal amphotericin B treatment for cryptococcal meningitis. New England Journal of Medicine 386 (12), 1109–1120. Available at https://doi.org/10.1056/NEJMoa2111904, http://www.nejm.org/medical-index.
Jarvis, J.N., Casazza, J.P., Stone, H.H., Meintjes, G., Lawn, S.D., Levitz, S.M., et al., 2013. The phenotype of the cryptococcus-specific CD^{4+} memory T-cell response is associated with disease severity and outcome in HIV-associated cryptococcal meningitis. Journal of Infectious Diseases 207 (12), 1817–1828. Available at https://doi.org/10.1093/infdis/jit099.
Jarvis, J.N., Chou, R., Harrison, T.S., Lawrence, D.S., Muthoga, C., Mupeli, K., et al., 2023. Translating evidence into global impact: lessons for HIV research and policy development from the AMBITION trial. The Lancet Global Health 11 (11), e1688. Available at https://doi.org/10.1016/S2214-109X(23)00412-6, http://www.elsevier.com/journals/the-lancet-global-health/2214-109x.
Jarvis, J.N., Meintjes, G., Bicanic, T., Buffa, V., Hogan, L., Mo, S., et al., 2015. Cerebrospinal fluid cytokine profiles predict risk of early mortality and immune reconstitution inflammatory syndrome in HIV-associated cryptococcal meningitis. PLoS Pathogens 11 (4), e1004754. Available at https://doi.org/10.1371/journal.ppat.1004754.
Jiang, Y.K., Zhou, L.H., Cheng, J.H., Zhu, J.H., Luo, Y., Li, L., et al., 2024. Anti-GM-CSF autoantibodies predict outcome of cryptococcal meningitis in patients not infected with HIV: a cohort study. Clinical Microbiology and Infection 30 (5), 660–665. Available at https://doi.org/10.1016/j.cmi.2024.01.018, https://www.sciencedirect.com/science/journal/1198743X.
Jiang, Y.-K., Wang, R.-Y., Zhou, L.-H., Cheng, J.-H., Luo, Y., Zhu, R.-S., et al., 2022. Cerebrospinal fluid cytokine and chemokine patterns correlate with prognosis of HIV-uninfected cryptococcal meningitis: a prospective observational study. Frontiers in Immunology 13. Available at https://doi.org/10.3389/fimmu.2022.993495, https://www.frontiersin.org/journals/immunology#.
Kalata, N., Ellis, J., Kanyama, C., Kuoanfank, C., Temfack, E., Mfinanga, S., et al., 2021. Short-term mortality outcomes of HIV-associated cryptococcal meningitis in antiretroviral therapy-naïve and -experienced patients in sub-saharan Africa. Open Forum Infectious Diseases 8 (10). Available at https://doi.org/10.1093/ofid/ofab397, https://academic.oup.com/ofid.
Kannambath, S., Jarvis, J.N., Wake, R.M., Longley, N., Loyse, A., Matzaraki, V., et al., 2020. Genome-wide association study identifies novel colony stimulating factor 1 locus conferring susceptibility to *Cryptococcosis* in human immunodeficiency virus-infected South Africans. Open Forum Infectious Diseases 7 (11). Available at https://doi.org/10.1093/ofid/ofaa489, https://academic.oup.com/ofid.
Larsen, R.A., Pappas, P.G., Perfect, J., Aberg, J.A., Casadevall, A., Cloud, G.A., et al., 2005. Phase I evaluation of the safety and pharmacokinetics of murine-derived anticryptococcal antibody 18B7 in subjects with treated cryptococcal meningitis. Antimicrobial Agents and Chemotherapy 49 (3), 952–958. Available at https://doi.org/10.1128/AAC.49.3.952-958.2005.
Lawrence, D.S., Muthoga, C., Meya, D.B., Tugume, L., Williams, D., Rajasingham, R., et al., 2022. Cost-effectiveness of single, high-dose, liposomal amphotericin regimen for HIV-associated cryptococcal meningitis in five countries in sub-Saharan Africa: an economic analysis of the AMBITION-cm trial. The Lancet Global Health 10 (12), e1845. Available at https://doi.org/10.1016/S2214-109X(22)00450-8, http://www.elsevier.com/journals/the-lancet-global-health/2214-109x.

Mashau, R.C., Meiring, S.T., Quan, V.C., Nel, J., Greene, G.S., Garcia, A., et al., 2022. Outcomes of flucytosine-containing combination treatment for cryptococcal meningitis in a South African national access programme: a cross-sectional observational study. The Lancet Infectious Diseases 22 (9), 1365–1373. Available at https://doi.org/10.1016/S1473-3099(22)00234-1, http://www.journals.elsevier.com/the-lancet-infectious-diseases.

Meya, D.B., Williamson, P.R., 2024. Cryptococcal disease in diverse hosts. New England Journal of Medicine 390 (17), 1597–1610. Available at https://doi.org/10.1056/NEJMra2311057, http://www.nejm.org/medical-index.

Molloy, S.F., Kanyama, C., Heyderman, R.S., Loyse, A., Kouanfack, C., Chanda, D., et al., 2018. Antifungal combinations for treatment of cryptococcal meningitis in Africa. New England Journal of Medicine 378 (11), 1004–1017. Available at https://doi.org/10.1056/NEJMoa1710922, http://www.nejm.org/medical-index.

Moyo, M., Lawrence, D.S., Jafali, J., Molloy, S.F., Kumwenda, J., Kanyama, C., et al., 2025. Recent antiretroviral therapy initiation is associated with increased mortality risk in HIV-associated cryptococcal meningitis: an analysis of clinical trial data from Africa. Clinical Infectious Diseases 81 (1), 75–83. Available at https://doi.org/10.1093/cid/ciae586.

Nassar, F., Brummer, E., Stevens, D.A., 1994. Effect of in vivo macrophage colony-stimulating factor on fungistasis of bronchoalveolar and peritoneal macrophages against *Cryptococcus neoformans*. Antimicrobial Agents and Chemotherapy 38 (9), 2162–2164. Available at https://doi.org/10.1128/AAC.38.9.2162, http://aac.asm.org/.

Nassar, F., Brummer, E., Stevens, D.A., 1995. Macrophage colony-stimulating factor (M-CSF) induction of enhanced anticryptococcal activity in human monocyte-derived macrophages: synergy with fluconazole for killing. Cellular Immunology 164 (1), 113–118. Available at https://doi.org/10.1006/cimm.1995.1149.

Nussbaum, J.C., Jackson, A., Namarika, D., Phulusa, J., Kenala, J., Kanyemba, C., et al., 2010. Combination flucytosine and high-dose fluconazole compared with fluconazole monotherapy for the treatment of cryptococcal meningitis: a randomized trial in malawi. Clinical Infectious Diseases 50 (3), 338–344. Available at https://doi.org/10.1086/649861.

Panackal, A.A., Wuest, S.C., Lin, Y.-C., Wu, T., Zhang, N., Kosa, P., et al., 2015. Paradoxical immune responses in non-HIV cryptococcal meningitis. PLoS Pathogens 11 (5), e1004884. Available at https://doi.org/10.1371/journal.ppat.1004884.

Pappas, P.G., Bustamante, B., Ticona, E., Hamill, R.J., Johnson, P.C., Reboli, A., et al., 2004. Recombinant interferon-γ1b as adjunctive therapy for AIDS-related acute cryptococcal meningitis. Journal of Infectious Diseases 189 (12), 2185–2191. Available at https://doi.org/10.1086/420829.

Rajasingham, R., Govender, N.P., Jordan, A., Loyse, A., Shroufi, A., Denning, D.W., et al., 2022. The global burden of HIV-associated cryptococcal infection in adults in 2020: a modelling analysis. The Lancet Infectious Diseases 22 (12), 1748–1755. Available at https://doi.org/10.1016/s1473-3099(22)00499-6.

Rhein, J., Hullsiek, K.H., Evans, E.E., Tugume, L., Nuwagira, E., Ssebambulidde, K., et al., 2018. Detrimental outcomes of unmasking cryptococcal meningitis with recent ART initiation. Open Forum Infectious Diseases 5 (8). Available at https://doi.org/10.1093/ofid/ofy122.

Rosen, L.B., Freeman, A.F., Yang, L.M., Jutivorakool, K., Olivier, K.N., Angkasekwinai, N., et al., 2013. Anti-GM-CSF autoantibodies in patients with cryptococcal meningitis. Journal of Immunology 190 (8), 3959–3966. Available at https://doi.org/10.4049/jimmunol.1202526, http://www.jimmunol.org/content/190/8/3959.full.pdf+html.

Roussey, J.A., Viglianti, S.P., Teitz-Tennenbaum, S., Olszewski, M.A., Osterholzer, J.J., 2017. Anti-PD-1 antibody treatment promotes clearance of persistent cryptococcal lung infection in mice. Journal of Immunology 199 (10), 3535–3546. Available at https://doi.org/10.4049/jimmunol.1700840, http://www.jimmunol.org/content/jimmunol/199/10/3535.full.pdf.

Samuels, T.H.A., Molloy, S.F., Lawrence, D.S., Loyse, A., Kanyama, C., Heyderman, R.S., et al., 2025. Personalised risk-prediction tools for cryptococcal meningitis mortality to guide treatment stratification in sub-Saharan Africa: a prognostic modelling study based on pooled analysis of two randomised controlled trials. The Lancet Global Health 13 (5), e920. Available at https://doi.org/10.1016/S2214-109X(25)00010-5, https://www.sciencedirect.com/science/journal/2214109X.

Shiri, T., Loyse, A., Mwenge, L., Chen, T., Lakhi, S., Chanda, D., et al., 2020. Addition of flucytosine to fluconazole for the treatment of cryptococcal meningitis in Africa: a multicountry cost-effectiveness analysis. Clinical Infectious Diseases 70 (1), 26–29. Available at https://doi.org/10.1093/cid/ciz163.

Siddiqui, A.A., Brouwer, A.E., Wuthiekanun, V., Jaffar, S., Shattock, R., Irving, D., et al., 2005. IFN-γ at the site of infection determines rate of clearance of infection in cryptococcal meningitis. Journal of Immunology 174 (3), 1746–1750. Available at https://doi.org/10.4049/jimmunol.174.3.1746, http://www.jimmunol.org/.

Ssebambulidde, K., Anjum, S.H., Hargarten, J.C., Chittiboina, P., Shoham, S., Seyedmousavi, S., et al., 2022. Treatment recommendations for non-HIV associated cryptococcal meningoencephalitis including management of post-infectious inflammatory response syndrome. Frontiers in Neurology 13. Available at https://doi.org/10.3389/fneur.2022.994396, http://www.frontiersin.org/Neurology.

Sun, H.Y., Alexander, B.D., Huprikar, S., Forrest, G.N., Bruno, D., Lyon, G.M., et al., 2015. Predictors of immune reconstitution syndrome in organ transplant recipients with cryptococcosis: implications for the management of immunosuppression. Clinical Infectious Diseases 60 (1), 36–44. Available at https://doi.org/10.1093/cid/ciu711, http://cid.oxfordjournals.org/content/by/year.

Tascini, C., Vecchiarelli, A., Preziosi, R., Francisci, D., Bistoni, F., Baldelli, F., 1999. Granulocyte-macrophage colony-stimulating factor and fluconazole enhance anti-cryptococcal activity of monocytes from AIDS patients. AIDS (London, England) 13 (1), 49–55. Available at https://doi.org/10.1097/00002030-199901140-00007.

Tenforde, M.W., Mokomane, M., Leeme, T., Patel, R.K.K., Lekwape, N., Ramodimoosi, C., et al., 2017. Advanced human immunodeficiency virus disease in Botswana following successful antiretroviral therapy rollout: incidence of and temporal trends in cryptococcal meningitis. Clinical Infectious Diseases 65 (5), 779–786. Available at https://doi.org/10.1093/cid/cix430, http://cid.oxfordjournals.org/content/by/year.

WHO, 2022. Guidelines for diagnosing, preventing and managing cryptococcal disease among adults, adolescents and children living with HIV. Geneva.

Xu, J., Neal, L.M., Ganguly, A., Kolbe, J.L., Hargarten, J.C., Elsegeiny, W., et al., 2020. Chemokine receptor CXCR3 is required for lethal brain pathology but not pathogen clearance during cryptococcal meningoencephalitis. Science Advances 6 (25). Available at https://doi.org/10.1126/sciadv.aba2502.

Yang, D.-H., England, M.R., Salvator, H., Anjum, S., Park, Y.-D., Marr, K.A., et al., 2021. *Cryptococcus gattii* species complex as an opportunistic pathogen: underlying medical conditions associated with the infection. MBio 12 (5). Available at https://doi.org/10.1128/mBio.02708-21.

CHAPTER

The role of interferon-gamma in invasive and chronic aspergillosis

4

Chris Kosmidis[1,2] and Stefano Colombo[3]

[1]*National Aspergillosis Centre, Manchester University NHS Foundation Trust, Manchester, United Kingdom,*
[2]*Faculty of Biology, Medicine, and Health, Manchester Fungal Infection Group, University of Manchester, Manchester, United Kingdom,*
[3]*Faculty of Biology, Medicine, and Health, Lydia Becker Institute of Immunology and Inflammation, University of Manchester, Manchester, United Kingdom*

Introduction

Interferon-gamma (IFN-γ) has long been of interest as an antifungal cytokine, due to its immunomodulatory properties, through synergism with antifungals as well as via direct antifungal activity (Stevens et al., 2006). IFN-γ led to more rapid clearance of fungi from the cerebrospinal fluid in a randomized trial of cryptococcal meningitis in HIV-positive patients, whereas ex vivo or animal models show encouraging findings in *Candida* and endemic mycoses (Jarvis et al., 2012; Brummer et al., 1988; Brummer et al., 1993; van Furth et al., 1993; Morrison et al., 1989). However, data on the role of IFN-γ in aspergillosis have only recently emerged. We discuss the cytokine response in invasive and chronic aspergillosis with a focus on IFN-γ, as well as in vitro, animal, and human studies exploring the role of IFN-γ in the treatment of these conditions. We explore the spectrum of *Aspergillus* disease manifestations, ranging from invasive aspergillosis (IA), which affects patients with significant immune compromise, to chronic pulmonary aspergillosis (CPA), which is seen in those with chronic lung conditions and no overt immune compromise.

Cytokine immunology of invasive and chronic aspergillosis

Given the interest in supplemental IFN-γ as a treatment modality in aspergillosis, it is essential to understand the role IFN-γ-driven immunity plays in the context of IA or CPA. However, in contrast to other disease settings, there is a significant limitation in the literature to-date in the characterization of the immune phenotype of patients with IA/CPA. In part, this is due to limited access to primary patient

Immunological Insights and Emerging Therapeutics in Medical Mycology. DOI: https://doi.org/10.1016/B978-0-443-23636-5.00003-4

samples for research. Additionally, where patient samples are available, these are typically from peripheral blood and/or bronchoalveolar lavage fluid (BALF), which, whilst informative, may only provide indirect insight into immune responses at the boundary of infection and the host. With these limitations in mind, we will discuss the current understanding of immunity to IA/CPA.

A number of studies have characterized the presence of cytokines in the serum and BALF of IA/CPA patients (Gonçalves et al., 2017; Salzer et al., 2018; Zhan et al., 2018; Heldt et al., 2017; Ren et al., 2023). Common to these studies are the elevated levels of IL-6 and IL-8 in the peripheral circulation and airways of IA/CPA patients relative to controls. However, it is unclear to what extent these observations are specific to pulmonary aspergillosis. One study of serum cytokines in CPA and tuberculosis patients observed that IL-6 and IL-8 were elevated in CPA patients compared to both the control group and tuberculosis patients, indicating that these cytokines may be suitable as discriminatory biomarkers for distinguishing CPA–tuberculosis coinfection from tuberculosis mono-infection (Ren et al., 2023). However, a previous study measuring cytokine concentration in the BALF found that elevated IL-6, IL-8, and IFN-γ observed in CPA patients were comparable to other non-CPA respiratory disorders, indicating that CPA may induce an inflammatory signature common to other pulmonary diseases (Salzer et al., 2018). IL-1β is also consistently observed to be elevated in the serum and plasma of IA/CPA patients, with one study identifying that the serum concentration of IL-1β correlated significantly with both aspergilloma size and cavity diameter (Zhan et al., 2018). Additionally, IL-17 has been observed to be elevated in the BALF of IA patients (Gonçalves et al., 2017). Whilst little attention has been paid to Th2-related cytokines in the context of IA/CPA, one study did note reduced concentrations of IL-4 and IL-5 in the serum of CPA patients relative to controls (Ren et al., 2023).

Elevated concentration of pro-inflammatory cytokines and reduced levels of Th2-associated cytokines are indicative of polarization towards a Th1 immune phenotype in IA/CPA patients. However, measurement of serum/BALF cytokine concentration only provides a limited picture of the functional potential of immune cells in infected patients. To elevate our depth of understanding in this key understudied area, we recently published a study characterizing cytokine production in CPA patients following whole blood culture with relevant fungal (zymosan, β-glucan) and bacterial (Lipopolysaccharide (LPS)) pathogen-associated molecular patterns (PAMPs), and cytokines (IL-12, IL-18) (Colombo et al., 2022). We observed that CPA patients had dramatically reduced potential to produce IFN-γ in response to stimulation compared to healthy controls under a range of stimulation conditions. Interestingly, patients who exhibited higher production of IFN-γ had longer survival (Colombo et al., 2022). These observations not only suggest a key role for IFN-γ and Th1 polarization in the control and resolution of CPA but also provide supporting evidence for the use of IFN-γ as an adjunct therapeutic in the treatment of patients who display resistance to frontline antifungal strategies.

The precise nature of the immune deficiency in the potential to produce IFN-γ in CPA patients remains unclear. Two likely possibilities present themselves: (1) effector T cells in CPA patients may become refractory to antigen exposure that would normally trigger IFN-γ production. T-cell exhaustion, characterized by suboptimal functionality and upregulation of immune checkpoint proteins such as programmed cell death protein 1 (PD1) and cytotoxic T lymphocyte antigen 4 (CTLA4), has become a hallmark of chronic inflammatory conditions, including cancer and chronic viral infection (Wherry and Kurachi, 2015). Confirmation that IFN-γ deficiency in CPA patients is a consequence of T-cell exhaustion would open up the exciting possibility for the application of checkpoint inhibitors as an adjunct immunotherapeutic strategy (Gaikwad et al., 2022). (2) Alternatively, IFN-γ deficiency in CPA patients may be a consequence of an impaired capacity of their innate immune cells to either present antigen to T cells and/or effectively trigger Th1 differentiation. Conventional dendritic cells (cDCs) play a crucial role in simultaneously presenting antigen to T cells and providing signals, via cytokine secretion, which trigger differentiation into specific Th cell subsets. Type-1 cDCs (cDC1s) are the primary cDC subset responsible for inducing Th1 differentiation through the production of IL-12 (Yin et al., 2021). Monocyte-derived DCs generated from peripheral blood mononuclear cells (PBMCs) isolated from healthy donors have a high capacity to generate IL-12 and TNF-α when exposed to *A. fumigatus* in culture in a Dectin-1-dependent manner (Yin et al., 2021), and have the capacity to prime Th1 cells (Gafa et al., 2006). It will be crucial going forward to determine whether DCs from CPA patients are dysfunctional in their ability to generate pro-inflammatory cytokines in response to fungal PAMPs.

Whilst the above data indicate a role for IFN-γ/Th1 immunity in control of IA/CPA, there is still a substantial gap in our mechanistic understanding of the role Th1 cells play in immunity to pulmonary aspergillosis. Data from a preclinical mouse model of IA using chimeric antigen receptor T cells specific to *A. fumigatus* indicates that antigen-specific $CD4^+$ T cells adopt a Th1 phenotype when exposed to *A. fumigatus* antigen, are host-protective in vivo, and enhance the potential of macrophages to directly target *A. fumigatus* hyphae in vitro (Seif et al., 2022). However, the picture in humans appears more complex. A study comparing the *Aspergillus*-specific T-cell response between PBMCs and cells isolated from resected lung tissue from donors without pulmonary aspergillosis indicated a clear distinction in the T-cell cytokine response between cells isolated from blood and lung. *Aspergillus*-pulsed blood T cells produced high levels of IFN-γ and did not produce IL-17. By contrast, lung T cells expressed high levels of IL-17 and only low levels of IFN-γ (Jolink et al., 2017). This would suggest that a healthy peripheral response to *Aspergillus* favors Th1 polarization whilst a lung response is Th17-inducing. As such, some caution must be taken when interpreting results from studies of IA/CPA patients reliant solely on peripheral blood samples. However, it also implies a dual necessity for both Th1 and Th17 immunity in the anti-*Aspergillus* immune response, with Th17 cells regulating immunity at the boundary of infection and Th1 cells potentially responsible for preventing dissemination into circulation or as sentinels against opportunistic bacterial pathogens.

Interferon-gamma as an antifungal agent

Role in invasive aspergillosis

Preclinical data

In vitro and animal studies have shown the potential for synergy between IFN-γ and antifungals, as well as the direct anti-*Aspergillus* activity of IFN-γ. Bouzani et al showed that the antifungal effect of NK cells on *Aspergillus* germlings is mediated at least partly by IFN-γ (Bouzani et al., 2011). In vitro IFN-γ had little antifungal activity against *A. fumigatus* or *A. flavus*, inhibiting growth by 6% and 11%, respectively (El-Khoury et al., 2017). However, when combined with amphotericin B, it enhanced its effect, suggesting a synergistic combination of IFN-γ with antifungals. Synergism between IFN-γ and a novel polyene macrolide antibiotic was also demonstrated in a mouse model of IA (Naik et al., 2011).

In a neutropenic mouse lung infection model, NK cells were shown to be the major source of IFN-γ during early IA, as depletion of NK cells resulted in a reduction of IFN-γ and increased susceptibility, whereas NK cell depletion did not increase susceptibility in IFN-γ-depleted mice (Park et al., 2009). In another report, IFN-γ in vitro significantly enhanced phagocytosis and killing function of neutrophils and alveolar macrophages in nonneutropenic mice with IA, but not in glucocorticoid-treated animals. However, in vivo administration did not improve mortality (Johnson et al., 2005). The way of administration may be important in achieving response: intranasal administration of a recombinant adenovirus vector carrying IFN-γ cDNA, followed by *Aspergillus* challenge 24 hours later, improved mortality (Shao et al., 2005).

Clinical data

A small number of case series on the outcomes of patients with IA treated with IFN-γ have been published. In the largest series, 26 hematopoietic stem cell transplant recipients received IFN-γ with antifungals to treat IA. Of these, 54% died. IFN-γ was well tolerated without serious adverse reactions. Interestingly, IFN-γ also improved graft-versus-host disease symptoms in some patients (Safdar et al., 2005). In a series of three renal transplant recipients with IA, including one with brain disease, clinical improvement was noted after the addition of IFN-γ to conventional antifungal treatment (Armstrong-James et al., 2010). No patient had a relapse during long-term follow-up. Case reports have been published in renal and liver transplant recipients with good outcomes (Estrada et al., 2012; Mezidi et al., 2014). An 8-year-old with leukemia developed *A. terreus* invasive disease and received IFN-γ after deterioration on antifungal therapy. She improved after 3 weeks with a reduction in serum galactomannan levels. In vitro studies suggested that IFN-γ increased the capacity of the patient's monocytes to kill *A. terreus* spores (Assendorp et al., 2018).

IFN-γ has been most widely used in chronic granulomatous disease (CGD) following a randomized controlled trial showing it prevents infective episodes, including fungal infections (International Chronic Granulomatous Disease Cooperative Study Group, 1991). As a result, several reports are available on the use of IFN-γ in this patient population. IFN-γ was shown to increase reactive oxygen species production in a CGD patient (Yamashita et al., 2013). Disseminated, brain or bone IA were treated successfully in such patients in combinations with antifungals (Darazam et al., 2014; Al-Tawfiq and Al-Abdely, 2010; Patiroglu et al., 2010). Finally, IFN-γ treatment has been described in a patient with COPD after ECMO treatment with a successful outcome (Parcell et al., 2014) and a patient with bronchiectasis and *Aspergillus* empyema (Bandera et al., 2008).

Randomized controlled trials of IFN-γ have been challenging to perform. Limitations may include the relative rarity of the condition, the need for subcutaneous administration, the side effect profile, and cost. A randomized controlled trial of IFN-γ was attempted in patients with candidiasis or aspergillosis, but only 6 patients were randomized. Therefore conclusions could not be made regarding efficacy. However, in vitro analysis showed that IL-17 and IL-22 production was increased on stimulation by phytohaemagglutinin or by fungal hyphae one day after IFN-γ was started, suggesting a beneficial immunomodulatory function (Delsing et al., 2014). This effect reverted to normal after 28 days.

Role in chronic pulmonary aspergillosis

IFN-γ production defects have been implicated in CPA (Colombo et al., 2022). Given the moderate effect of antifungals in CPA, the need for prolonged courses, and the frequent emergence of resistance, INF-γ has attracted interest as a supplementary treatment to antifungals.

The first report on the use of IFN-γ in CPA included two patients. Both patients had a marked reduction in IFN-γ production in peripheral blood after stimulation by the T-cell mitogen phytohemagglutinin. None of the patients produced neutralizing IFN-γ autoantibodies (Kelleher et al., 2006). Both patients deteriorated on antifungals alone but exhibited clinical improvement upon addition of IFN-γ. Another patient with CPA did not improve on itraconazole but did improve after the addition of IFN-γ. It was stopped after 48 days due to side effects (Bandera et al., 2008).

In the largest retrospective series, 36 patients received IFN-γ as salvage therapy due to failure of azole treatment (Monk et al., 2020). Twenty patients received IFN-γ for more than 12 months; eight stopped due to side effects after a mean duration of 2.5 months, and eight patients died within a year of starting. Most patients also continued antifungal treatment. Patients who were able to tolerate IFN-γ for more than a year had a significantly reduced rate of acute exacerbations and hospital admissions compared to the year prior to IFN-γ treatment (Monk et al., 2020). Therefore IFN-γ shows promise as adjunctive treatment in CPA, however the tolerability profile may make administration challenging, as prolonged courses are usually considered, given the chronicity of the condition. A randomized controlled trial of IFN-γ in CPA is currently underway (NCT05653193, clintrials.gov).

Conclusion

There is significant scope for future research to expand our understanding of the role of IFN-γ and Th1 immunity in invasive and CPA. Deep immune phenotyping of cells isolated from the periphery and from the lungs of patients will be essential in defining how the immune system is changed in the context of infection. Additionally, there is an urgent need for larger-scale trials of IFN-γ as an adjunct therapeutic to confirm its efficacy. Such trials should be paired with immune profiling to provide a mechanistic understanding of how IFN-γ supports an effective anti-*Aspergillus* immune response. Such studies have the potential to dramatically transform strategies for the treatment of pulmonary aspergillosis and fungal infection more broadly.

References

Al-Tawfiq, J.A., Al-Abdely, H.M., 2010. Vertebral osteomyelitis due to *Aspergillus fumigatus* in a patient with chronic granulomatous disease successfully treated with antifungal agents and interferon-gamma. Medical Mycology 48 (3), 537–541. Available at https://doi.org/10.3109/13693780903325290.

Armstrong-James, D., Teo, I.A., Shrivastava, S., Petrou, M.A., Taube, D., Dorling, A., et al., 2010. Exogenous interferon-γ immunotherapy for invasive fungal infections in kidney transplant patients. American Journal of Transplantation 10 (8), 1796–1803. Available at https://doi.org/10.1111/j.1600-6143.2010.03094.x.

Assendorp, E.L., Gresnigt, M.S., Sprenkeler, E.G.G., Meis, J.F., Dors, N., van der Linden, J.W.M., et al., 2018. Adjunctive interferon-γ immunotherapy in a pediatric case of *Aspergillus terreus* infection. European Journal of Clinical Microbiology and Infectious Diseases 37 (10), 1915–1922. Available from: Available at https://doi.org/10.1007/s10096-018-3325-4, link.springer.de/link/service/journals/10096/index.htm.

Bandera, A., Trabattoni, D., Ferrario, G., Cesari, M., Franzetti, F., Clerici, M., et al., 2008. Interferon-γ and granulocyte-macrophage colony stimulating factor therapy in three patients with pulmonary aspergillosis. Infection 36 (4), 368–373. Available at https://doi.org/10.1007/s15010-008-7378-7.

Bouzani, M., Ok, M., McCormick, A., Ebel, F., Kurzai, O., Morton, C.O., et al., 2011. Human NK cells display important antifungal activity against aspergillus fumigatus, which is directly mediated by IFN-γ release. The Journal of Immunology 187 (3), 1369–1376. Available at https://doi.org/10.4049/jimmunol.1003593.

Brummer, E., Hanson, L.H., Restrepo, A., Stevens, D.A., 1988. In vivo and in vitro activation of pulmonary macrophages by IFN-γ for enhanced killing of *Paracoccidioides brasiliensis* of *Blastomyces dermatitidis*. Journal of Immunology 140 (8), 2786–2789.

Brummer, E., Hanson, L.H., Stevens, D.A., 1993. IL-4, IgE, and interferon-γ production in pulmonary blastomycosis: comparison in mice untreated, immunized, or treated with an antifungal (SCH 39304). Cellular Immunology 149 (2), 258–267. Available at https://doi.org/10.1006/cimm.1993.1153.

Colombo, S.A.P., Hashad, R., Denning, D.W., Kumararatne, D.S., Ceron-Gutierrez, L., Barcenas-Morales, G., et al., 2022. Defective interferon-gamma production is common in chronic pulmonary aspergillosis. Journal of Infectious Diseases 225 (10), 1822–1831. Available at https://doi.org/10.1093/infdis/jiab583. Available from: http://jid.oxfordjournals.org/content/current.

Darazam, I.A., Zanjani, H.A., Sanaee, D., Tabarsi, P., Moghadam, M.A., Mansouri, D., 2014. Disseminated aspergillosis as the herald manifestation of chronic granulomatous disease in an adult patient. Iranian journal of allergy, asthma, and immunology 13 (1), 66–70. Available from: http://ijaai.tums.ac.ir/index.php/ijaai/article/view/637/618.

Delsing, C.E., Gresnigt, M.S., Leentjens, J., Preijers, F., Frager, F.A., Kox, M., et al., 2014. Interferon-gamma as adjunctive immunotherapy for invasive fungal infections: a case series. BMC infectious diseases 14 (1). Available at https://doi.org/10.1186/1471-2334-14-166. Available from: http://www.biomedcentral.com/1471-2334/14/166.

El-Khoury, M., Ligot, R., Mahoney, S., Stack, C.M., Perrone, G.G., Morton, C.O., 2017. The in vitro effects of interferon-gamma, alone or in combination with amphotericin B, tested against the pathogenic fungi *Candida albicans* and *Aspergillus fumigatus*. BMC Research Notes 10 (1). Available at https://doi.org/10.1186/s13104-017-2696-4. Available from: http://www.biomedcentral.com/bmcresnotes/.

Estrada, C., Desai, A.G., Chirch, L.M., Suh, H., Seidman, R., Darras, F., et al., 2012. Invasive aspergillosis in a renal transplant recipient successfully treated with interferon-gamma. Case Reports in Transplantation 2012, 1–5. Available at https://doi.org/10.1155/2012/493758.

van Furth, R., Kullberg, B.J., van't Wout, J.W., Hoogstraten, C., 1993. Recombinant interferon-γ enhances resistance to acute disseminated *Candida albicans* infection in mice. Journal of Infectious Diseases 168 (2), 436–443. Available at https://doi.org/10.1093/infdis/168.2.436.

Gafa, V., Lande, R., Gagliardi, M.C., Severa, M., Giacomini, E., Remoli, M.E., et al., 2006. Human dendritic cells following *Aspergillus fumigatus* infection express the CCR7 receptor and a differential pattern of interleukin-12 (IL-12), IL-23, and IL-27 cytokines, which lead to a Th1 response. Infection and Immunity 74 (3), 1480–1489. Available at https://doi.org/10.1128/iai.74.3.1480-1489.2006.

Gaikwad, S., Agrawal, M.Y., Kaushik, I., Ramachandran, S., Srivastava, S.K., 2022. Immune checkpoint proteins: signaling mechanisms and molecular interactions in cancer immunotherapy. Seminars in Cancer Biology 86, 137–150. Available at https://doi.org/10.1016/j.semcancer.2022.03.014. Available from: http://www.elsevier.com/inca/publications/store/6/2/2/9/4/3/index.htt.

Gonçalves, S.M., Lagrou, K., Rodrigues, C.S., Campos, C.F., Bernal-Martínez, L., Rodrigues, F., et al., 2017. Evaluation of bronchoalveolar lavage fluid cytokines as biomarkers for invasive pulmonary aspergillosis in at-risk patients. Frontiers in Microbiology 8. Available at https://doi.org/10.3389/fmicb.2017.02362. Available from: https://www.frontiersin.org/articles/10.3389/fmicb.2017.02362/full.

Heldt, S., Eigl, S., Prattes, J., Flick, H., Rabensteiner, J., Prüller, F., et al., 2017. Levels of interleukin (IL)-6 and IL -8 are elevated in serum and bronchoalveolar lavage fluid of haematological patients with invasive pulmonary aspergillosis. Mycoses 60 (12), 818–825. Available at https://doi.org/10.1111/myc.12679.

International Chronic Granulomatous Disease Cooperative Study Group, 1991. A controlled trial of interferon gamma to prevent infection in chronic granulomatous disease. New England Journal of Medicine. 324 (8), 509–516, doi: 10.1056/nejm199102213240801.

Jarvis, J.N., Meintjes, G., Rebe, K., Williams, G.N., Bicanic, T., Williams, A., et al., 2012. Adjunctive interferon-γ immunotherapy for the treatment of HIV-associated cryptococcal meningitis: a randomized controlled trial. AIDS (London, England) 26 (9), 1105–1113. Available at https://doi.org/10.1097/QAD.0b013e3283536a93.

Johnson, C.P., Edmiston, C.E., Zhu, Y.R., Adams, M.B., Roza, A.M., Kurup, V., 2005. A murine model of invasive aspergillosis: variable benefit of interferon-gamma administration under in vitro and in vivo conditions. Surgical infections 6 (4), 397–407. Available at https://doi.org/10.1089/sur.2005.6.397.

Jolink, H., de Boer, R., Hombrink, P., Jonkers, R.E., van Dissel, J.T., Falkenburg, J.H.F., et al., 2017. Pulmonary immune responses against *Aspergillus fumigatus* are characterized by high frequencies of IL-17 producing T-cells. Journal of Infection 74 (1), 81–88. Available at https://doi.org/10.1016/j.jinf.2016.10.010.

Kelleher, P., Goodsall, A., Mulgirigama, A., Kunst, H., Henderson, D.C., Wilson, R., et al., 2006. Interferon-γ therapy in two patients with progressive chronic pulmonary aspergillosis. European Respiratory Journal 27 (6), 1307–1310. Available at https://doi.org/10.1183/09031936.06.00021705.

Mezidi, M., Belafia, F., Nougaret, S., Pageaux, G.P., Conseil, M., Panaro, E., et al., 2014. Interferon gamma in association with immunosuppressive drugs withdrawal and antifungal combination as a rescue therapy for cerebral invasive aspergillosis in a liver transplant recipient. Minerva Anestesiologica 80 (12), 1359–1360. Available from: http://www.minervamedica.it/en/journals/minerva-anestesiologica/archive.php.

Monk, E.J.M., Harris, C., Döffinger, R., Hayes, G., Denning, D.W., Kosmidis, C., 2020. Interferon gamma replacement as salvage therapy in chronic pulmonary aspergillosis: effects on frequency of acute exacerbation and all-cause hospital admission. Thorax 75 (6), 513–516. Available at https://doi.org/10.1136/thoraxjnl-2019-213606. Available from: http://thorax.bmj.com/.

Morrison, C.J., Brummer, E., Stevens, D.A., 1989. In vivo activation of peripheral blood polymorphonuclear neutrophils by gamma interferon results in enhanced fungal killing. Infection and Immunity 57 (10), 2953–2958. Available at https://doi.org/10.1128/iai.57.10.2953-2958.1989.

Naik, S.R., Thakare, V.N., Desai, S.K., Rahalkar, P.R., 2011. Study of immunological aspects of aspergillosis in mice and effect of polyene macrolide antibiotic (SJA-95) and IFN-γ: a possible role of IFN-γ as an adjunct in antifungal therapy. Immunology Letters 141 (1), 68–73. Available at https://doi.org/10.1016/j.imlet.2011.07.008.

Parcell, B.J., Pavan, P.K., Johnson, E.M., Fardon, T.C., Olver, W.J., 2014. Invasive pulmonary aspergillosis post extracorporeal membrane oxygenation support and literature review. Medical Mycology Case Reports 4 (1), 12–15. Available at https://doi.org/10.1016/j.mmcr.2014.01.003. Available from: http://www.journals.elsevier.com/medical-mycology-case-reports/.

Park, S.J., Hughes, M.A., Burdick, M., Strieter, R.M., Mehrad, B., 2009. Early NK cell-derived IFN-γ is essential to host defense in neutropenic invasive aspergillosis. Journal of

Immunology 182 (7), 4306–4312. Available at https://doi.org/10.4049/jimmunol.0803462. Available from: http://www.jimmunol.org/cgi/reprint/182/7/4306.

Patiroglu, T., Unal, E., Yikilmaz, A., Koker, M.Y., Ozturk, M.K., 2010. Atypical presentation of chronic granulomatous disease in an adolescent boy with frontal lobe located *Aspergillus abscess* mimicking intracranial tumor. Child's Nervous System 26 (2), 149–154. Available at https://doi.org/10.1007/s00381-009-1003-7.

Ren, W., Li, H., Guo, C., Shang, Y., Wang, W., Zhang, X., et al., 2023. Serum cytokine biomarkers for use in diagnosing pulmonary tuberculosis versus chronic pulmonary aspergillosis. Infection and Drug Resistance 16, 2217–2226. Available at https://doi.org/10.2147/IDR.S403401. Available from: https://www.dovepress.com/getfile.php?fileID=88973.

Safdar, A., Rodriguez, G., Ohmagari, N., Kontoyiannis, D.P., Rolston, K.V., Raad, I.I., et al., 2005. The safety of interferon-γ-1b therapy for invasive fungal infections after hematopoietic stem cell transplantation. Cancer 103 (4), 731–739. Available at https://doi.org/10.1002/cncr.20883.

Salzer, H.J.F., Prattes, J., Flick, H., Reimann, M., Heyckendorf, J., Kalsdorf, B., et al., 2018. Evaluation of galactomannan testing, the aspergillus-specific lateral-flow device test and levels of cytokines in bronchoalveolar lavage fluid for diagnosis of chronic pulmonary aspergillosis. Frontiers in Microbiology 9 Available from: Available at https://doi.org/10.3389/fmicb.2018.02223, www.frontiersin.org/Microbiology.

Seif, M., Kakoschke, T.K., Ebel, F., Bellet, M.M., Trinks, N., Renga, G., et al., 2022. CAR T cells targeting *Aspergillus fumigatus* are effective at treating invasive pulmonary aspergillosis in preclinical models. Science Translational Medicine 14 (664). Available at https://doi.org/10.1126/scitranslmed.abh1209. Available from: https://www.science.org/doi/10.1126/scitranslmed.abh1209.

Shao, C., Qu, J., He, L., Zhang, Y., Wang, J., Wang, Y., et al., 2005. Transient overexpression of γ interferon promotes *Aspergillus* clearance in invasive pulmonary aspergillosis. Clinical and Experimental Immunology 142 (2), 233–241. Available at https://doi.org/10.1111/j.1365-2249.2005.02828.x.

Stevens, D.A., Brummer, E., Clemons, K.V., 2006. 9 15 2006/09/15 Journal of Infectious Diseases 10.1086/505357 00221899 1 S33-S37S33 United States Interferon-γ as an antifungal 194.

Wherry, E.J., Kurachi, M., 2015. Molecular and cellular insights into T cell exhaustion. Nature reviews. Immunology 15 (8), 486–499. Available at https://doi.org/10.1038/nri3862. Available from: http://www.nature.com/nri/index.html.

Yamashita, K., Miyoshi, T., Arai, Y., Mizugishi, K., Takaori-Kondo, A., Ueyama, T., 2013. Enhanced generation of reactive oxygen species by interferon-γ may have contributed to successful treatment of invasive pulmonary aspergillosis in a patient with chronic granulomatous disease. International Journal of Hematology 97 (4), 505–510. Available at https://doi.org/10.1007/s12185-013-1315-y.

Yin, X., Chen, S., Eisenbarth, S.C., 2021. Dendritic cell regulation of T helper cells. Annual Review of Immunology 39, 759–790. Available at https://doi.org/10.1146/annurev-immunol-101819-025146. Available from: http://www.annualreviews.org/journal/immunol.

Zhan, M., Xu, B., Zhao, L., Li, B., Xu, L., Sun, Q., et al., 2018. The serum level of IL-1B correlates with the activity of chronic pulmonary aspergillosis. Canadian Respiratory Journal 2018, 1–9. Available at https://doi.org/10.1155/2018/8740491.

CHAPTER

Breaches in antifungal immunity and viral-associated aspergillosis

5

Simon Feys[1,2], Laura Seldeslachts[3], Greetje Vande Velde[3] and Joost Wauters[1,2]

[1]*Department of Microbiology, Immunology and Transplantation, Leuven, Flemish Brabant, Belgium,*
[2]*Medical Intensive Care, University Hospitals Leuven, Leuven, Flemish Brabant, Belgium,*
[3]*Department of Imaging & Pathology, KU Leuven, Leuven, Flemish Brabant, Belgium*

The clinical picture of viral-associated pulmonary aspergillosis

The spectrum of patients prone to develop invasive aspergillosis has been rapidly expanding, in part due to the introduction of a wide array of immunosuppressive therapies (Latgé and Chamilos, 2019). In the past decades, autopsy studies revealed that nonneutropenic patients requiring intensive care were also prone to develop aspergillosis (Meersseman et al., 2007). Among these critically ill patients, a special category at risk for aspergillosis is constituted by patients with severe viral pneumonia. Cases of invasive pulmonary aspergillosis have been described as early as 1952 in critically ill patients with influenza without preexisting immunosuppression (Abbott et al., 1952). However, it would take until the 2009 H1N1 pandemic to recognize influenza-associated pulmonary aspergillosis (IAPA) as a distinct, frequently occurring superinfection (Schauwvlieghe et al., 2018; Wauters et al., 2012; Van De Veerdonk et al., 2017b). When coronavirus disease 2019 (COVID-19) emerged, COVID-19–associated pulmonary aspergillosis (CAPA) was rapidly recognized as well (Wasylyshyn et al., 2021; Coste et al., 2021; Lahmer et al., 2021; Huang et al., 2020). IAPA and CAPA are collectively called viral-associated pulmonary aspergillosis (VAPA).

IAPA and CAPA share similarities, but also distinct clinical features (Fig. 5.1). For both superinfections, reported incidences vary between less than 1% to more than 30% in patients admitted to ICU with severe influenza or COVID-19, due to several diagnostic reasons (Feys et al., 2024b). However, true incidences probably lie around 10%–20% in critically ill patients (Feys et al., 2024b). IAPA tends to occur soon during ICU stay, and is often already detectable at time of admission (Vanderbeke et al., 2021), while CAPA tends to occur later, typically between 3 and 9 days after ICU admission (Gangneux et al., 2022; Prattes et al., 2022; Janssen et al., 2021). VAPA is challenging to diagnose, with clinical features and radiological findings often being nonspecific. Diagnosis mainly relies on bronchoscopy with

Immunological Insights and Emerging Therapeutics in Medical Mycology. DOI: https://doi.org/10.1016/B978-0-443-23636-5.00002-2

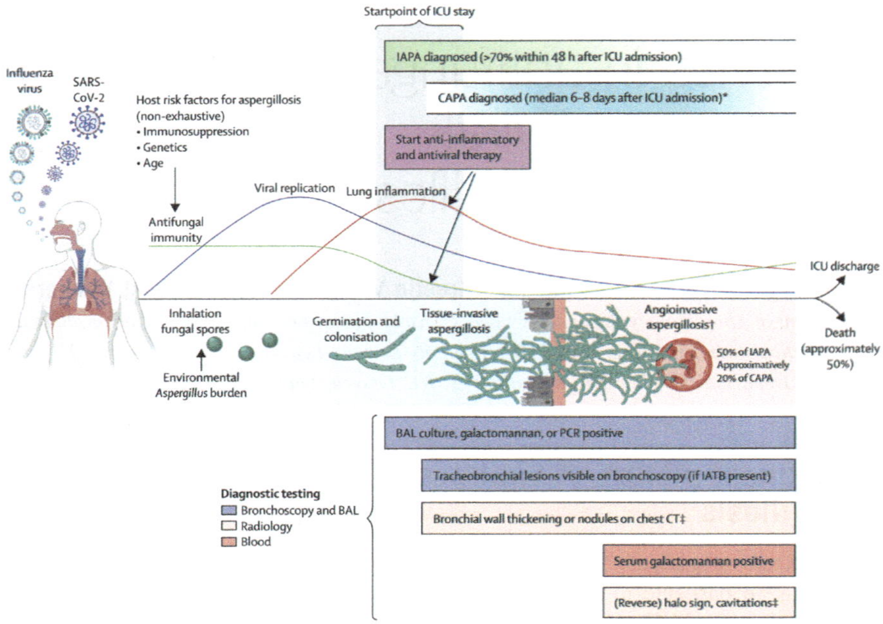

FIGURE 5.1 Clinical disease course of influenza-associated (IAPA) and COVID-19–associated pulmonary aspergillosis (CAPA).

Summary of the disease course and diagnostic findings throughout disease of IAPA and CAPA. The disease course is highly variable in patients (e.g., some patients might have angio-invasive aspergillosis already upon ICU admission).

Modified from Feys, S., Carvalho, A., Clancy, C. J., Gangneux, J.-P., Hoenigl, M., Lagrou, K., Rijnders, B. J. A., Seldeslachts, L., Vanderbeke, L., van de Veerdonk, F. L., Verweij, P. E. & Wauters, J. (2024). Influenza-associated and COVID-19-associated pulmonary aspergillosis in critically ill patients. The Lancet. Respiratory Medicine. https://doi.org/10.1016/S2213-2600(24)00151-6. Panel originally created with Biorender.com.

bronchoalveolar lavage (BAL) sampling to detect the fungus through culture, galactomannan (an *Aspergillus* antigen), or polymerase chain reactions testing (Verweij et al., 2020; Koehler et al., 2021). Positivity of galactomannan in serum, which reflects angioinvasion of *Aspergillus* hyphae, is rarely detected in VAPA (Schauwvlieghe et al., 2018; Ergün et al., 2021; Dellière et al., 2022). Despite antifungal therapy, both IAPA and CAPA are associated with an overall mortality rate of approximately 50%, which is 2 to 3 times higher than that of patients with severe viral pneumonia without VAPA (Lu et al., 2024; Shi et al., 2022; Chen et al., 2022; Krzych et al., 2022).

Insight into the mechanisms behind VAPA, and in the differences between patients with severe viral pneumonia who do and who do not develop VAPA, is key to improving our diagnostic, prognostic, and therapeutic toolbox. Many hypotheses on the mechanism of VAPA have been raised (Salazar et al., 2022), and several groups have started to investigate the pathophysiology of VAPA, using in vitro set-ups, animal models, and patient samples.

Primer on severe viral pneumonia

Currently, severe viral pneumonias caused by two distinct respiratory viruses have been described to provoke VAPA in multiple observational studies: influenza virus and severe acute respiratory syndrome coronavirus 2 (SARS-CoV-2).

Influenza viruses are negative-sense, single-stranded RNA viruses (Flerlage et al., 2021). They are enveloped viruses, subtyped based on two surface glycoproteins: hemagglutinin (H) and neuraminidase (N). Hemagglutinin is involved in binding to sialic acids and subsequent cell entry, and neuraminidase mediates release from infected cells. Influenza A virus and influenza B virus are the two genera of main concern for humans (Uyeki et al., 2022). Currently, influenza A(H1N1)pdm09 and A(H3N2) are the most common influenza strains causing disease in people worldwide (Uyeki et al., 2022).

SARS-CoV-2 is a positive-sense, single-stranded RNA virus (Yang and Rao, 2021). Several variants of concern have established worldwide or regional dominance since SARS-CoV-2 first occurred. After the ancestral strain, the alpha, beta, gamma, and delta variants became the most important variants of concern, outcompeting previous variants. In late 2021, the omicron variant emerged and soon established worldwide dominance. Since then, many omicron subvariants have appeared, often existing in parallel, with varying dominance (Carabelli et al., 2023). Several receptors have been described for SARS-CoV-2, with the ACE2 receptor being the most prominent one. ACE2 is found abundantly in the lungs, but also in vascular endothelium (Hamming et al., 2004). This may in part explain the tropism of the virus for nonrespiratory organs, and may explain the immunothrombotic disorders often encountered in severe COVID-19 (Bourgonje et al., 2020).

Airborne virus transmission leads to epithelial infection in the upper respiratory tract, which may descend to the lower respiratory tract in case of severe viral infection. In severe disease, hyperinflammation is the result of a dysregulated immune response to pulmonary viral replication. Viral RNA is sensed through several pattern recognition receptors, which induce an interferon response and an inflammatory response. For instance, RNA of both viruses is detected by retinoic acid inducible gene I, and by distinct Toll-like receptors in infected cells and/or in immune cells (Iwasaki and Pillai, 2014). This mounts an interferon response, which is characterized by transcription of interferon-stimulated genes (ISGs). These ISGs lead to an antiviral state that aims to restrict viral replication (Iwasaki and Pillai, 2014). Additionally, a pro-inflammatory response is induced through activation of the nuclear factor-κB (NF-κB) pathway and of the NLR family pyrin domain-containing 3 inflammasome (Niu and Meng, 2023; Potere et al., 2022). Damage-associated molecular patterns released upon infection may further drive the pro-inflammatory response (Land, 2021). Severe viral pneumonia is associated with excessive complement activation, albeit more pronounced in severe COVID-19, which may contribute to lung tissue damage and the production of pro-inflammatory substances (Xiao et al., 2024; Carvelli et al., 2020).

Neutrophils and monocytes are recruited to the viral-infected lungs in response to pro-inflammatory cytokines and chemokines, and other chemotactic molecules such as complement C5a. In the meantime, dendritic cells take up viral antigens and are subsequently triggered to migrate to the lymph nodes for antigen presentation to T lymphocytes, with subsequent B cell activation (Alon et al., 2021). In severe viral pneumonia, an excessive influx of hyperinflammatory neutrophils and monocytes occurs, which is associated with collateral tissue damage. Hence, high levels of pro-inflammatory cytokines such as IL-1ß, IL-6, or TNF-α in the lungs of these patients, as well as higher viral loads, are associated with increased mortality in patients with severe influenza or COVID-19 (Pronier et al., 2021; Fajnzylber et al., 2020; Lobo et al., 2019; Gao et al., 2013; Del Valle et al., 2020).

Multilevel disruption of anti-*Aspergillus* immunity in severe viral pneumonia

Several layers of antifungal immunity are affected by severe viral pneumonia Fig. 5.2. Severe influenza and severe COVID-19 share many similarities but also some differences regarding their effect on the immune response directed against *Aspergillus*.

Multiple strategies have been used to gain deeper insight into the clinical observations and pathophysiology of VAPA. BAL samples from patients with severe influenza or COVID-19 with or without aspergillosis have been investigated using multiomics approaches, and antifungal effector functions of blood cells from these patients have been assessed (Feys et al., 2022, 2023, 2024a,b; Tappe et al., 2022). Moreover, in vitro models and murine models of VAPA have been established (Nicolas de Lamballerie et al., 2020; König et al., 2024; Tobin et al., 2020; Seldeslachts et al., 2021, 2022; Liu et al., 2022; Sarden et al., 2022; Lee et al., 2023; Wurster et al., 2023). Among the animal models, five mimic the development of IAPA in previously healthy hosts (Tobin et al., 2020; Seldeslachts et al., 2021, 2022; Liu et al., 2022; Sarden et al., 2022; Lee et al., 2023), one model employs corticosteroid induction for IAPA simulation (Wurster et al., 2023), and one murine model used a SARS-CoV-2 pseudovirus to establish CAPA (Sarden et al., 2022). Consistent with clinical observations, both immunocompetent and immunosuppressed mice with a severe viral infection showed heightened susceptibility to aspergillosis due to different viral-induced modulations in the antifungal host immunity.

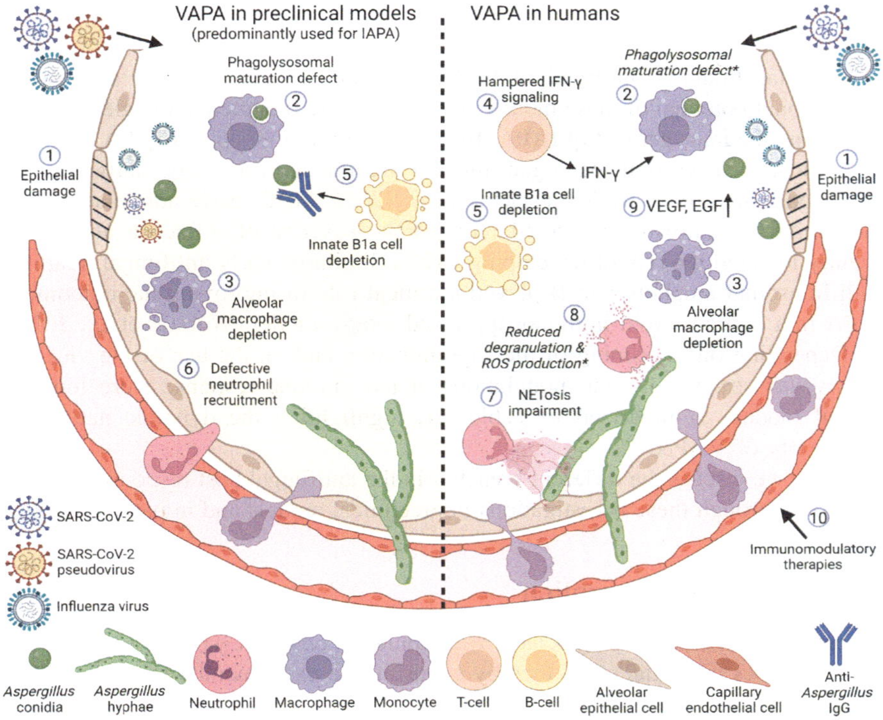

FIGURE 5.2 Breaches in antifungal immunity in viral-associated pulmonary aspergillosis (VAPA).

Observations made in preclinical mouse and in vitro models of VAPA, and in patients with severe viral pneumonia with or without VAPA, are depicted in an alveolus. Viral-induced epithelial barrier disruption paves the way for *Aspergillus* to become tissue-invasive, and may impair mucociliary clearance, resulting in reduced clearance of inhaled *Aspergillus* conidia (1). Phagocytosis and clearance of the conidia may be impaired through phagolysosomal maturation defects in phagocytes (2), alveolar macrophage depletion with replacement by hyperinflammatory monocytes that are not very effective at phagocytosis (3), impaired interferon-gamma (IFN-γ) signaling (4), and innate B1a cell depletion with resulting lack of natural antibodies against *Aspergillus*, or through other defects in recognition of *Aspergillus* (5). Defective neutrophil recruitment has been described in a mouse model of influenza-associated pulmonary aspergillosis (IAPA) (6). Neutrophil effector functions such as production of neutrophil extracellular traps (NETs) (7) and neutrophil degranulation or production of reactive oxygen species (ROS) (8) might be impaired as well in patients with VAPA compared to severe viral pneumonia patients without VAPA. Increased levels of growth factors such as vascular endothelial growth factor (VEGF) and epidermal growth factor (EGF) are observed in bronchoalveolar lavage fluid of patients with VAPA, and might be associated with increased fibrosis of the lungs (9). Lastly, immunomodulatory therapies (such as corticosteroids) may further hamper the antifungal host response in VAPA (10). *Defects in italics depicted with an asterisk are only indirectly observed in humans (for instance through transcriptomics), more mechanistic in-depth research is required to confirm these observations. Figure made with Biorender.com.

No Permission Required.

The similar findings observed in IAPA mice and patient samples suggest the translational potential of these mouse models to assess treatment strategies aimed at improving the management of IAPA. Indeed, two mouse models of IAPA evaluated the efficacy of current pathogen-directed treatments involving antivirals and antifungals. In studies by Seldeslachts et al. (2021, 2022) early administration of oseltamivir or baloxavir marboxil reduced the severity of influenza and consequently lowered the risk of developing IAPA. Similarly, early antifungal treatment with liposomal amphotericin B played a critical role in improving the outcome of IAPA in a corticosteroid-immunosuppressed mouse model (Wurster et al., 2023).

Depending on the timing of the superinfection and on the use of the viral and *Aspergillus* strain, different modulations of the immune response were found in animal models, summarized in Table 5.1, highlighting the dynamic nature and complexity of VAPA.

Next, we discuss the different breaches in the antifungal host response observed in VAPA through these investigations in preclinical models and in patient samples.

Epithelial barrier disruption

Severe viral pneumonia is associated with epithelial erosions. The lytic effect of the virus damages epithelial cells, thereby exposing the basal membrane to the airway lumen (Flerlage et al., 2021; Ackermann et al., 2020). Both in a human biopsy sample of invasive *Aspergillus* tracheobronchitis in a patient with CAPA, and in mouse models of IAPA, this epithelial barrier disruption has been shown to serve as a port-of-entry for tissue-invasive *Aspergillus* hyphae (Feys et al., 2022; Seldeslachts et al., 2021, 2022). Moreover, viral infection may lead to impaired mucociliary clearance (Pittet et al., 2010; Robinot et al., 2021), which might lead to reduced removal of *Aspergillus* conidia from the lower airways. Mucociliary clearance could potentially be further aggravated when aspergillosis is established, as shown in an in vitro human airway epithelial model of CAPA (Nicolas de Lamballerie et al., 2020).

Defective conidial phagocytosis and killing

In healthy lungs, *Aspergillus* conidia that escape mucociliary clearance are phagocytosed and killed by phagocytes, primarily alveolar macrophages (Van De Veerdonk et al., 2017a). These alveolar macrophages are partially depleted in both humans and in mouse models of severe influenza, COVID-19, and IAPA (Tobin et al., 2020; Seldeslachts et al., 2022; Ghoneim et al., 2013; Wauters et al., 2021). In severe viral pneumonia, there is an influx of hyperinflammatory monocytes (Ghoneim et al., 2013; Wauters et al., 2021), and in COVID-19 patients, these monocytes have been observed to show reduced differentiation towards well-functioning macrophages (Wauters et al., 2021). These macrophage and monocyte-related changes could contribute to hampered phagocytosis and killing of

Table 5.1 Mouse models of viral-associated pulmonary aspergillosis.

Study	Virus	*Aspergillus*	Day of superinfection	*Aspergillus*germination	Immunosuppression	Main findings
(Tobin et al., 2020)	Influenza A H1N1 PR/ 8/34	ATCC	5	Yes	No	– Reduced CXCL1 and CXCL2 levels in lungs of IAPA mice compared to influenza-only mice. – Reduced neutrophil recruitment to the lungs of IAPA mice. – Deletion of STAT1 results in decreased fungal burden, increased CXCL1, and increased airway and lung neutrophils in IAPA mice.
(Seldeslachts et al., 2022, 2021)	Influenza A H3N2 Ishikawa/ 7/82	CBS144.89	4	Yes	No	– Viral-inducedepithelial damage paves the way for tissue-invasive aspergillosis. – Macrophages are depleted in IAPA mice. – Early treatment with oseltamivir or baloxavir marboxil reduces macrophage depletion, epithelial damage, and neutrophilic inflammation in superinfected mice.
		CEA10	6	Yes	No	

(*Continued*)

Table 5.1 Mouse models of viral-associated pulmonary aspergillosis. (*Continued*)

Study	Virus	*Aspergillus*	Day of superinfection	*Aspergillus*germination	Immunosuppression	Main findings
(Liu et al., 2022)	Influenza A H1N1 PR/8/34					– No differences in inflammatory cell recruitment in IAPA mice compared to *Aspergillus*-only infected controls. – Neutrophil and monocyte conidial uptake and killing defects. – Killing defect in part due to reduced phagolysosome maturation.
(Sarden et al., 2022)	Influenza A H1N1 PR/8/34 - SARS-CoV-2 pseudovirus (VSV-GS)	Af293	5	Yes	No	– Circulating innate B1a cells are depleted in the setting of influenza, COVID-19 and dexamethasone treatment. – This results in reduced levels of anti-*Aspergillus fumigatus* natural immunoglobulin G. – This leads to impaired recognition of *Aspergillus* conidia by neutrophils. – Transfer of B1a-derived antibodies improves SARS-CoV-2 pseudovirus

Table 5.1 Mouse models of viral-associated pulmonary aspergillosis. (*Continued*)

Study	Virus	*Aspergillus*	Day of superinfection	*Aspergillus*germination	Immunosuppression	Main findings
						induced susceptibility to *Aspergillus fumigatus*.
(Lee et al., 2023)	Influenza A H1N1 PR/8/34	CEA10	2/5/8/14	Minimal	No	– Increased inflammatory cytokines in IAPA mice compared to *Aspergillus*-only or influenza-only mice. – No increased inflammation on histopathological analysis. – Dampened neutrophil recruitment to the lungs if *Aspergillus* was administered early during influenza infection. – No major effect of influenza infection on neutrophil phagocytosis and killing of *Aspergillus* conidia.
(Wurster et al., 2023)	Influenza A H3N2 mouse-adapted Hong Kong 1968	Af293	9	Yes	Corticosteroids	– Early administration of liposomal amphotericin B improves outcomes of IAPA in mice immunosuppressed with corticosteroids.

IAPA: influenza-associated pulmonary aspergillosis; *SARS-CoV-2*: severe acute respiratory syndrome coronavirus 2; *VSV-GS*: vesicular stomatitis virus expressing its natural glycoprotein and SARS-CoV-2 S protein.

Aspergillus conidia. Indeed, reduced phagocytosis of conidia and subsequent phagolysosomal fusion have been described in monocytes in one of the two mouse studies of IAPA in which these mechanisms were investigated (Liu et al., 2022; Lee et al., 2023). An interesting observation related to this matter is the downregulation of several genes linked to LC3-associated phagocytosis, a noncanonical form of autophagy implicated in phagolysosomal fusion and subsequent killing of *Aspergillus* conidia, in BAL fluid of IAPA patients compared to that of patients with influenza only (Feys et al., 2022). The exact mechanisms driving these observations have not been elucidated yet.

Immunometabolic dysregulation could be a potential driver for disturbed antifungal macrophage effector functions in severe viral pneumonia. In a single-cell RNA sequencing study of BAL fluid, monocytes and macrophages of patients with CAPA compared to non-CAPA COVID-19 patients showed increased expression of genes linked to oxidative phosphorylation, and reduced expression of genes encoding proteins with functions in glycolysis (Feys et al., 2024c). Expression of genes related to the mTOR pathway was reduced as well, providing a possible upstream mechanism for the reduced transcription of glycolysis-related genes (Feys et al., 2024c). Macrophages normally upregulate glycolysis in response to *Aspergillus* conidia, a mechanism that aids them in killing phagocytosed spores (Gonçalves et al., 2020). Therefore the observations in CAPA patients could imply hampered phagolysosomal killing of spores, predisposing these patients to develop aspergillosis. More in-depth research regarding immunometabolism in VAPA is required to further delineate its role in the mechanism behind these superinfections.

Interferon-gamma (IFN-γ) produced by T- and NK-cells (especially Th1 cells) may boost phagocytosis and killing by phagocytes (Van De Veerdonk et al., 2017a). While early excessive IFN-γ has been implicated in the pathogenesis of severe disease in both influenza and COVID-19 (Sun and Metzger, 2008; Grant et al., 2021), potentially predisposing to more secondary infections (Sun and Metzger, 2008), several patient observations point to a potentially harmful role for a later diminished response to IFN-γ (Feys et al., 2024a,b; Tappe et al., 2022). Indeed, IAPA and CAPA patients show reduced transcriptional responses to IFN-γ in BAL fluid compared to patients with severe viral pneumonia without VAPA. In CAPA patients, reduced differentiation along the Th1 maturation trajectory was observed in BAL fluid, potentially leading to reduced IFN-γ production (Feys et al., 2024a,b), and in patients with COVID-19 in general, an almost complete abrogation of IFN-γ production by peripheral blood mononuclear cells was observed in response to *Aspergillus* (Tappe et al., 2022). In contrast, in one IAPA mouse model, IFN-γ signaling did not play a significant role in driving murine IAPA, as gene expression levels of IFN (including IFN-γ) were increased, and deletion of STAT1, a mediator of IFN responses, resulted in decreased fungal burden (Tobin et al., 2020). More research into IFN-γ kinetics, including the influence of the timing difference observed between late-stage human disease (with excessive hyphae) and early-stage mouse models (with mainly germinating conidia and limited hyphae), and the potential of blocking or boosting IFN-γ to counter VAPA, will be necessary.

Hampered killing of *Aspergillus* hyphae by neutrophils

Neutrophils are the main effector cells against hyphae, using several strategies such as production of reactive oxygen species, expulsion of neutrophil extracellular traps (NETs), and degranulation of antimicrobial peptides, enzymes, and other substances such as lactoferrin stored within their granules to tackle these large fungal structures (Van De Veerdonk et al., 2017a; Ballard et al., 2020). As such, most patients with VAPA showed a neutrophilic necrotizing inflammation surrounding *Aspergillus* hyphae, impeding the growth of these hyphae in an autopsy study (Vanderbeke et al., 2023).

The relevance of neutrophils in VAPA has been underscored by the observation that CAPA patients show higher NET production in the lungs compared to patients with severe COVID-19 without CAPA, and by the observation that CAPA patients with lower BAL NET levels showed reduced 90-day survival rates compared to CAPA patients with higher NET levels (Feys et al., 2024c). Moreover, hybrid neutrophils become the dominant neutrophil phenotype in the lungs of CAPA patients (Feys et al., 2024c). These hybrid neutrophils express genes related to major histocompatibility complex II, which is normally seen on antigen-presenting cells, and have been described to emerge during other diseases such as lung cancer (Vono et al., 2017; Matsushima et al., 2013; Singhal et al., 2016). Hybrid neutrophils have been studied in mouse models of fungal disease and were shown to exert increased antifungal effector functions in comparison to regular neutrophils (Fites et al., 2018). The emergence and dominance of hybrid neutrophils in CAPA lungs could therefore constitute a specialized response towards the presence of *Aspergillus* hyphae. More research into the functions of hybrid neutrophils in VAPA is required, for instance, to determine whether these neutrophils participate in antigen presentation or whether they directly tackle the fungal structures.

In humans, most observations have been obtained for CAPA patients. However, there is indirect evidence for more outspoken defective neutrophil responses in IAPA compared to CAPA. First, transcription of genes related to neutrophil degranulation was significantly downregulated in BAL fluid of patients with IAPA compared to influenza-only patients, but not in BAL fluid of CAPA versus COVID-19-only patients (Feys et al., 2022). Second, the decrease in neutrophil fraction in BAL fluid observed in CAPA patients, caused by increased destruction due to NETosis, is not seen in IAPA patients, implying hampered production of NETs in response to the fungus in these patients (Feys et al., 2022, 2024a,b). NET-level assessment in BAL samples from IAPA patients will be necessary to confirm this hypothesis and to open the door to more in-depth analyses as to why neutrophils do not respond as they should in the setting of IAPA.

Reduced *Aspergillus* recognition

Several direct and indirect arguments for reduced recognition of *Aspergillus* have been observed in the setting of VAPA. First, the reduction in lung neutrophils in mice with IAPA compared to mice with *Aspergillus* infection only, observed in two studies (Tobin et al., 2020; Lee et al., 2023), could potentially, in part, be explained by reduced *Aspergillus* recognition in the setting of severe influenza.

Second, in an elegant study with human samples and mouse models infected with the influenza virus or a SARS-CoV-2 pseudovirus, levels of anti-*Aspergillus fumigatus* natural immunoglobulin G (IgG) were shown to be reduced in the context of viral pneumonia (Sarden et al., 2022). Viral pneumonia (as well as dexamethasone) led to depletion of circulating innate B1a cells, which are responsible for the production of these natural antibodies. Consequently, there is less opsonization of *Aspergillus* conidia, leading to reduced uptake and killing of conidia by neutrophils. Importantly, repletion of anti-*Aspergillus* natural IgG in mice infected by SARS-CoV-2 pseudovirus showed improved outcomes, including survival, when challenged with *Aspergillus fumigatus* (Sarden et al., 2022). Later, studying severe COVID-19 patients, innate B1a cells were found to be almost completely absent in BAL fluid as well (Feys et al., 2024a,b).

Third, downregulation of genes encoding proteins that bind to *Aspergillus* has been observed in BAL fluid of patients with IAPA who succumbed compared to those who survived (Feys et al., 2023). Of the 11 significantly downregulated genes observed in these patients, eight were implicated in anti-*Aspergillus* immunity, including *CLEC7A* (encoding Dectin-1), *LGALS3* (encoding Galectin-3), and *SIGLEC15* (encoding SIGLEC15). Dectin-1 recognizes ß-1,3-glucan, which is present on the surface of growing *Aspergillus* conidia, and has pleiotropic functions in anti-*Aspergillus* immunity, including cytokine production, induction of phagocytosis, and respiratory burst (Brown, 2006). Galectin-3 binds *Aspergillus* and has been shown to induce neutrophil chemotaxis to the lungs during aspergillosis in a mouse model outside the setting of viral pneumonia (Snarr et al., 2020). SIGLEC15 may bind *Aspergillus fumigatus* sialic acids and seems to be implicated in mounting a cytokine response to aspergillosis (Dewi et al., 2021). The observation that downregulation of the expression of *CLEC7A*, *LGALS3,* and *SIGLEC15* at the time of IAPA diagnosis predisposes to poor outcome (Feys et al., 2023), stresses the importance of proper *Aspergillus* recognition by immune cells even when aspergillosis has already been established. The mechanism behind this downregulation in certain patients should be investigated. Based on these observations, host-directed biomarkers could potentially be useful in prognostication of these patients, or even for diagnostic tools.

The role of the long pentraxin-3 (PTX3) in aspergillosis has been extensively studied in the setting of severe immunosuppression (Cunha et al., 2014; Garianda et al., 2002). PTX3 opsonizes *Aspergillus*, after which it binds to the complement receptor 3 and Fcγ receptor, leading to phagocytosis of conidia and initiation of a targeted immune response against hyphae. Single nucleotide polymorphisms (SNPs) in the gene encoding PTX3 have been implicated in increased risk of invasive pulmonary aspergillosis in groups of patients, including those who received an allogeneic stem cell transplantation or a solid organ transplantation and patients with acute leukemia or chronic obstructive pulmonary disease (Cunha et al., 2014; Wójtowicz et al., 2015; Brunel et al., 2018; He et al., 2018). Whether PTX3 SNPs could predispose to the development of IAPA or CAPA remains to be investigated. However, it is possible that there is no association at all between these SNPs and IAPA or CAPA occurrence. Indeed, although patients with IAPA showed reduced gene expression of *PTX3* in BAL fluid compared to severe influenza patients without aspergillosis, patients with severe influenza or COVID-19 displayed high protein levels of PTX3, irrespective of the presence of aspergillosis (Feys et al., 2022). Given the abundance of PTX3 in these patients, it is less likely that PTX3 or the underlying SNPs have a big impact on the pathogenesis and occurrence of VAPA, but this needs further investigation.

Lung vascular and mesenchymal growth factors in viral-associated pulmonary aspergillosis

An interesting finding is the significantly increased levels of growth factors such as vascular endothelial growth factor (VEGF) or epidermal growth factor in BAL fluid of patients with VAPA compared to patients with severe viral pneumonia without aspergillosis (Feys et al., 2022). These growth factors are implicated in the genesis of lung fibrosis (Barratt et al., 2018; Schramm et al., 2022), and therefore these increased levels in VAPA patients might be implicated in further lung function impairment in these patients. This could potentially partly address why half of VAPA patients die despite initiation of antifungal therapy. Indeed, both VEGF levels and downstream VEGF signaling were increased in BAL fluid of patients with IAPA who died compared to those who survived (Feys et al., 2023). One hypothesis could be that micro-infarctions caused by angio-invasive hyphae lead to increased VEGF production, thereby driving angiogenesis, but also the progression of lung fibrosis. More mechanistic insight into the reason for the increase of these growth factors in the lungs of these patients is required.

Direct *Aspergillus*-viral interactions

The direct interaction of the influenza virus with *Aspergillus*, without the presence of human cells, was shown to induce fungal growth during superinfection (König et al., 2024). In addition, coinfection of influenza virus and *Aspergillus* resulted in reduced viral replication but also reduced the expression of cytokines and chemokines important in the antiviral host immune response (König et al., 2024). These observations align with the general attenuation of transcriptional responses seen to pro-inflammatory substances, such as IL-1ß and TNF-α signaling in BAL fluid of IAPA compared to influenza-only patients (Feys et al., 2022).

Iatrogenic attenuation of antifungal immunity

Besides viral-induced changes to the antifungal host response, iatrogenic impairment of antifungal immunity plays a role in the pathophysiology of VAPA. Modulating the hyperinflammatory immune response seen in severe viral pneumonia has become a mainstay of treatment in critically ill patients with COVID-19 (van de Veerdonk et al., 2022).

Several randomized controlled trials (RCTs) investigating immunomodulatory treatments were performed during the first years of the COVID-19 pandemic. Corticosteroids have been recommended for the treatment of severe COVID-19 since the open-label Randomised Evaluation of COVID-19 Therapy (RECOVERY) RCT, which showed a reduction in 28-day mortality with dexamethasone among COVID-19 patients requiring respiratory support ("Dexamethasone in Hospitalized Patients with Covid-19," 2021). However, later placebo-controlled RCTs could not show a clear mortality benefit by using corticosteroids (Sweeney et al., 2024; Dequin et al., 2020; Jeronimo et al., 2021). Baricitinib, a Janus kinase inhibitor that inhibits interferon signaling, demonstrated benefit in three double-blind placebo-controlled RCTs, implying that targeted immunomodulation might be more beneficial (Sweeney et al., 2024; Ely et al., 2022; Marconi et al., 2021; Kalil et al., 2021). Conflicting results were obtained for other frequently used immunomodulatory agents in placebo-controlled RCTs (for instance, anti-IL-6 therapy) (Sweeney et al., 2024; Shankar-Hari et al., 2021), and larger trials are warranted to confirm promising results obtained in smaller RCTs (for instance, anti-C5a therapy) (Sweeney et al., 2024; Vlaar et al., 2022).

A commonality of the mentioned immunomodulatory agents is their demonstrated or presumed ability to impair antifungal immunity, thereby increasing susceptibility to aspergillosis. Corticosteroids have pleiotropic effects on the antifungal host response, including inhibition of NF-κB transcription, LC3-associated phagocytosis, and the NADPH-oxidase, and depletion of circulating innate B1a cells (Sarden et al., 2022; Lewis and Kontoyiannis, 2009; Kyrmizi et al., 2013). Loss of IL-6 signaling (which is caused by tocilizumab) and type I interferon signaling (which is caused by baricitinib) has been implicated in disrupted LC3-associated phagocytosis (Akoumianaki et al., 2021) and in inappropriate inflammatory and neutrophil responses and to aspergillosis (Peng et al., 2023; Wang et al., 2020; Espinosa et al., 2017), respectively, whereas complement C5a inhibition could potentially lead to reduced neutrophil effector functions against *Aspergillus* (Feys et al., 2024a,b). It is therefore not surprising that a large systematic review and metaanalysis of CAPA literature found a significant association between use of corticosteroids and use of tocilizumab as treatment for COVID-19 and increased incidence of CAPA (Gioia et al., 2024). Baricitinib and anti-C5a inhibitors require more research to establish whether they are risk factors for development of CAPA. Importantly, none of the large RCTs published on immunomodulation for COVID-19 reported fungal infection rates specifically. In influenza patients, prolonged use of corticosteroids before ICU admission was also found to be linked to a heightened incidence of IAPA in a systematic review and metaanalysis (Lu et al., 2024), but more research regarding the role of corticosteroids and other immunomodulatory treatments in ICU and IAPA incidence is required.

Therapies administered in the ICU without the intention to modulate the immune response may nevertheless influence the antifungal host response. The best example is oseltamivir, a neuraminidase inhibitor that acts as an antiviral agent against influenza.

Oseltamivir was shown to influence the host response against *Aspergillus fumigatus* in vitro and increase susceptibility to pulmonary aspergillosis in a mouse model (Dewi et al., 2021). Mechanistically, it may impair phagocytic killing capacity, presumably through reduced recognition of sialic acids of *Aspergillus* by the immune system (Dewi et al., 2021). Timing is important: if given early during influenza, it may mitigate severe disease and therefore mitigate IAPA occurrence (Seldeslachts et al., 2021). The immunomodulatory effect of oseltamivir on the antifungal host response mainly warrants caution when starting oseltamivir upon ICU admission, although research into the clinical relevance of this mechanistic observation is warranted.

Conclusion

In summary, VAPA poses a significant threat to patients admitted to the ICU with severe viral pneumonia. Several layers of the antifungal host response are affected by the viral infection and by therapies administered in ICU to curb viral replication or hyperinflammation. As the field of VAPA is still very young, much remains to be investigated. More insight into the pathophysiology will undoubtedly lead to improved prognostic, diagnostic, and therapeutic tools for fungal (super)infection, and will prove valuable not only for influenza and COVID-19, but also for future respiratory viral pandemics.

References

Abbott, J.D., Fernando, H.V.J., Gurling, K., Meade, B.W., 1952. Pulmonary aspergillosis following post-influenzal bronchopneumonia treated with antibiotics. British Medical Journal 1 (4757), 523–525. Available at https://doi.org/10.1136/bmj.1.4757.523.

Ackermann, M., Verleden, S.E., Kuehnel, M., Haverich, A., Welte, T., Laenger, F., et al., 2020. Pulmonary vascular endothelialitis, thrombosis, and angiogenesis in Covid-19. Journal of Medicine 383 (2), 120–128. Available at https://doi.org/10.1056/NEJMoa2015432. Available from: http://www.nejm.org/medical-index.

Akoumianaki, T., Vaporidi, K., Diamantaki, E., Pène, F., Beau, R., Gresnigt, M.S., et al., 2021. Uncoupling of IL-6 signaling and LC3-associated phagocytosis drives immunoparalysis during sepsis. Cell Host & Microbe 29 (8), 1277. Available at https://doi.org/10.1016/j.chom.2021.06.002.

Alon, R., Sportiello, M., Kozlovski, S., Kumar, A., Reilly, E.C., Zarbock, A., et al., 2021. Leukocyte trafficking to the lungs and beyond: lessons from influenza for COVID-19. Nature reviews. Immunology 21 (1), 49–64. Available at https://doi.org/10.1038/s41577-020-00470-2. Available from: http://www.nature.com/nri/index.html.

Ballard, E., Yucel, R., Melchers, W.J.G., Brown, A.J.P., Verweij, P.E., Warris, A., 2020. Antifungal activity of antimicrobial peptides and proteins against *Aspergillus fumigatus*. Journal of Fungi 6 (2). Available at https://doi.org/10.3390/jof6020065. Available from: https://www.mdpi.com/2309-608X/6/2/65/pdf.

Barratt, S.L., Flower, V.A., Pauling, J.D., Millar, A.B., 2018. VEGF (Vascular endothelial growth factor) and fibrotic lung disease. International Journal of Molecular Sciences 19 (5). Available at https://doi.org/10.3390/ijms19051269. Available from: http://www.mdpi.com/1422-0067/19/5/1269/pdf.

Bourgonje, A.R., Abdulle, A.E., Timens, W., Hillebrands, J.L., Navis, G.J., Gordijn, S.J., et al., 2020. Angiotensin-converting enzyme 2 (ACE2), SARS-CoV-2 and the pathophysiology of coronavirus disease 2019 (COVID-19). Journal of Pathology 251 (3), 228–248. Available at https://doi.org/10.1002/path.5471. Available from: http://onlinelibrary.wiley.com/journal/10.1002/(ISSN)1096-9896.

Brown, G.D., 2006. Dectin-1: a signalling non-TLR pattern-recognition receptor. Nature Reviews. Immunology 6 (1), 33–43. Available at https://doi.org/10.1038/nri1745.

Brunel, A.S., Wójtowicz, A., Lamoth, F., Spertini, O., Neofytos, D., Calandra, T., et al., 2018. Pentraxin-3 polymorphisms and invasive mold infections in acute leukemia patients receiving intensive chemotherapy. Haematologica 103 (11), e527. Available at https://doi.org/10.3324/haematol.2018.195453. http://www.haematologica.org/content/haematol/103/11/e527.full.pdf.

Carabelli, A.M., Peacock, T.P., Thorne, L.G., Harvey, W.T., Hughes, J., de Silva, T.I., et al., 2023. SARS-CoV-2 variant biology: immune escape, transmission and fitness. Nature Reviews. Microbiology 21 (3), 162–177. Available at https://doi.org/10.1038/s41579-022-00841-7. https://www.nature.com/nrmicro/.

Carvelli, J., Demaria, O., Vély, F., Batista, L., Chouaki Benmansour, N., Fares, J., et al., 2020. Association of COVID-19 inflammation with activation of the C5a–C5aR1 axis. Nature 588 (7836), 146–150. Available at https://doi.org/10.1038/s41586-020-2600-6.

Chen, W., Yin, C., Zhong, M., Hu, B., Gao, X., Zhang, K., et al., 2022. Incidence and outcomes of patients with COVID-19 associated pulmonary aspergillosis (CAPA) in intensive care units: a systematic review and meta-analysis of 31 cohort studies. Annals of Palliative Medicine 11 (7), 2202–2209. Available at https://doi.org/10.21037/apm-21-2043.

Coste, A., Frérou, A., Raute, A., Couturaud, F., Morin, J., Egreteau, P.Y., et al., 2021. The extent of aspergillosis in critically Ill patients with severe influenza pneumonia: a multicenter cohort study. Critical Care Medicine 49 (6), 934–942. Available at https://doi.org/10.1097/CCM.0000000000004861. http://journals.lww.com/ccmjournal/pages/default.aspx.

Cunha, C., Aversa, F., Lacerda, J.F., Busca, A., Kurzai, O., Grube, M., et al., 2014. Genetic PTX3 deficiency and aspergillosis in stem-cell transplantation. New England Journal of Medicine 370 (5), 421–432. Available at https://doi.org/10.1056/NEJMoa1211161. http://www.nejm.org/doi/pdf/10.1056/NEJMoa1211161.

Del Valle, D.M., Kim-Schulze, S., Huang, H.H., Beckmann, N.D., Nirenberg, S., Wang, B., et al., 2020. An inflammatory cytokine signature predicts COVID-19 severity and survival. Nature Medicine 26 (10), 1636–1643. Available at https://doi.org/10.1038/s41591-020-1051-9. http://www.nature.com/nm/index.html.

Dellière, S., Dudoignon, E., Voicu, S., Collet, M., Fodil, S., Plaud, B., et al., 2022. Combination of mycological criteria: a better surrogate to identify COVID-19-associated pulmonary aspergillosis patients and evaluate prognosis? Journal of Clinical Microbiology 60 (3). Available at https://doi.org/10.1128/jcm.02169-21.

Dequin, P.F., Heming, N., Meziani, F., Plantefève, G., Voiriot, G., Badié, J., et al., 2020. Effect of hydrocortisone on 21-day mortality or respiratory support among critically Ill patients with COVID-19: a randomized clinical trial. JAMA - Journal of the American Medical Association 324 (13), 1298–1306. Available at https://doi.org/10.1001/jama.2020.16761. http://jama.jamanetwork.com/journal.aspx.

Dewi, I.M.W., Cunha, C., Jaeger, M., Gresnigt, M.S., Gkountzinopoulou, M.E., Garishah, F.M., et al., 2021. Neuraminidase and SIGLEC15 modulate the host defense against pulmonary aspergillosis. Cell Reports Medicine 2 (5). Available at https://doi.org/10.1016/j.xcrm.2021.100289, www.cell.com/cell-reports-medicine.

Dexamethasone in Hospitalized Patients with Covid-19, 2021. New England Journal of Medicine. 384 (8), 693–704, doi: 10.1056/nejmoa2021436.

Ely, E.W., Ramanan, A.V., Kartman, C.E., de Bono, S., Liao, R., Piruzeli, M.L.B., et al., 2022. Efficacy and safety of baricitinib plus standard of care for the treatment of critically ill hospitalised adults with COVID-19 on invasive mechanical ventilation or extracorporeal membrane oxygenation: an exploratory, randomised, placebo-controlled trial. The Lancet Respiratory Medicine 10 (4), 327–336. Available at https://doi.org/10.1016/S2213-2600(22)00006-6. https://www.sciencedirect.com/science/journal/22132600.

Ergün, M., Brüggemann, R.J.M., Alanio, A., Dellière, S., van Arkel, A., Bentvelsen, R.G., et al., 2021. Aspergillus test profiles and mortality in critically ill covid-19 patients. Journal of Clinical Microbiology 59 (12). Available at https://doi.org/10.1128/JCM.01229-21. https://journals.asm.org/doi/pdf/10.1128/JCM.01229-21.

Espinosa, V., Dutta, O., McElrath, C., Du, P., Chang, Y.J., Cicciarelli, B., et al., 2017. Type III interferon is a critical regulator of innate antifungal immunity. Science Immunology 2 (16). Available at https://doi.org/10.1126/sciimmunol.aan5357. http://immunology.sciencemag.org/content/immunology/2/16/eaan5357.full.pdf.

Fajnzylber, J., Regan, J., Coxen, K., Corry, H., Wong, C., Rosenthal, A., et al., 2020. Zhu, SARS-CoV-2 viral load is associated with increased disease severity and mortality. Nature Communications 11 (1). Available at https://doi.org/10.1038/s41467-020-19057-5.

Feys, S., Carvalho, A., Clancy, C.J., Gangneux, J.-P., Hoenigl, M., Lagrou, K., et al., 2024a. Influenza-associated and COVID-19-associated pulmonary aspergillosis in critically ill patients. The Lancet. Respiratory medicine. Available at https://doi.org/10.1016/S2213-2600(24)00151-6.

Feys, S., Gonçalves, S.M., Khan, M., Choi, S., Boeckx, B., Chatelain, D., et al., 2022. Lung epithelial and myeloid innate immunity in influenza-associated or COVID-19-associated pulmonary aspergillosis: an observational study. The Lancet Respiratory Medicine 10 (12), 1147–1159. Available at https://doi.org/10.1016/S2213-2600(22)00259-4. http://www.elsevier.com/journals/the-lancet-respiratory-medicine/2213-2600.

Feys, S., Heylen, J., Carvalho, A., Van Weyenbergh, J., Wauters, J., Gonçalves, S.M., et al., 2023. A signature of differential gene expression in bronchoalveolar lavage fluid predicts mortality in influenza-associated pulmonary aspergillosis. Intensive Care Medicine 49 (2), 254–257. Available at https://doi.org/10.1007/s00134-022-06958-w. https://www.springer.com/journal/134.

Feys, S., Hoenigl, M., Gangneux, J.P., Verweij, P.E., Wauters, J., 2024b. Fungal fog in viral storms: necessity for rigor in aspergillosis diagnosis and research. American Journal of Respiratory and Critical Care Medicine 209 (6), 631–633. Available at https://doi.org/10.1164/rccm.202310-1815VP.

Feys, S., Vanmassenhove, S., Kraisin, S., Yu, K., Jacobs, C., Boeckx, B., et al., 2024c. Lower respiratory tract single-cell RNA sequencing and neutrophil extracellular trap profiling of COVID-19-associated pulmonary aspergillosis: a single centre, retrospective, observational study. The Lancet Microbe 5 (3), e247. Available at https://doi.org/10.1016/s2666-5247(23)00368-3.

Fites, J.S., Gui, M., Kernien, J.F., Negoro, P., Dagher, Z., Sykes, D.B., et al., 2018. An unappreciated role for neutrophil-DC hybrids in immunity to invasive fungal infections. PLoS pathogens 14 (5), e1007073. Available at https://doi.org/10.1371/journal.ppat.1007073.

Flerlage, T., Boyd, D.F., Meliopoulos, V., Thomas, P.G., Schultz-Cherry, S., 2021. Influenza virus and SARS-CoV-2: pathogenesis and host responses in the respiratory tract. Nature Reviews. Microbiology 19 (7), 425–441. Available at https://doi.org/10.1038/s41579-021-00542-7. http://www.nature.com/nrmicro/index.html.

Gangneux, J.P., Dannaoui, E., Fekkar, A., Luyt, C.E., Botterel, F., De Prost, N., et al., 2022. Fungal infections in mechanically ventilated patients with COVID-19 during the first wave: the French multicentre MYCOVID study. The Lancet Respiratory Medicine 10 (2), 180–190. Available at https://doi.org/10.1016/S2213-2600(21)00442-2. http://www.elsevier.com/journals/the-lancet-respiratory-medicine/2213-2600.

Gao, R., Bhatnagar, J., Blau, D.M., Greer, P., Rollin, D.C., Denison, A.M., et al., 2013. Cytokine and chemokine profiles in lung tissues from fatal cases of 2009 pandemic influenza A (H1N1): role of the host immune response in pathogenesis. American Journal of Pathology 183 (4), 1258–1268. Available at https://doi.org/10.1016/j.ajpath.2013.06.023.

Garianda, C., Hirsch, E., Bozza, S., Salustri, A., De Acetis, M., Nota, R., et al., 2002. Non-redundant role of the long pentraxin PTX3 in anti-fungal innate immune response. Nature 420 (6912), 182–186. Available at https://doi.org/10.1038/nature01195.

Ghoneim, H.E., Thomas, P.G., McCullers, J.A., 2013. Depletion of alveolar macrophages during influenza infection facilitates bacterial superinfections. Journal of Immunology 191 (3), 1250–1259. Available at https://doi.org/10.4049/jimmunol.1300014UnitedStates. http://www.jimmunol.org/content/191/3/1250.full.pdf+html.

Gioia, F., Walti, L.N., Orchanian-Cheff, A., Husain, S., 2024. Risk factors for COVID-19-associated pulmonary aspergillosis: a systematic review and meta-analysis. The Lancet Respiratory Medicine 12 (3), 207–216. Available at https://doi.org/10.1016/S2213-2600(23)00408-3. https://www.sciencedirect.com/science/journal/22132600.

Gonçalves, S.M., Duarte-Oliveira, C., Campos, C.F., Aimanianda, V., ter Horst, R., Leite, L., et al., 2020. Phagosomal removal of fungal melanin reprograms macrophage metabolism to promote antifungal immunity. Nature Communications 11 (1). Available at https://doi.org/10.1038/s41467-020-16120-z. http://www.nature.com/ncomms/index.html.

Grant, R.A., Morales-Nebreda, L., Markov, N.S., Swaminathan, S., Querrey, M., Guzman, E.R., et al., 2021. Circuits between infected macrophages and T cells in SARS-CoV-2 pneumonia. Nature 590 (7847), 635–641. Available at https://doi.org/10.1038/s41586-020-03148-w. http://www.nature.com/nature/index.html.

Hamming, I., Timens, W., Bulthuis, M.L.C., Lely, A.T., Navis, G.J., van Goor, H., 2004. Tissue distribution of ACE2 protein, the functional receptor for SARS coronavirus. A first step in understanding SARS pathogenesis. The Journal of Pathology 203 (2), 631–637. Available at https://doi.org/10.1002/path.1570.

He, Q., Li, H., Rui, Y., Liu, L., He, B., Shi, Y., et al., 2018. Pentraxin 3 gene polymorphisms and pulmonary aspergillosis in chronic obstructive pulmonary disease patients. Clinical Infectious Diseases 66 (2), 261–267. Available at https://doi.org/10.1093/cid/cix749.

Huang, L., Zhai, T., Hua, L., Zhan, Q., 2020. Early identification of patients with severe influenza-associated aspergillosis (IAA) in the intensive care unit——an IAA prediction score system (Asper-PreSS). Journal of Infection 81 (4), 639–646. Available at https://doi.org/10.1016/j.jinf.2020.07.036.

Iwasaki, A., Pillai, P.S., 2014. Innate immunity to influenza virus infection. Nature reviews. Immunology 14 (5), 315–328. Available at https://doi.org/10.1038/nri3665.

Janssen, N.A.F., Nyga, R., Vanderbeke, L., Jacobs, C., Ergün, M., Buil, J.B., et al., 2021. Multinational observational cohort study of covid-19-associated pulmonary aspergillosis1. Emerging Infectious Diseases 27 (11), 2892–2898. Available at https://doi.org/10.3201/eid2711.211174. https://search.bvsalud.org/global-literature-on-novel-coronavirus-2019-ncov/resource/en/covidwho-1406813.

Jeronimo, C.M.P., Farias, M.E.L., Val, F.F.A., Sampaio, V.S., Alexandre, M.A.A., Melo, G.C., et al., 2021. Methylprednisolone as adjunctive therapy for patients hospitalized with coronavirus disease 2019 (COVID-19; Metcovid): a randomized, double-blind, phase IIb, placebo-controlled trial. Clinical Infectious Diseases 72 (9). Available at https://doi.org/10.1093/cid/ciaa1177. E373, http://cid.oxfordjournals.org/content/by/year.

Kalil, A.C., Patterson, T.F., Mehta, A.K., Tomashek, K.M., Wolfe, C.R., Ghazaryan, V., et al., 2021. Baricitinib plus remdesivir for hospitalized adults with Covid-19. New England Journal of Medicine 384 (9), 795–807. Available at https://doi.org/10.1056/NEJMoa2031994. http://www.nejm.org/medical-index.

Koehler, P., Bassetti, M., Chakrabarti, A., Chen, S.C.A., Colombo, A.L., Hoenigl, M., et al., 2021. Defining and managing COVID-19-associated pulmonary aspergillosis: the 2020 ECMM/ISHAM consensus criteria for research and clinical guidance. The Lancet Infectious Diseases 21 (6), e149. Available at https://doi.org/10.1016/S1473-3099(20)30847-1. http://www.journals.elsevier.com/the-lancet-infectious-diseases.

König, S., Schroeder, J., Nietzsche, S., Heinekamp, T., Brakhage, A.A., Zell, R., et al., 2024. The influenza A virus promotes fungal growth of *Aspergillus fumigatus* via direct interaction in vitro. Microbes and Infection 26 (3). Available at https://doi.org/10.1016/j.micinf.2023.105264. https://www.sciencedirect.com/science/journal/12864579.

Krzych, Ł.J., Putowski, Z., Gruca, K., Pluta, M.P., 2022. Mortality in critically ill COVID-19 patients with fungal infections: a comprehensive systematic review and meta-analysis. Polish Archives of Internal Medicine 132 (5). Available at https://doi.org/10.20452/pamw.16221. https://www.mp.pl/paim/issue/article/16221/.

Kyrmizi, I., Gresnigt, M.S., Akoumianaki, T., Samonis, G., Sidiropoulos, P., Boumpas, D., et al., 2013. Corticosteroids block autophagy protein recruitment in *Aspergillus fumigatus* Phagosomes via targeting dectin-1/Syk kinase signaling. The Journal of Immunology 191 (3), 1287–1299. Available at https://doi.org/10.4049/jimmunol.1300132.

Lahmer, T., Kriescher, S., Herner, A., Rothe, K., Spinner, C.D., Schneider, J., et al., 2021. Invasive pulmonary aspergillosis in critically ill patients with severe COVID-19 pneumonia: results from the prospective AspCOVID-19 study. PLoS ONE 16 (3), e0238825. Available at https://doi.org/10.1371/journal.pone.0238825.

Land, W.G., 2021. Role of DAMPs in respiratory virus-induced acute respiratory distress syndrome—with a preliminary reference to SARS-CoV-2 pneumonia. Genes and Immunity 22 (3), 141–160. Available at https://doi.org/10.1038/s41435-021-00140-w. https://www.nature.com/gene/.

Latgé, J.-P., Chamilos, G., 2019. *Aspergillus fumigatus* and aspergillosis in 2019. Clinical Microbiology Reviews 33 (1). Available at https://doi.org/10.1128/cmr.00140-18.

Lee, C.K., Oliveira, L.V.N., Akalin, A., Specht, C.A., Lourenco, D., Gomez, C.L., et al., 2023. Dysregulated pulmonary inflammatory responses exacerbate the outcome of secondary aspergillosis following influenza. American Society for Microbiology, United States mBio 14 (5). Available at https://doi.org/10.1128/mbio.01633-23. https://journals.asm.org/toc/mbio/14/5.

Lewis, R.E., Kontoyiannis, D.P., 2009. Invasive aspergillosis in glucocorticoid-treated patients. Medical Mycology 47 (1), S271. Available at https://doi.org/10.1080/13693780802227159.

Liu, K.W., Grau, M.S., Jones, J.T., Wang, X., Vesely, E.M., James, M.R., et al., 2022. Postinfluenza environment reduces *Aspergillus fumigatus* conidium clearance and facilitates invasive aspergillosis in vivo. mBio 13 (6). Available at https://doi.org/10.1128/mbio.02854-22. https://journals.asm.org/doi/10.1128/mbio.02854-22.

Lobo, S.M., Watanabe, A.S.A., Salomão, M.L.M., Queiroz, F., Gandolfi, J.V., de Oliveira, N.E., et al., 2019. Excess mortality is associated with influenza A (H1N1) in patients with severe acute respiratory illness. Journal of Clinical Virology 116, 62–68. Available from. Available at https://doi.org/10.1016/j.jcv.2019.05.003, www.elsevier.com/inca/publications/store/5/2/4/0/6/2.

Lu, L.Y., Lee, H.M., Burke, A., Li Bassi, G., Torres, A., Fraser, J.F., et al., 2024. Prevalence, risk factors, clinical features, and outcome of influenza-associated pulmonary aspergillosis in critically ill patients: a systematic review and meta-analysis. Chest 165 (3), 540–558. Available at https://doi.org/10.1016/j.chest.2023.09.019. https://www.sciencedirect.com/science/journal/00123692.

Marconi, V.C., Ramanan, A.V., de Bono, S., Kartman, C.E., Krishnan, V., Liao, R., et al., 2021. Efficacy and safety of baricitinib for the treatment of hospitalised adults with COVID-19 (COV-BARRIER): a randomised, double-blind, parallel-group, placebo-controlled phase 3 trial. The Lancet Respiratory Medicine 9 (12), 1407–1418. Available at https://doi.org/10.1016/s2213-2600(21)00331-3.

Matsushima, H., Geng, S., Lu, R., Okamoto, T., Yao, Y., Mayuzumi, N., et al., 2013. Neutrophil differentiation into a unique hybrid population exhibiting dual phenotype and functionality of neutrophils and dendritic cells. Blood 121 (10), 1677–1689. Available at https://doi.org/10.1182/blood-2012-07-445189.

Meersseman, W., Lagrou, K., Maertens, J., Wijngaerden, E.V., 2007. Invasive aspergillosis in the intensive care unit. Clinical Infectious Diseases 45 (2), 205–216. Available at https://doi.org/10.1086/518852.

Nicolas de Lamballerie, C., Pizzorno, A., Fouret, J., Szpiro, L., Padey, B., Dubois, J., et al., 2020. Transcriptional profiling of immune and inflammatory responses in the context of SARS-CoV-2 fungal superinfection in a human airway epithelial model. Microorganisms 8 (12), 1974. Available at https://doi.org/10.3390/microorganisms8121974.

Niu, J., Meng, G., 2023. Roles and mechanisms of NLRP3 in influenza viral infection. Viruses 15 (6), 1339. Available at https://doi.org/10.3390/v15061339.

Peng, M., Li, X., Zhang, X., Peng, L., 2023. Inhibition of cGAS aggravated the host inflammatory response to *Aspergillus fumigatus*. Experimental Lung Research 49 (1), 86–100. Available at https://doi.org/10.1080/01902148.2023.2211663.

Pittet, L.A., Hall-Stoodley, L., Rutkowski, M.R., Harmsen, A.G., 2010. Influenza virus infection decreases tracheal mucociliary velocity and clearance of *Streptococcus pneumoniae*. American Journal of Respiratory Cell and Molecular Biology 42 (4), 450–460. Available at https://doi.org/10.1165/rcmb.2007-0417OCUnitedStates. http://ajrcmb.atsjournals.org/cgi/reprint/42/4/450.

Potere, N., Del Buono, M.G., Caricchio, R., Cremer, P.C., Vecchié, A., Porreca, E., et al., 2022. Interleukin-1 and the NLRP3 inflammasome in COVID-19: pathogenetic and therapeutic implications. EBioMedicine 85, 104299. Available at https://doi.org/10.1016/j.ebiom.2022.104299.

Prattes, J., Wauters, J., Giacobbe, D.R., Salmanton-García, J., Maertens, J., Bourgeois, M., et al., 2022. Risk factors and outcome of pulmonary aspergillosis in critically ill coronavirus disease 2019 patients—a multinational observational study by the European confederation of medical mycology. Clinical Microbiology and Infection 28 (4), 580–587. Available at https://doi.org/10.1016/j.cmi.2021.08.014. https://www.journals.elsevier.com/clinical-microbiology-and-infection.

Pronier, C., Gacouin, A., Lagathu, G., Le Tulzo, Y., Tadié, J.-M., Thibault, V., 2021. Respiratory influenza viral load as a marker of poor prognosis in patients with severe symptoms. Journal of Clinical Virology 136, 104761. Available at https://doi.org/10.1016/j.jcv.2021.104761.

Robinot, R., Hubert, M., de Melo, G.D., Lazarini, F., Bruel, T., Smith, N., et al., 2021. SARS-CoV-2 infection induces the dedifferentiation of multiciliated cells and impairs mucociliary clearance. Nature Communications 12 (1). Available at https://doi.org/10.1038/s41467-021-24521-x. http://www.nature.com/ncomms/index.html.

Salazar, F., Bignell, E., Brown, G.D., Cook, P.C., Warris, A., 2022. Pathogenesis of respiratory viral and fungal coinfections. Clinical Microbiology Reviews 35 (1). Available at https://doi.org/10.1128/CMR.00094-21. https://journals.asm.org/doi/10.1128/CMR.00094-21.

Sarden, N., Sinha, S., Potts, K.G., Pernet, E., Hiroki, C.H., Hassanabad, M.F., et al., 2022. A B1a-natural IgG-neutrophil axis is impaired in viral- and steroid-associated aspergillosis. Science Translational Medicine 14 (674). Available at https://doi.org/10.1126/scitranslmed.abq6682. https://www.science.org/doi/epdf/10.1126/scitranslmed.abq6682.

Schauwvlieghe, A.F.A.D., Rijnders, B.J.A., Philips, N., Verwijs, R., Vanderbeke, L., Van Tienen, C., et al., 2018. Invasive aspergillosis in patients admitted to the intensive care unit with severe influenza: a retrospective cohort study. The Lancet Respiratory Medicine 6 (10), 782–792. Available at https://doi.org/10.1016/S2213-2600(18)30274-1. http://www.elsevier.com/journals/the-lancet-respiratory-medicine/2213-2600.

Schramm, F., Schaefer, L., Wygrecka, M., 2022. EGFR signaling in lung fibrosis. Cells 11 (6), 986. Available at https://doi.org/10.3390/cells11060986.

Seldeslachts, L., Jacobs, C., Tielemans, B., Vanhoffelen, E., Van der Sloten, L., Humblet-Baron, S., et al., 2022. Overcome double trouble: baloxavir marboxil suppresses influenza thereby mitigating secondary invasive pulmonary aspergillosis. Journal of Fungi 8 (1), 1. Available at https://doi.org/10.3390/jof8010001.

Seldeslachts, L., Vanderbeke, L., Fremau, A., Reséndiz-Sharpe, A., Jacobs, C., Laeveren, B., et al., 2021. Early oseltamivir reduces risk for influenza-associated aspergillosis in a double-hit murine model. Virulence 12 (1), 2493–2508. Available at https://doi.org/10.1080/21505594.2021.1974327.

Shankar-Hari, M., Vale, C.L., Godolphin, P.J., Fisher, D., Higgins, J.P.T., Spiga, F., et al., 2021. J.A.C. Sterne, association between administration of IL-6 antagonists and mortality among patients hospitalized for COVID-19: a meta-analysis. JAMA - Journal of the American Medical Association 326 (6), 499–518. Available at https://doi.org/10.1001/jama.2021.11330. http://jama.jamanetwork.com/journal.aspx.

Shi, C., Shan, Q., Xia, J., Wang, L., Wang, L., Qiu, L., et al., 2022. Incidence, risk factors and mortality of invasive pulmonary aspergillosis in patients with influenza: a systematic review and meta-analysis. Mycoses 65 (2), 152–163. Available at https://doi.org/10.1111/myc.13410.

Singhal, S., Bhojnagarwala, P.S., O'Brien, S., Moon, E.K., Garfall, A.L., Rao, A.S., et al., 2016. Origin and role of a subset of tumor-associated neutrophils with antigen-presenting cell features in early-stage human lung cancer. Cancer cell 30 (1), 120–135. Available at https://doi.org/10.1016/j.ccell.2016.06.001. https://www.journals.elsevier.com/cancer-cell.

Snarr, B.D., St-Pierre, G., Ralph, B., Lehoux, M., Sato, Y., Rancourt, A., et al., 2020. Galectin-3 enhances neutrophil motility and extravasation into the airways during *Aspergillus fumigatus* infection. PLoS pathogens 16 (8). Available at https://doi.org/10.1371/JOURNAL.PPAT.1008741. https://dx.plos.org/10.1371/journal.ppat.1008741.

Sun, K., Metzger, D.W., 2008. Inhibition of pulmonary antibacterial defense by interferon-γ during recovery from influenza infection. Nature Medicine 14 (5), 558–564. Available at https://doi.org/10.1038/nm1765.

Sweeney, D.A., Lobo, S.M., Póvoa, P., Kalil, A.C., 2024. Choosing immunomodulating therapies for the treatment of COVID-19: recommendations based on placebo-controlled trial evidence. Clinical Microbiology and Infection. Available at https://doi.org/10.1016/j.cmi.2023.12.028. https://www.sciencedirect.com/science/journal/1198743X.

Tappe, B., Lauruschkat, C.D., Strobel, L., Pantaleón García, J., Kurzai, O., Rebhan, S., et al., 2022. COVID-19 patients share common, corticosteroid-independent features of impaired host immunity to pathogenic molds. Frontiers in immunology 13. Available at https://doi.org/10.3389/fimmu.2022.954985. https://www.frontiersin.org/journals/immunology#.

Tobin, J.M., Nickolich, K.L., Ramanan, K., Pilewski, M.J., Lamens, K.D., Alcorn, J.F., et al., 2020. Influenza suppresses neutrophil recruitment to the lung and exacerbates secondary invasive pulmonary aspergillosis. Journal of Immunology 205 (2), 480–488. Available at https://doi.org/10.4049/jimmunol.2000067. https://www.jimmunol.org/content/jimmunol/205/2/480.full.pdf.

Uyeki, T.M., Hui, D.S., Zambon, M., Wentworth, D.E., Monto, A.S., Influenza, 2022. The Lancet 400, 982–985. Available at https://doi.org/10.1016/S0140-6736(222022.

Vanderbeke, L., Jacobs, C., Feys, S., Reséndiz-Sharpe, A., Debaveye, Y., Hermans, G., et al., 2023. A pathology-based case series of influenza- and COVID-19–associated pulmonary aspergillosis: the proof is in the tissue. American Journal of Respiratory and Critical Care Medicine 208 (3), 301–311. Available at https://doi.org/10.1164/rccm.202208-1570oc.

Vanderbeke, L., Janssen, N.A.F., Bergmans, D.C.J.J., Bourgeois, M., Buil, J.B., Debaveye, Y., et al., 2021. Posaconazole for prevention of invasive pulmonary aspergillosis in critically ill influenza patients (POSA-FLU): a randomised, open-label, proof-of-concept trial. Intensive Care Medicine 47 (6), 674–686. Available at https://doi.org/10.1007/s00134-021-06431-0, link.springer.de/link/service/journals/00134/index.htm.

Van De Veerdonk, F.L., Gresnigt, M.S., Romani, L., Netea, M.G., Latgé, J.P., 2017a. *Aspergillus fumigatus* morphology and dynamic host interactions. Nature Reviews. Microbiology 15 (11), 661–674. Available at https://doi.org/10.1038/nrmicro.2017.90, http://www.nature.com/nrmicro/index.html.

Van De Veerdonk, F.L., Kolwijck, E., Lestrade, P.P.A., Hodiamont, C.J., Rijnders, B.J.A., Van Paassen, J., et al., 2017b. Influenza-associated aspergillosis in critically ill patients. American Journal of Respiratory and Critical Care Medicine 196 (4), 524–527. Available at https://doi.org/10.1164/rccm.201612-2540LE, http://www.atsjournals.org/doi/pdf/10.1164/rccm.201612-2540LE.

van de Veerdonk, F.L., Giamarellos-Bourboulis, E., Pickkers, P., Derde, L., Leavis, H., van Crevel, R., et al., 2022. A guide to immunotherapy for COVID-19. Nature Medicine 28 (1), 39–50. Available at https://doi.org/10.1038/s41591-021-01643-9, http://www.nature.com/nm/index.html.

Verweij, P.E., Rijnders, B.J.A., Brüggemann, R.J.M., Azoulay, E., Bassetti, M., Blot, S., et al., 2020. Review of influenza-associated pulmonary aspergillosis in ICU patients and proposal for a case definition: an expert opinion link.springer.de/link/service/journals/00134/index.htm. Intensive Care Medicine 46 (8), 1524–1535. Available at https://doi.org/10.1007/s00134-020-06091-6.

Vlaar, A.P.J., Witzenrath, M., van Paassen, P., Heunks, L.M.A., Mourvillier, B., de Bruin, S., et al., 2022. Anti-C5a antibody (vilobelimab) therapy for critically ill, invasively mechanically ventilated patients with COVID-19 (PANAMO): a multicentre, double-blind, randomised, placebo-controlled, phase 3 trial. The Lancet Respiratory Medicine 10 (12), 1137–1146. Available at https://doi.org/10.1016/S2213-2600(22)00297-1, https://www.sciencedirect.com/science/journal/22132600.

Vono, M., Lin, A., Norrby-Teglund, A., Koup, R.A., Liang, F., Loré, K., 2017. Neutrophils acquire the capacity for antigen presentation to memory CD4+ T cells in vitro and ex vivo. American Society of Hematology, Sweden Blood 129 (14), 1991–2001. Available at https://doi.org/10.1182/blood-2016-10-744441, http://www.bloodjournal.org/content/bloodjournal/129/14/1991.full.pdf.

Wang, X., Caffrey-Carr, A.K., Liu, K.W., Espinosa, V., Croteau, W., Dhingra, S., et al., 2020. MDA5 is an essential sensor of a pathogen-associated molecular pattern associated with vitality that is necessary for host resistance against aspergillus fumigatus. Journal of Immunology 205 (11), 3058–3070. Available at https://doi.org/10.4049/jimmunol.2000802, https://www.jimmunol.org/content/205/11/3058.

Wasylyshyn, A.I., Wasylyshyn, G.R., Linder, K.A., Miceli, M.H., 2021. COVID-19-associated pulmonary aspergillosis at an academic medical center in the Midwestern United States. Mycopathologia 186 (4), 499–505. Available at https://doi.org/10.1007/s11046-021-00564-y, https://rd.springer.com/journal/11046.

Wauters, J., Baar, I., Meersseman, P., Meersseman, W., Dams, K., De Paep, R., et al., 2012. Invasive pulmonary aspergillosis is a frequent complication of critically ill H1N1 patients: a retrospective study. Intensive Care Medicine 38 (11), 1761–1768. Available at https://doi.org/10.1007/s00134-012-2673-2.

Wauters, E., Van Mol, P., Garg, A.D., Jansen, S., Van Herck, Y., Vanderbeke, L., et al., 2021. Discriminating mild from critical COVID-19 by innate and adaptive immune single-cell profiling of bronchoalveolar lavages. Cell Research 31 (3), 272–290. Available at https://doi.org/10.1038/s41422-020-00455-9, http://www.nature.com/cr/index.html.

Wójtowicz, A., Lecompte, T.D., Bibert, S., Manuel, O., Rüeger, S., Berger, C., et al., 2015. PTX3 polymorphisms and invasive mold infections after solid organ transplant. Clinical Infectious Diseases 61 (4), 619–622. Available at https://doi.org/10.1093/cid/civ386, http://cid.oxfordjournals.org/content/by/year.

Wurster, S., Pantaleón García, J., Albert, N.D., Jiang, Y., Bhoda, K., Kulkarni, V.V., et al., 2023. Development of a corticosteroid-immunosuppressed mouse model to study the pathogenesis and therapy of influenza-associated pulmonary aspergillosis. Journal of Infectious Diseases 227 (7), 901–906. Available at https://doi.org/10.1093/infdis/jiad001, http://jid.oxfordjournals.org/content/current.

Xiao, M.T., Ellsworth, C.R., Qin, X., 2024. Emerging role of complement in COVID-19 and other respiratory virus diseases. Cellular and Molecular Life Sciences 81 (1). Available at https://doi.org/10.1007/s00018-024-05157-8, https://www.springer.com/journal/18.

Yang, H., Rao, Z., 2021. Structural biology of SARS-CoV-2 and implications for therapeutic development. Nature Reviews. Microbiology 19 (11), 685–700. Available at https://doi.org/10.1038/s41579-021-00630-8.

CHAPTER

6

Immune mechanisms underlying airway mycosis–related allergic airway diseases

Amber U. Luong[1], Farrah Kheradmand[2], John M. Knight[3], Hua Sun[1] and David B. Corry[2]

[1]Department of Otorhinolaryngology–Head and Neck Surgery, McGovern Medical School, The University of Texas Health Science Center at Houston, Houston, TX, United States,
[2]Departments of Medicine and Pathology & Immunology, Dan L. Duncan Comprehensive Cancer Center, Michael E. DeBakey VA Center for Translational Research in Inflammatory Diseases, Baylor College of Medicine, Houston, TX, United States,
[3]Department of Pathology & Immunology, Baylor College of Medicine, Houston, TX, United States

Introduction

Allergic airway diseases comprise diverse disorders affecting the upper and lower airways, including the paranasal sinuses and lungs. These disorders share numerous inflammatory features, including peripheral blood and airway mucosal eosinophilia, elevated serum or mucosal IgE, goblet cell metaplasia with mucus hyperproduction, and a stereotypical pattern of T-helper (Th) effector cells and innate lymphoid cells (ILCs) recruited to the airway mucosa that produce the signature cytokines IL-4, IL-5, IL-13, IL-6, IL-17, and others. Not all affected individuals express all inflammatory features; moreover, the relative expression of cytokines can vary over time within individuals and across clinically distinct groups, giving rise to unique disease endotypes.

Despite these immunological differences, the allergic airway diseases share characteristic features that include, most prominently, airway congestion leading to upper airway obstruction and associated facial pain and pressure, headaches, and reduced olfaction (in chronic rhinosinusitis [CRS]) and cough, dyspnea, and wheezing (asthma) if affecting the lungs. Death is fortunately rare, but it is an inescapable threat to those suffering from severe disease. Recent research suggests that underlying the more severe forms of allergic airway disease is airway mycosis, the noninvasive infection of the upper or lower airways with diverse fungi. With the realization that fungi are major causes of these disorders has come focused research on the unique pathogenesis of the airway mycosis-related allergic airway diseases

Immunological Insights and Emerging Therapeutics in Medical Mycology. DOI: https://doi.org/10.1016/B978-0-443-23636-5.00005-8

(AMRAADs), which has uncovered new insights into the host response to airway mycosis and how this drives disease expression. This has, in turn, led to improved disease management strategies. In this chapter, we review the fungal basis of the allergic airway diseases, emphasizing the immune response to airway mycosis and the therapeutic advances that build on these discoveries.

Fungal links to allergic airway disease

Fungi have been linked to the expression of allergic airway diseases for many decades and have likely been suspected of playing a role in these disorders far longer. Evidence for the involvement of fungi includes serological, epidemiological, and microbiological findings complemented more recently by animal model data in which fungi isolated from the human airway have been shown to replicate key disease features. These four separate lines of evidence, most recently complemented by positive antifungal clinical trials, establish the fungal infectious basis of the allergic airway diseases.

Serological and cellular immune evidence of airway mycosis in allergic airway disease

A key distinction between pathogen infection and commensalism is whether the organism is immunologically "silent" or whether it induces B- or T-cell-based specific recall responses, the latter usually indicative of true infection. Soon after its discovery in 1966, IgE antibodies were linked to asthma and only much later to CRS, especially to specific subtypes of CRS, including central compartment atopic disease and allergic fungal rhinosinusitis (AFRS). AFRS is a clinically defined subtype of CRS characterized by sinonasal polyps, an accumulation of mucin containing degranulated eosinophils and fungal hyphae within inflamed and expanded sinus cavities, elevated serum IgE levels, and evidence of hypersensitivity to fungi. Indeed, having IgE-based reactivity to one or more fungi (i.e., fungal allergy) is required as part of the most widely used AFRS clinical definition (Bent and Kuhn, 1996). Similarly, a well-described subset of severe asthma is severe asthma with fungal sensitization (SAFS) (Denning et al., 2009), in which severe asthmatics show serum IgE reactivity to one or more fungi. Among other clinical utilities, having a diagnosis of SAFS indicates the need for, and favorable responsiveness to, antifungals.

However, only approximately 16% of patients with fungal culture-proven airway mycosis demonstrate fungal allergy (Porter et al., 2014). In part, this extreme insensitivity is due to the dozens and potentially more fungi capable of causing airway mycosis (Agbetile et al., 2012; Porter et al., 2014), only a small fraction of which are tested for IgE reactivity through commonly available clinical assays. A more sensitive method for detecting fungus-specific allergic reactivity is to assess for T-cell—specifically Th cell type 2 (Th2)—reactivity to fungi using an enzyme-linked immunocell spot (ELISpot)-based assay. This assay shows greater sensitivity for detecting allergic airway disease (sensitivity 73% and specificity 100% versus 50% and 77% with IgE testing) when performed against a panel of only nine fungal allergens (Porter et al., 2014). When performed against a fungus specifically cultured from the airway, the fungus-specific Th2 ELISpot was nearly 100% sensitive and specific for detecting AFRS (Porter et al., 2014). The major drawback of this assay is that it has only been performed in research contexts and is not available commercially.

Although not epidemiologically related to AFRS, allergic bronchopulmonary mycosis (ABPM) (more often termed allergic bronchopulmonary aspergillosis [ABPA] in Europe) is in several respects the lower airway equivalent of AFRS. ABPM typically evolves from asthma as a more clinically virulent disease with more overt lower airway fungal burdens and more robust fungus-specific IgE, IgG, and eosinophilic inflammation, and typically involves airway remodeling changes that include physical airway obstruction (likely due to fibrin and mucus deposition), bronchiectasis (abnormal airway dilation), and bronchial wall thickening (Agarwal et al., 2024).

Epidemiological evidence of airway mycosis in allergic airway disease

In addition to the seroepidemiologic evidence briefly summarized above, the presence of mold and mold spores in and outside home and work environments correlates with diagnoses of allergic airway diseases in the occupants as documented by numerous studies (Kumar et al., 1990; O'Hollaren et al., 1991; Güneser et al., 1994; Fairs et al., 2013; Li et al., 1995; Licorish et al., 1985; Chen et al., 2014). Additionally, specific environmental phenomena and disruptions to the built environment that favor the overgrowth and wide dispersal of fungal spores, such as thunderstorms occurring in desert environments and water damage to homes and businesses, are very strongly linked to the induction and exacerbation, at times fatal, of allergic airway disease (Dales et al., 1991; Pulimood et al., 2007; Dales et al., 2003; Quansah et al., 2012; Oshikata et al., 2017). Similarly, remediation of mold contamination in households has been shown to improve respiratory health (Johnson et al., 2009).

Mycological evidence of airway mycosis in allergic airway disease

As part of the overall burden of proof of infection, the etiologic organism must be found in the target organ of the proposed infectious disease. For the allergic airway diseases, it should be possible to regularly culture fungi from respiratory secretions or at least visualize fungi on histologic examination of airway tissue and mucus. For AFRS and ABPA, disorders with characteristically higher airway fungal burdens, fungi have long been demonstrable in airway specimens (Bent and Kuhn, 1994; Friedman et al., 1991;

Manning et al., 1991; Imbeau et al., 1978; Sandhu et al., 1979). For asthma and chronic rhinosinusitis with nasal polyps (CRSwNP), which are very similar disorders to ABPA and AFRS, respectively, greater sensitivity is required to reveal the substantially lower airway fungal burdens. Culture of respiratory mucus specimens (sputum) is typically fruitless (Pashley et al., 2012) because respiratory mucus is potently antimicrobial (McGuckin et al., 2011; Sheng and Hasnain, 2022), preventing the growth of both fungi and bacteria. This is a serious worldwide problem for microbiological laboratories that limits the ability of clinicians to diagnose any infectious disease of the respiratory tract and has impaired the widespread recognition of the fungal infectious nature of allergic airway diseases. The insensitivity of sputum culture can be overcome by chemical treatment to liquefy the mucus, which can then be separated from the fungal elements to allow their efficient growth in culture (Mak et al., 2013). This improved culture technique increases fungal culture yields in diseased patients from 11%–16% to 84%–87% with a single culture attempt (Li et al., 2018). Similarly, the culture of sinus lavage fluid obtained at the time of endoscopic sinus surgery yields fungi in most patients having CRSwNP, but in only a few patients with nonallergic sinus disease (Porter et al., 2014).

Evidence from animal models

Another critical element to defining the putative infectious role of a pathogen is to determine whether the organism reproduces key disease features when given to experimental animals. Many viable fungi and extracts from fungi have now been given experimentally to mice and other rodents and shown to reproduce key features of both asthma and CRSwNP, including airway hyperresponsiveness, goblet cell metaplasia, peribronchial and sinonasal eosinophil, Th2, Th17, and ILC accumulation, elevated total and specific IgE, and airway mucus plugging (Kheradmand et al., 2002; Instanes et al., 2004; Sun et al., 2022; Porter et al., 2009; Corry et al., 1998; Murali et al., 1992; Mehlhop et al., 1997; Murai et al., 2012; Kobayashi et al., 2009). In contrast, other putative infectious causes of asthma and sinusitis, such as bacteria and viruses, induce patterns of inflammation, lung pathology, and physiological changes that fail to mimic most asthma and sinusitis features (Jupelli et al., 2013; Newcomb et al., 2008; Roy et al., 2014; Richmond et al., 2016; Yoo et al., 2013). The only other credible organism capable of inducing asthma-like disease in animals is lung-migratory parasites such as *Ascaris suum* (Weatherhead et al., 2018). Such infections certainly occur in humans, but are relatively rare events and cannot explain the high prevalence of asthma in the United States.

Fungal pathogenesis of allergic airway disease

CRS describes inflammation of the mucosal lining of the upper airway, which is characterized by type 1 (T1), type 2 (T2), type 3 (T3), or mixed immunologic profiles. Phenotypically, CRS is described in terms of the absence or presence of nasal polyps. Some patients with polyps have been further subcategorized into AFRS, aspirin-exacerbated respiratory disease, and cystic fibrosis based on specific clinical criteria. Nearly 90% of the 12.5 million US CRS patients with polyps express a primarily T2 or mixed sinonasal mucosal immunologic profile, which includes T2 inflammation (Stevens et al., 2019).

Numerous fungal components are immunogenic, including the β-glucans, chitin, mannans, and galactosaminogalactans derived from the fungal cell wall (Fig. 6.1). Within both the innate and adaptive immune systems, molecular immunologic pathways have been described linking fungal exposure to T2 immune responses. Although the focus here will be on the fungus-induced T2 immune response, fungi are linked to different disease presentations in the upper airway. In a nonatopic immunocompetent individual, fungal spores can be trapped within sinus cavities that are conducive to germination. An ensuing inflammatory reaction occurs without sinus polyps, creating a fungus ball, and is limited to the sinus cavity in which the fungal spores were trapped. This mycetoma or fungus ball represents an accumulation of fibrinous, typically necrotic, sinus mucosal exudate and tightly packed fungal hyphae. In the ethmoid sinuses, where the anatomy does not create a closed cavity and the underlying mucosa has been exposed to extended courses of

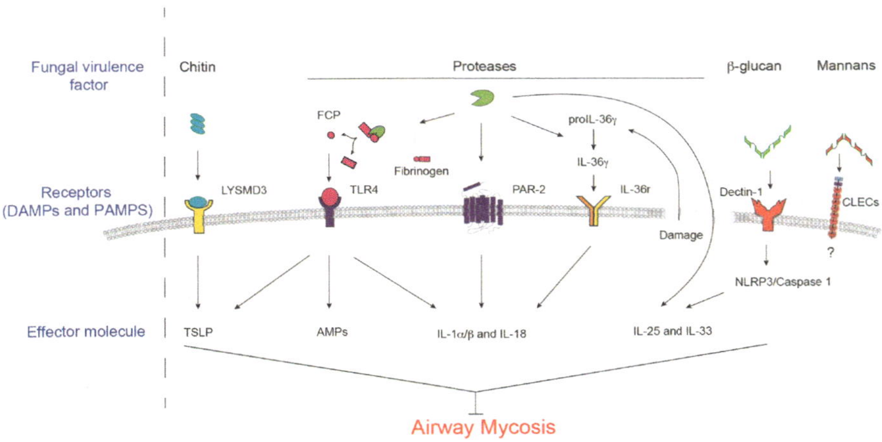

FIGURE 6.1 Innate immune activation during airway mycosis.

Depicted are major innate immune effector pathways activated by fungi during airway mycosis. Fungal virulence factors that have been studied in detail include the cell wall components chitin, β-glucan, and mannans, and secreted proteinases. Each of these factors is recognized either directly or indirectly through pathogen-associated molecular pattern (PAMP) or danger-associated molecular pattern (DAMP) receptors that promote the secretion of effector cytokines and antimicrobial peptides (AMPs) that directly or indirectly inhibit fungal growth.

antibiotics, fungi can colonize the mucosa without inciting a significant inflammatory response. Such saprophytic fungal disease typically resolves with removal of the debris followed by saline irrigations. By contrast, immunocompromised patients, such as those on immunosuppressant medications or experiencing diabetic ketoacidosis or COVID-19, exposure to fungi can lead to invasive fungal sinusitis, which is a life-threatening condition (Kaur et al., 2024). As such, the state of the host immune system dictates the disease that can manifest with fungal exposure in the sinus cavities.

Fungus-induced innate immune mechanisms

A central task of the airway immune system is the early recognition of airway fungi to initiate neutralizing antifungal responses, including downstream effector Th cell responses, if needed. In immunocompetent patients, the pathophysiology of fungal-mediated inflammation includes disruption of the mucosal barrier and fungus-induced molecular signaling that activates both innate and adaptive effector cells and coordinate a robust T2/T17 immune response. In addition to the detection of pathogen-associated molecular patterns, airway immune cells have evolved distinct mechanisms for detecting signature biochemical, especially proteinase, activity of fungi.

Respiratory epithelial cells

Both CRS and asthma have been associated with loss of epithelial barrier integrity. Tight junction (TJ) proteins, such as members of the zonula occludens and claudin families, establish robust physical connections between adjacent epithelial cells and regulate the permeability of the epithelial barrier (Fanning et al., 2012). Decreased expression or integrity of these TJ proteins and consequently decreased barrier resistance have been found in patients with CRS and allergic asthma and in experimental models (Herbert et al., 1995; Xiao et al., 2011; Ohashi et al., 1992; Wan et al., 1999; de Boer et al., 2008; Sweerus et al., 2017; Srisomboon et al., 2020). Defective barrier function is a critical issue in the pathophysiology leading to CRS and asthma (Sun et al., 2024). In addition to the T2 cytokine milieu contributing to the breakdown of the epithelial barrier, fungal proteases can also degrade these TJ proteins (Barros et al., 2022). The resulting defects in the epithelial barrier enhance antigen capture and subsequent presentation to adaptive immune cells via epithelial dendritic cells (DCs), thus establishing a positive feedback loop in fungus-induced T2 and T17 inflammation (Bartemes and Kita, 2018) (Fig. 6.2).

Pattern recognition receptors on epithelial cells recognize fungal protein components, including Toll-like receptors (TLRs), protease-activated receptors (PARs), C-type lectin receptors, and the receptor for advanced glycation end products (Bartemes and Kita, 2018; Crossen et al., 2023). In response to airway mycosis or airway challenge with fungal products, especially proteinases and cell

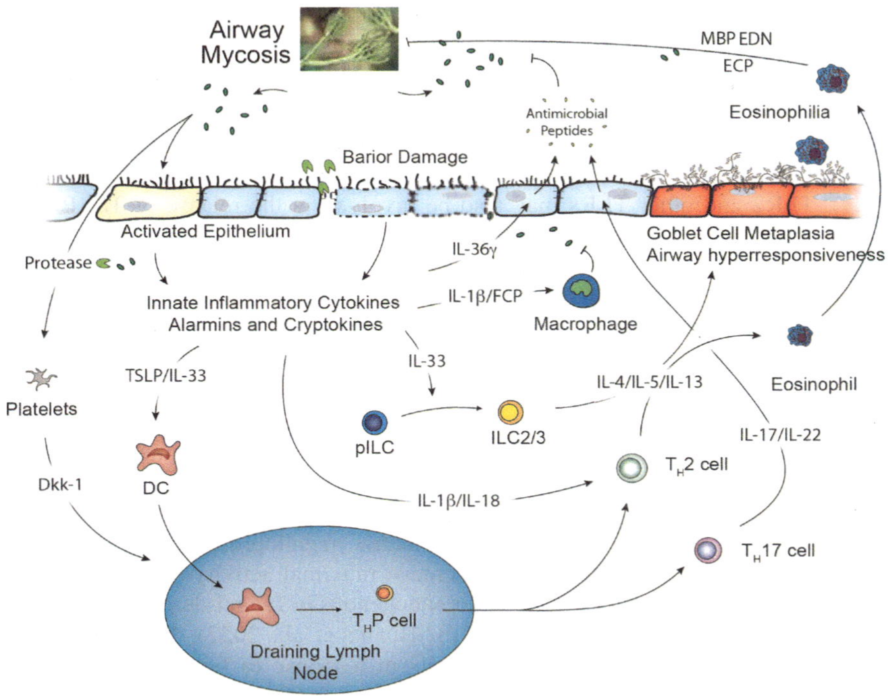

FIGURE 6.2 Cellular immune response to airway mycosis.

The airway epithelium plays a central role in detecting airway mycosis, releasing cytokines, alarmins, and cryptokines that activate downstream effector cells that include macrophages, precursor innate lymphoid cells (pILC), platelets, and dendritic cells (DCs). T-helper precursor cells differentiate into T-helper type 2 (Th2) and Th17 through signals derived from both platelets [Dickkopf-1 (Dkk-1)] and DCs. Th2 and Th17 cytokines activate diverse additional cells, including eosinophils, macrophages, and airway epithelial cells, primarily through their secreted cytokines. Fungal growth is inhibited through a multilayered effector program that includes the release of antimicrobial peptides, toxic cellular products such as major basic protein (MBP), eosinophil-derived neurotoxin (EDN), and eosinophil cationic protein (ECP), airway goblet cell-derived mucus, and physiological changes that include exaggerated bronchoconstriction (airway hyperresponsiveness).

wall products that include β-glucans, chitin, and mannans, the airway epithelium and other innate airway cells respond rapidly with the production of many cytokines, including IL-33, IL-25, and thymic stromal lymphopoietin (TSLP); IL-1 family cytokines that include IL-1α/β, IL-18, and IL-36; IL-6; many chemokines; and cytokine-like fibrinogen cleavage products (cryptokines) that shape downstream inflammatory events and, often but not always, pave the way for effective antifungal responses (Fig. 6.1).

Immediate early airway epithelial cytokines produced in response to fungal challenge include TSLP, IL-33, and IL-25. TSLP is produced in response to chitin (Khosravi et al., 2016) (a polymers of N-acetylglucosamine, the major structural component of the fungal cell wall) and fungal proteinases, the latter acting in part through PAR-2 (Hiraishi et al., 2018). The most important airway receptor regulating chitin-dependent cytokine production is probably LYSMD3 (He et al., 2021). TLR2 and other TLRs may also be involved in the release of TSLP from airway epithelial cells activated by fungi (Shin et al., 2016). TSLP drives eosinophilic airway inflammation through DCs by enhancing the NF-κB-dependent surface expression of OX40L that enhances Th2 differentiation and the activation of the transcription factor signal transducer and activator of transcription 6 to promote secretion of chemokines that promote allergic effector cell recruitment (Ito et al., 2005; Seshasayee et al., 2007) (Fig. 6.1).

Fungal proteinases also elicit secretion of IL-25 and IL-33 the from airway epithelium by activating PAR-2 (Hiraishi et al., 2018). Both cytokines function in parallel with TSLP to drive allergic airway inflammation in response to fungal signals, but uniquely undergo proteolytic cleavage to achieve maximal biological activity. IL-25 is proteolytically cleaved by matrix metalloproteinase 7, which is in turn induced by fungal proteinases, to achieve maximal activity (Goswami et al., 2009), whereas IL-33 is cleaved by either endogenous or fungal-derived proteinases to become activated (Cayrol et al., 2018; Huang et al., 2022). IL-33 is rapidly released from mouse airway epithelial cells in response to fungal proteases and fungal-antigen-dependent ATP release and activates ILCs to secrete IL-5 and IL-13 as part of the early innate response to fungal challenge (Heyen et al., 2016; Srisomboon et al., 2020; Kouzaki et al., 2011), with ILC-derived IL-5 driving the early innate airway eosinophil response (Anderson et al., 2016). IL-33 appears to play a similar role in pediatric SAFS (Castanhinha et al., 2015).

Surprisingly, IL-33 also plays an immunosuppressive role during airway fungal challenge, acting via prostaglandin E2 to limit IL-17 and IL-22 production. The net effect of cytokine inhibition by IL-33 is to reduce airway fungal clearance early during infection (Garth et al., 2017). However, unlike TSLP and IL-25, enhanced IL-33 secretion triggered by chitin also enhances Th2 responses by promoting the release of IL-1β from airway DCs (Arae et al., 2018). Combined with IL-6-dependent Th17 responses, the coordinated Th2/Th17 response to airway mycosis creates a hostile airway environment that, in otherwise normal mice, leads to the resolution of the fungal infection. It should be noted, however, that this generally protective immunological paradigm is not invariantly so. Despite triggering an identical airway immune response to that induced by molds and Candida *albicans*, the encapsulated fungus *Cryptococcus neoformans* gains a survival advantage in the lung that promotes brain dissemination and early death of the host (Hansakon et al., 2023).

The inflammasome-related cytokines IL-1α, IL-1β, and IL-18 are also critically important for controlling airway mycosis innately and driving downstream adaptive immune responses. Fungal β-glucan, but likely also secreted fungal proteinases, activate the NLRP3 inflammasome that, in turn, activates caspase-1 to convert latent cytoplasmic pro-forms of IL-1α, IL-1β, and IL-18 into their mature secreted forms (Huang et al., 2018; Pericolini et al., 2015). IL-1α and IL-1β appear to play nonredundant roles, with IL-1α regulating airway chemokine production, especially CXCL1, to drive recruitment of antifungal effector cells, whereas IL-1β acts directly on macrophages to enhance antifungal activity (Caffrey et al., 2015). IL-1β and IL-18 both promote Th2 development and recruitment to the airways (Murai et al., 2012) (Fig. 6.1, Fig. 6.2).

Two additional cytokines or cytokine-like molecules are uniquely induced in the context of enhanced airway proteinase activity, seen during airway mycosis. IL-36γ is an airway epithelial cytokine that accumulates in the cytoplasm in a pro-form and does not enter the canonical secretory system, controlling the release of many other cytokines. Rather, pro-IL-36γ is released only after cellular injury and cell membrane disruption, as may occur through the action of secreted proteinases, lytic toxins such as the *C. albicans* product candidalysin (Moyes et al., 2016), or perhaps the mechanical extension of hyphae through epithelial cells. After liberation from the cytoplasm, pro-IL-36γ is cleaved by fungal proteinases into the fully active cytokine (Macleod et al., 2020). It remains unclear what the precise functions of IL-36γ are in the context of airway mycosis, but they likely parallel the previously described functions of IL-36γ in the skin, which include promoting the secretion of itself, IL-1α/β, IL-17, and the chemokines IL-8 and CCL2. These cytokines, in turn, enhance the expression of the antimicrobial peptides (AMPs) cathelicidin (LL-37), human β-defensins 2 and 3, and S100 proteins (Johnston et al., 2011; Carrier et al., 2011; Foster et al., 2014) (Fig. 6.1).

Fungal proteinases also act to posttranslationally modify immunologically inactive proteins constitutively present in the airway lining fluid, such as the clotting protein fibrinogen. Mold (Landers et al., 2019), but not *C. albicans* (Wu et al., 2021), proteinases selectively remove the alpha chain from the fibrinogen D domain to expose the globular and somewhat proteinase-resistant D domain core consisting of the remaining β- and γ-chains chains. This residual β-γ "cryptokine" becomes competent to bind to the Mac-1 integrin complex (CD18/CD11b) that can then ligate TLR4 expressed on airway macrophages and epithelial cells, enhancing antifungal immunity, airway eosinophilia, airway hyperresponsiveness, and cytokine receptor expression (Landers et al., 2019; Millien et al., 2013) (Fig. 6.1, Fig. 6.2).

As illustrated in the preceding paragraphs, a key effector outcome of fungus-associated airway cytokine production is the induction of AMPs. Defensins, cathelicidins, and histatins are the three main AMP classes expressed in the human airways. Although all have antifungal activity, histatins are particularly known for their antifungal potency (Hof et al., 2000; Lupetti et al., 2008; Oppenheim et al., 2012; da Rocha Curvelo et al., 2018). Decreased expression of several AMPs, including human β-defensins 2 and 3 and LL-37 (derived from cathelicidin) (Dürr et al., 2006), has been noted in diseased sinus mucosa (Huang et al., 2021; Viksne et al., 2023). AFRS is a clinical subtype of CRS with nasal polyps characterized by an accumulation of mucin containing degranulated eosinophils and fungal hyphae within inflamed and expanded sinus cavities. Molecularly, AFRS patients have significantly depressed levels of histatins and Th17 cells that are critical for promoting AMP expression within inflamed sinus mucosa as compared to other nonAFRS CRSwNP patients (Sun et al., 2024). As evidenced, lack of histatin and other AMPs explains both the exaggerated airway mycosis and disease indices of AFRS (Fig. 6.1).

Innate effector cells responding to fungal exposure

Eosinophils are critical in defending against various microbes, including parasites and fungi, and are associated with allergic T2 diseases such as allergic rhinitis, allergic asthma, and CRSwNP (Ramirez et al., 2018). Upon activation by fungi, eosinophils release cytokines and chemokines that contribute to the coordinated antifungal activity with other immune cells. In addition, eosinophils contain numerous granules that contain cytotoxic and inflammatory proteins such as major basic protein, eosinophil-derived neurotoxin (EDN), eosinophil cationic protein (ECP), and eosinophil peroxidase. The highly cationic EDN and ECP exhibit potent ribonuclease activity (Gleich et al., 1986) that may contribute to the antifungal activity of eosinophils, as shown in vitro and in vivo, a contact-dependent response that requires the integrin CD11b (Porter et al., 2009; Yoon et al., 2008; Lilly et al., 2014). Elevated serum and/or tissue eosinophils are a signature feature of AMRAADs (Tyler et al., 2021) (Fig. 6.2).

In addition to the release of cytotoxic antifungal enzymes, eosinophils exert antifungal activity via the release of extracellular traps (ETs) consisting of DNA and eosinophil granule proteins in response to fungal contact. Although these ETs have not demonstrated direct enzymatic antifungal activity, they serve to immobilize and limit fungi from invading the nearby tissue (Silva et al., 2021). Pathologically, excessive release of eosinophil ETs into bronchial and sinus secretions can contribute to the pathology of chronic allergic airway diseases such as AFRS by promoting the generation of thick mucus (Tyler et al., 2021).

At the mucosal barrier, type 2 innate lymphoid cells (ILC2s) are another innate effector cell type that can also be activated by fungi, typically via epithelial cell-derived cytokines. ILC2s are present within the diseased mucosa of CRSwNP patients (Stevens and Kato, 2021) and are central effectors driving type 2 inflammation. The expression of both IL-33 and IL-25 from respiratory epithelial cells can be driven by fungi (Dietz et al., 2019; Patel et al., 2019). In CRSwNP, IL-33-activated ILC2s are significant sources of the type 2 cytokine IL-13 (Shaw et al., 2013). Although ILC2s do not have direct antifungal activity, these cells drive a type 2 response contributing to allergic airway pathology that underlies a complex, multilayered antifungal program (Porter et al., 2011, 2009) (Fig. 6.2).

Fungus-induced adaptive immune mechanisms

When innate antifungal immune responses are insufficient to eradicate incipient airway mycosis, adaptive immune responses are elicited and become dominant disease features. Within mucosal surfaces, Th17 cells play a crucial role in defending against airway mycosis (Tangye and Puel, 2023). Fungal antigens captured and expressed by airway DCs in the appropriate costimulatory contexts induce differentiation of naive T cells into Th17 cells and reactivation of resident memory T cells, leading to the release of the cytokines IL-17, IL-22, and IL-17F. These cytokines act directly on respiratory epithelial cells to recruit neutrophils, activate expression and release of AMPs, and promote tissue repair and epithelial barrier restoration (McAleer and Kolls, 2011) (Fig. 6.2). Several fungus-driven diseases have been shown to be critically linked to defects in the Th17 activation pathway including chronic mucocutaneous candidiasis and autosomal dominant hyperIgE syndrome (Job's syndrome) (Holland et al., 2007). AFRS is found to have significant deficiencies in mucosal Th17 cells and AMPs, thus existing within the same immunologic continuum as these disorders (Sun et al., 2024).

During airway mycosis, impaired recruitment or development of Th17 cells can shift an immune profile toward a Th1- and Th2-dominant response. In AFRS, fungal exposure enhances allergen-driven Th2 activation, leading to the exaggerated inflammation that in part distinguishes AFRS from CRSwNP. Unlike a balanced T2/T17 response, unbalanced responses involving excessive Th2 activation are characterized by reduced AMP-dependent antifungal activity and excessive inflammation. Presumably, to compensate for the lack of AMPs, activated fungus-specific IgE bound to mast cells and eosinophils contributes to containing fungal infections via phagocytosis and release of mediators that help clear fungi either directly or via recruitment of other cells. However, most patients with severe, fungus-driven allergic asthma exhibit a balanced Th17 and Th2 profile or a Th17- and neutrophil-predominant profile that contains, but fails to clear the airway mycosis. In these instances, excessive inflammation is again seen and is associated with steroid resistance (Zhang et al., 2017). It remains unclear why, in these instances, the airway mycosis is not resolved, but it is possible that subtle, yet undefined immunodeficiencies may be involved.

Platelets and Dickkopf-1

The signature immunological profile of the allergic airway diseases involving the nonstochastic recruitment of T2 and T17 cells to the airway suggests that fungi specifically elicit these cells through molecular signals detected by the innate immune system. Advances in the understanding of fungus-derived virulence factors eventually led to the discovery that platelets, and therefore their precursor cells, megakaryocytes, are key immunological effectors that coordinate the generation and recruitment of Th2 and Th17 cells to the asthmatic airway. Candidalysin was found to bind the von Willebrand factor receptor GP1Bα, found exclusively on platelets and megakaryocytes. Engagement of GP1Bα with candidalysin results in platelet degranulation and the release of the Wnt pathway antagonist protein Dickkopf-1 (Dkk-1), which acts, either directly or indirectly, on developing Th cells to drive Th2 and Th17 differentiation (Wu et al., 2021). More research is needed to know if Dkk-1 is a final common effector of Th2 and Th17 differentiation and recruitment in response to diverse fungi causing airway mycosis (Fig. 6.2).

Clinical implications

Role of surgery in fungi-driven allergic airway diseases

The complex anatomy of the paranasal sinuses hinders the ability to deliver topical antifungal and antiinflammatory therapy in CRS. In addition, sinus anatomy inhibits the clearance of inflammatory triggers such as fungi and the viscous mucus and inflammatory debris they elicit. Although surgery is not a curative therapeutic option, functional endoscopic sinus surgery (FESS) plays a critical role in clearing trapped fungal-laden mucinous debris and obstructing nasal polyps. In addition to providing postoperative access for topical medications, FESS serves to reduce the inflammatory burden and triggers within the diseased sinus cavities. As such, FESS is recommended as a critical component of the management of severe CRSwNP and AFRS after failed topical and systemic medical therapy.

On the other hand, surgery plays a very limited role in the lower airway, being rarely used in ABPA to resect aspergillomas causing hemoptysis or other life-threatening complications. In severe allergic asthma recalcitrant to medical therapy, bronchial thermoplasty may be offered with the goal of ablating smooth muscle that constrict airways. In a longitudinal prospective cohort study involving eight academic centers, baseline CT imaging parameters were identified that predicted response to bronchial thermoplasty in severe asthmatic patients (Samant et al., 2024). As such, surgery can only serve as one, if any, component of the management of these chronic inflammatory respiratory diseases.

Targeted inhibition of critical immune pathways

Numerous asthma and CRS clinical trials have now been conducted to evaluate the efficacy of biologic agents that interrupt the key inflammatory pathways linked to airway mycosis as described earlier. For most clinical trials, a specific effort to identify airway mycosis was not made, but the common nature of airway mycosis in these conditions suggests that most patients had underlying airway fungal infections.

AFRS and ABPM patients are usually excluded from clinical trials of biologics; thus there are no published results from randomized studies of biologics involving these important patient subsets. There is one randomized trial with anti-IL-4Rα that was completed specifically for AFRS patients whose data is expected by the end of 2025 (NCT04684524). A retrospective analysis of ABPM patients found that up to 65% respond favorably to anti-IgE, anti-IL-5/IL-5Rα, or anti-IL-4Rα therapy

(Carter et al., 2025). Numerous smaller studies indicate that biologics, with the exception of anti-IgE, reduce disease exacerbations and glucocorticoid use in greater than 85% of patients (Moss, 2023). Furthermore, Phase II studies of anti-IgE and anti-IL-5/IL-5Rα in SAFS show that these agents are as effective in patients with SAFS as in asthma patients without fungal sensitization (Dhariwal et al., 2021; Wark et al., 2020). Similarly, Phase III studies of anti-IgE, anti-IL-5/IL-5Rα, and anti-IL-4Rα have proven highly successful in CRSwNP, leading to FDA approval of these agents. Smaller studies of AFRS patients suggest that these agents are likely to be equally effective (Luong et al., 2022). While generally safe, an important exception is anaphylaxis, which can occur with anti-IgE therapies; fungal overgrowth syndromes involving the skin and mucous membranes are increasingly being reported with multiple biologics (Chong et al., 2024).

Antifungal clinical trials in allergic airway diseases

The efficacy of antifungals has been extensively explored in SAFS and ABPM, although no Phase III clinical trials have yet been conducted. At least 13 Phase II clinical trials have explored the efficacy of diverse antifungals in SAFS and ABPM (Denning and Pfavayi, 2023). Nine of these studies were unequivocally positive, demonstrating statistically significant improvements in symptoms, lung function, and/or reductions in oral glucocorticoid requirements, findings that were also observed in a retrospective study (Li et al., 2018).

Topically applied antifungals have been studied in several small studies of AFRS and CRSwNP, generally with negative results, perhaps due to inadequate contact time with the fungi or the inability to penetrate thick mucus to reach sinus fungi when administered through this route (Weschta et al., 2004; Ebbens et al., 2006; Weschta et al., 2006; Ebbens et al., 2009; Isaacs et al., 2011). In contrast, retrospective and prospective studies of itraconazole given together with glucocorticoids and following endoscopic surgery suggest that adjunctive antifungal therapy might reduce the need for revision surgery and provide additional symptomatic relief (Patro et al., 2015; Rains and Mineck, 2003), observations that are further supported by a retrospective analysis of terbinafine and other oral antifungals in CRSwNP (Li et al., 2021). Larger clinical trials involving oral antifungals given to well-defined and controlled CRS subsets are needed to rigorously address the value of this treatment modality.

Summary

Environmental fungi are now recognized as critically important causes of AMRAADs, especially severe forms of asthma and CRSwNP that include ABPA and AFRS. Intensive analysis of key fungal virulence factors, such as their secreted proteinases, cell surface-associated polysaccharides, and unique factors such as candidalysin from *C. albicans,* has led to the discovery of the mammalian substrates and receptors that initiate the airway innate and adaptive immune responses that mediate control and, ideally, resolution of airway mycosis. Such knowledge has led to an expanded arsenal of biologic agents that interrupt pertinent signaling pathways that drive disease symptoms, but also disrupt antifungal immunity. Not surprisingly, while effective in relieving symptoms, biologics are increasingly being linked to fungal overgrowth syndromes, and a major concern is that chronic use of these agents and glucocorticoids in isolation will lead to a gradually expanding airway fungal biomass and worsening airway mycosis, resulting in progressively more severe and ultimately treatment-resistant AMRAADs. As newer biologic agents and antifungals are individually explored in the context of AMRAADs, the need to study combinations of these agents will likely become increasingly evident.

References

Agarwal, R., Muthu, V., Sehgal, I.S., 2024. Clinical manifestation and treatment of allergic bronchopulmonary aspergillosis. Seminars in Respiratory and Critical Care Medicine 45 (1), 114–127. Available at https://doi.org/10.1055/s-0043–1776912, http://www.thieme-connect.com/ejournals/toc/srccm.

Agbetile, J., Fairs, A., Desai, D., Hargadon, B., Bourne, M., Mutalithas, K., et al., 2012. Isolation of filamentous fungi from sputum in asthma is associated with reduced post-bronchodilator FEV1. Clinical and Experimental Allergy Journal of the British Society for Allergy and Clinical Immunology 42 (5), 782–791. Available at https://doi.org/10.1111/j.1365-2222.2012.03987.x.

Anderson, E.L., Kobayashi, T., Iijima, K., Bartemes, K.R., Chen, C.-C., Kita, H., 2016. IL -33 mediates reactive eosinophilopoiesis in response to airborne allergen exposure. Allergy 71 (7), 977–988. Available at https://doi.org/10.1111/all.12861.

Arae, K., Morita, H., Unno, H., Motomura, K., Toyama, S., Okada, N., et al., 2018. Chitin promotes antigen-specific Th2 cell-mediated murine asthma through induction of IL-33-mediated IL-1β production by DCs. Scientific Reports 8 (1). Available at https://doi.org/10.1038/s41598-018-30259-2.

Barros, B.C.S.C., Almeida, B.R., Barros, D.T.L., Toledo, M.S., Suzuki, E., 2022. Respiratory epithelial cells: more than just a physical barrier to fungal infections. Journal of Fungi 8 (6). Available at https://doi.org/10.3390/jof8060548, https://www.mdpi.com/2309-608X/8/6/548/pdf?version=1653365163.

Bartemes, K.R., Kita, H., 2018. Innate and adaptive immune responses to fungi in the airway. Journal of Allergy and Clinical Immunology 142 (2), 353–363. Available at https://doi.org/10.1016/j.jaci.2018.06.015, http://www.elsevier.com/inca/publications/store/6/2/3/3/6/8/index.htt.

Bent, J.P., Kuhn, F.A., 1994. Diagnosis of allergic fungal sinusitis. Otolaryngology–Head and Neck Surgery Official Journal of American Academy of Otolaryngology-Head and Neck Surgery 111 (5), 580–588. Available at https://doi.org/10.2500/108854196778662273.

Bent, J.P., Kuhn, F.A., 1996. Allergic fungal sinusitis/polyposis. Allergy and Asthma Proceedings 17 (5), 259–268. Available at https://doi.org/10.2500/108854196778662273.

Caffrey, A.K., Lehmann, M.M., Zickovich, J.M., Espinosa, V., Shepardson, K.M., Watschke, C.P., et al., 2015. IL-1α signaling is critical for leukocyte recruitment after pulmonary *Aspergillus fumigatus* challenge. PLoS Pathogens 11 (1). Available at https://doi.org/10.1371/journal.ppat.1004625.

Carrier, Y., Ma, H.-L., Ramon, H.E., Napierata, L., Small, C., O'Toole, M., et al., 2011. Interregulation of Th17 cytokines and the IL-36 cytokines in vitro and in vivo: implications in psoriasis pathogenesis. The Journal of Investigative Dermatology 131 (12), 2428–2437. Available at https://doi.org/10.1038/jid.2011.234.

Carter, C., Torre, I.B., Blackburn, S., Nwankwo, L., Semple, T., Rawal, B., et al., 2025. Real-world effectiveness of biologic therapy in allergic bronchopulmonary *Aspergillosis*. Journal of Allergy and Clinical Immunology: In Practice 13 (5), 1094. Available at https://doi.org/10.1016/j.jaip.2025.03.006.

Castanhinha, S., Sherburn, R., Walker, S., Gupta, A., Bossley, C.J., Buckley, J., et al., 2015. Pediatric severe asthma with fungal sensitization is mediated by steroid-resistant IL-33. Journal of Allergy and Clinical Immunology 136 (2), 312. Available at https://doi.org/10.1016/j.jaci.2015.01.016.

Cayrol, C., Duval, A., Schmitt, P., Roga, S., Camus, M., Stella, A., et al., 2018. Environmental allergens induce allergic inflammation through proteolytic maturation of IL-33. Nature Immunology 19 (4), 375–385. Available at https://doi.org/10.1038/s41590-018-0067-5.

Chen, C.H., Chao, H.J., Chan, C.C., Chen, B.Y., Guo, Y.L., 2014. Current asthma in schoolchildren is related to fungal spores in classrooms. Chest 146 (1), 123–134. Available at https://doi.org/10.1378/chest.13-2129, http://journal.publications.chestnet.org/data/Journals/CHEST/930460/chest_146_1_123.pdf.

Chong, A.C., Navarro-Triviño, F.J., Su, M., Park, C.O., 2024. Fungal head and neck dermatitis: current understanding and management. Clinical Reviews in Allergy and Immunology 66 (3), 363–375. Available at https://doi.org/10.1007/s12016-024-09000-7, https://www.springer.com/journal/12016.

Corry, D.B., Grünig, G., Hadeiba, H., Kurup, V.P., Warnock, M.L., Sheppard, D., et al., 1998. Requirements for allergen-induced airway hyperreactivity in T and B cell-deficient mice. Molecular Medicine 4 (5), 344–355. Available at https://doi.org/10.1007/bf03401741, https://molmed.biomedcentral.com/.

Crossen, A.J., Ward, R.A., Reedy, J.L., Surve, M.V., Klein, B.S., Rajagopal, J., et al., 2023. Human airway epithelium responses to invasive fungal infections: a critical partner in innate immunity. Journal of Fungi 9 (1). Available at https://doi.org/10.3390/jof9010040, www.mdpi.com/journal/jof.

Dales, R.E., Cakmak, S., Judek, S., Dann, T., Coates, F., Brook, J.R., et al., 2003. The role of fungal spores in thunderstorm asthma. Chest 123 (3), 745–750. Available at https://doi.org/10.1378/chest.123.3.745, http://www.chestjournal.org/.

Dales, Burnett, Zwanenburg, 1991. Adverse health effects among adults exposed to home dampness and molds. American Review of Respiratory Disease 143 (3 I), 505–509. Available at https://doi.org/10.1164/ajrccm/143.3.505.

de Boer, W.I., Sharma, H.S., Baelemans, S.M.I., Hoogsteden, H.C., Lambrecht, B.N., Braunstahl, G.J., 2008. Altered expression of epithelial junctional proteins in atopic asthma: possible role in inflammation. Canadian Journal of Physiology and Pharmacology 86 (3), 105–112. Available at https://doi.org/10.1139/y08-004.

Denning, D.W., O'Driscoll, B.R., Powell, G., Chew, F., Atherton, G.T., Vyas, A., et al., 2009. Randomized controlled trial of oral antifungal treatment for severe asthma with fungal sensitization: the fungal asthma sensitization Trial (FAST) study. American Journal of Respiratory and Critical Care Medicine 179 (1), 11–18. Available at https://doi.org/10.1164/rccm.200805-737OC, http://ajrccm.atsjournals.org/cgi/reprint/179/1/11.

Denning, D.W., Pfavayi, L.T., 2023. Poorly controlled asthma – easy wins and future prospects for addressing fungal allergy. Allergology International 72 (4), 493–506. Available at https://doi.org/10.1016/j.alit.2023.07.003.

da Rocha Curvelo, J.A., Reis de Sá, L.F., Moraes, D.C., Soares, R.M., Ferreira-Pereira, A., 2018. Histatin-5 induces the reversal of Pdr5p mediated fluconazole resistance in *Saccharomyces cerevisae*. Journal de Mycologie Médicale 28 (1), 137–142. Available at https://doi.org/10.1016/j.mycmed.2017.11.002.

Dhariwal, J., Hearn, A.P., Kavanagh, J.E., d'Ancona, G., Green, L., Fernandes, M., et al., 2021. Real-world effectiveness of anti–IL-5/5 R therapy in severe atopic eosinophilic asthma with fungal sensitization. Journal of Allergy and Clinical Immunology: In Practice 9 (6). Available at https://doi.org/10.1016/j.jaip.2021.02.048.

Dietz, C.J., Sun, H., Yao, W.C., Citardi, M.J., Corry, D.B., Luong, A.U., 2019. *Aspergillus fumigatus* induction of IL-33 expression in chronic rhinosinusitis is PAR2-dependent. The Laryngoscope 129 (10), 2230–2235. Available at https://doi.org/10.1002/lary.28000, http://onlinelibrary.wiley.com/journal/10.1002/(ISSN)1531-4995.

Dürr, U.H.N., Sudheendra, Ramamoorthy, A., 2006. LL-37, the only human member of the cathelicidin family of antimicrobial peptides. Biochimica et Biophysica Acta - Biomembranes 1758 (9), 1408–1425. Available at https://doi.org/10.1016/j.bbamem.2006.03.030.

Ebbens, F.A., Scadding, G.K., Badia, L., Hellings, P.W., Jorissen, M., Mullol, J., et al., 2006. Amphotericin B nasal lavages: not a solution for patients with chronic rhinosinusitis. Journal of Allergy and Clinical Immunology 118 (5), 1149–1156. Available at https://doi.org/10.1016/j.jaci.2006.07.058.

Ebbens, F.A., Georgalas, C., Luiten, S., Van Dru Nen, C.M., Badia, L., Scadding, G.K., et al., 2009. The effect of topical amphotericin B on inflammatory markers in patients with chronic rhinosinusitis: a multicenter randomized controlled study. The Laryngoscope 119 (2), 401–408. Available at https://doi.org/10.1002/lary.20064.

Fairs, A., Agbetile, J., Bourne, M., Hargadon, B., Monteiro, W.R., Morley, J.P., et al., 2013. Isolation of *Aspergillus* fumigatus from sputum is associated with elevated airborne levels in homes of patients with asthma. Indoor Air 23 (4), 275–284. Available at https://doi.org/10.1111/ina.12020.

Fanning, A.S., Van Itallie, C.M., Anderson, J.M., 2012. Zonula occludens-1 and -2 regulate apical cell structure and the zonula adherens cytoskeleton in polarized epithelia. Molecular Biology of the Cell 23 (4), 577–590. Available at https://doi.org/10.1091/mbc.E11-09-0791.

Foster, A.M., Baliwag, J., Chen, C.S., Guzman, A.M., Stoll, S.W., Gudjonsson, J.E., et al., 2014. IL-36 promotes myeloid cell infiltration, activation, and inflammatory activity in skin. Journal of Immunology 192 (12), 6053–6061. Available at https://doi.org/10.4049/jimmunol.1301481, http://www.jimmunol.org/content/192/12/6053.full.pdf+html.

Friedman, G.C., Hartwick, R.W.J., Ro, J.Y., Saleh, G.Y., Tarrand, J.J., Ayala, A.G., 1991. Allergic fungal sinusitis: report of three cases associated with dematiaceous fungi. American Journal of Clinical Pathology 96 (3), 368–372. Available at https://doi.org/10.1093/ajcp/96.3.368.

Garth, J.M., Reeder, K.M., Godwin, M.S., Mackel, J.J., Dunaway, C.W., Blackburn, J.P., et al., 2017. IL-33 signaling regulates innate IL-17A and IL-22 production via suppression of prostaglandin E2 during lung fungal infection. Journal of Immunology 199 (6), 2140–2148. Available at https://doi.org/10.4049/jimmunol.1602186, http://www.jimmunol.org/content/jimmunol/199/6/2140.full.pdf.

Gleich, G.J., Loegering, D.A., Bell, M.P., Checkel, J.L., Ackerman, S.J., McKean, D.J., 1986. Biochemical and functional similarities between human eosinophil-derived neurotoxin and eosinophil cationic protein: homology with ribonuclease. Proceedings of the National Academy of Sciences 83 (10), 3146–3150. Available at https://doi.org/10.1073/pnas.83.10.3146.

Goswami, S., Angkasekwinai, P., Shan, M., Greenlee, K.J., Barranco, W.T., Polikepahad, S., et al., 2009. Divergent functions for airway epithelial matrix metalloproteinase 7 and retinoic acid in experimental asthma. Nature Immunology 10 (5), 496–503. Available at https://doi.org/10.1038/ni.1719.

Güneser, S., Atici, A., Köksal, F., Yaman, A., 1994. Mold allergy in Adana, Turkey. Allergologia et Immunopathologia 22 (2), 52–54.

Hansakon, A., Jeerawattanawart, S., Angkasekwinai, P., 2023. Differential and cooperative effects of IL-25 and IL-33 on T helper cells contribute to cryptococcal virulence and brain infection. Scientific reports 13 (1). Available at https://doi.org/10.1038/s41598-023-37158-1.

He, X., Howard, B.A., Liu, Y., Neumann, A.K., Li, L., Menon, N., et al., 2021. LYSMD3: a mammalian pattern recognition receptor for chitin. Cell Reports 36 (3), 109392. Available at https://doi.org/10.1016/j.celrep.2021.109392.

Herbert, King, Ring, Holgate, Stewart, Thompson, et al., 1995. Augmentation of permeability in the bronchial epithelium by the house dust mite allergen Der p1. American Journal of Respiratory Cell and Molecular Biology 12 (4), 369–378. Available at https://doi.org/10.1165/ajrcmb.12.4.7695916.

Heyen, L., Müller, U., Siegemund, S., Schulze, B., Protschka, M., Alber, G., et al., 2016. Lung epithelium is the major source of IL-33 and is regulated by IL-33-dependent and IL-33-independent mechanisms in pulmonary cryptococcosis. Pathogens and Disease 74 (7), ftw086. Available at https://doi.org/10.1093/femspd/ftw086.

Hiraishi, Y., Yamaguchi, S., Yoshizaki, T., Nambu, A., Shimura, E., Takamori, A., et al., 2018. IL-33, IL-25 and TSLP contribute to development of fungal-associated protease-induced innate-type airway inflammation. Scientific Reports 8 (1). Available at https://doi.org/10.1038/s41598-018-36440-x.

Hof, W.van't, Reijnders, I.M., Helmerhorst, E.J., Walgreen-Weterings, E., Simoons-Smit, I.M., Veerman, E.C.I., et al., 2000. Synergistic effects of low doses of histatin 5 and its analogues on amphotericin B anti-mycotic activity. International Journal of General and Molecular Microbiology 78 (2), 163–169. Available at https://doi.org/10.1023/A:1026572128004.

Holland, S.M., DeLeo, F.R., Elloumi, H.Z., Hsu, A.P., Uzel, G., Brodsky, N., et al., 2007. STAT3 mutations in the hyper-IgE syndrome. New England Journal of Medicine 357 (16), 1608–1619. Available at https://doi.org/10.1056/NEJMoa073687, http://content.nejm.org/cgi/reprint/357/16/1608.pdf.

Huang, Y., Li, X., Zhu, L., Huang, C., Chen, W., Ling, Z., et al., 2022. Thrombin cleaves IL-33 and modulates IL-33-activated allergic lung inflammation. Allergy: European Journal of Allergy and Clinical Immunology 77 (7), 2104–2120. Available at https://doi.org/10.1111/all.15210, http://onlinelibrary.wiley.com/journal/10.1111/(ISSN)1398-9995.

Huang, Y., Wang, M., Hong, Y., Bu, X., Luan, G., Wang, Y., et al., 2021. Reduced expression of antimicrobial protein secretory leukoprotease inhibitor and clusterin in chronic rhinosinusitis with nasal polyps. Journal of immunology research 2021, 1. Available at https://doi.org/10.1155/2021/1057186.

Huang, Y., Hua, M., Cui, X., 2018. Fungal β-Glucan activates the NLRP3 inflammasome in human bronchial epithelial cells through ROS production. Inflammation 41 (1), 164–173. Available at https://doi.org/10.1007/s10753-017-0674-6.

Imbeau, S.A., Nichols, D., Flaherty, D., Dickie, H., Reed, C., 1978. Relationships between prednisone therapy, disease activity, and the total serum IgE level in allergic bronchopulmonary aspergillosis. Journal of Allergy and Clinical Immunology 62 (2), 91–95. Available at https://doi.org/10.1016/0091-6749(78)90084-2.

Instanes, C., Ormstad, Rydjord, Wiker, Hetland, 2004. Mould extracts increase the allergic response to ovalbumin in mice. Clinical and Experimental Allergy 34 (10), 1634–1641. Available at https://doi.org/10.1111/j.1365-2222.2004.02076.x.

Isaacs, S., Fakhri, S., Luong, A., Citardi, M.J., 2011. A meta-analysis of topical amphotericin B for the treatment of chronic rhinosinusitis. International Forum of Allergy and Rhinology 1 (4), 250–254. Available at https://doi.org/10.1002/alr.20056.

Ito, T., Wang, Y.-H., Duramad, O., Hori, T., Delespesse, G.J., Watanabe, N., et al., 2005. TSLP-activated dendritic cells induce an inflammatory T helper type 2 cell response through OX40 ligand. Journal of Experimental Medicine 202 (9), 1213–1223. Available at https://doi.org/10.1084/jem.20051135.

Johnson, L., Ciaccio, C., Barnes, C.S., Kennedy, K., Forrest, E., Gard, L.C., et al., 2009. Low-cost interventions improve indoor air quality and children's health. Allergy and Asthma Proceedings the Official Journal of Regional and State Allergy Societies 30 (4), 377–385. Available at https://doi.org/10.2500/aap.2009.30.3257.

Johnston, A., Xing, X., Guzman, A.M., Riblett, M.B., Loyd, C.M., Ward, N.L., et al., 2011. IL-1F5, -F6, -F8, and -F9: A novel IL-1 family signaling system that is active in psoriasis and promotes keratinocyte antimicrobial peptide expression. Journal of Immunology 186 (4), 2613–2622. Available at https://doi.org/10.4049/jimmunol.1003162.

Jupelli, M., Shimada, K., Chiba, N., Slepenkin, A., Alsabeh, R., Jones, H.D., et al., 2013. *Chlamydia pneumoniae* infection in mice induces chronic lung inflammation, iBALT formation, and fibrosis. PLoS One 8 (10), e77447. Available at https://doi.org/10.1371/journal.pone.0077447.

Kaur, M., Thakur, P., Verma, N., Choksket, S., Harshvardhan, Korpole, S., et al., 2024. Invasive fungal infections in immunocompromised conditions: emphasis on COVID-19. Current Microbiology 81 (11). Available at https://doi.org/10.1007/s00284-024-03916-1.

Kheradmand, F., Kiss, A., Xu, J., Lee, S.-H., Kolattukudy, P.E., Corry, D.B., 2002. A protease-activated pathway underlying Th cell type 2 activation and allergic lung disease. Journal of Immunology 169 (10), 5904–5911. Available at https://doi.org/10.4049/jimmunol.169.10.5904.

Khosravi, A.R., Erle, D.J., Zissel, G., 2016. Chitin-induced airway epithelial cell innate immune responses are inhibited by carvacrol/thymol. PLoS One 11 (7), e0159459. Available at https://doi.org/10.1371/journal.pone.0159459.

Kobayashi, T., Iijima, K., Radhakrishnan, S., Mehta, V., Vassallo, R., Lawrence, C.B., et al., 2009. Asthma-related environmental fungus, alternaria, activates dendritic cells and produces potent Th2 adjuvant activity. The Journal of Immunology 182 (4), 2502–2510. Available at https://doi.org/10.4049/jimmunol.0802773.

Kouzaki, H., Iijima, K., Kobayashi, T., O'Grady, S.M., Kita, H., 2011. The danger signal, extracellular ATP, is a sensor for an airborne allergen and triggers IL-33 release and innate Th2-type responses. Journal of Immunology 186 (7), 4375–4387. Available at https://doi.org/10.4049/jimmunol.1003020, http://www.jimmunol.org/content/186/7/4375.full.pdf+html.

Kumar, P., Lopez, M., Fan, W., Cambre, K., Elston, R.C., 1990. Mold contamination of automobile air conditioner systems. Annals of Allergy 64 (2 Pt 1), 174–177.

Landers, C.T., Tung, H.Y., Knight, J.M., Madison, M.C., Wu, Y., Zeng, Z., et al., 2019. Selective cleavage of fibrinogen by diverse proteinases initiates innate allergic and antifungal immunity through CD11b. Journal of Biological Chemistry 294 (22), 8834–8847. Available at https://doi.org/10.1074/jbc.RA118.006724, http://www.jbc.org/content/294/22/8834.full.pdf.

Li, C.S., Hsu, L.Y., Chou, C.C., Hsieh, K.H., 1995. Fungus allergens inside and outside the residences of atopic and control children. Archives of Environmental Health 50 (1), 38–43. Available at https://doi.org/10.1080/00039896.1995.9955011.

Li, E., Scheurer, M., Kheradmand, F., Luong, A.U., Corry, D.B., 2021. Computer-assisted analysis of oral antifungal therapy in chronic rhinosinusitis with airway mycosis: a retrospective cohort analysis. Antimicrobial Agents and Chemotherapy 65 (11). Available at https://doi.org/10.1128/AAC.01697-21, https://journals.asm.org/doi/10.1128/AAC.01697-21.

Li, E., Tsai, C.-L., Maskatia, Z.K., Kakkar, E., Porter, P., Rossen, R.D., et al., 2018. Benefits of antifungal therapy in asthma patients with airway mycosis: a retrospective cohort analysis. Immunity, Inflammation and Disease 6 (2), 264–275. Available at https://doi.org/10.1002/iid3.215.

Licorish, K., Novey, H.S., Kozak, P., Fairshter, R.D., Wilson, A.F., 1985. Role of altemaria and penicillium spores in the pathogenesis of asthma. Journal of Allergy and Clinical Immunology 76 (6), 819–825. Available at https://doi.org/10.1016/0091-6749(85)90755-9.

Lilly, L.M., Scopel, M., Nelson, M.P., Burg, A.R., Dunaway, C.W., Steele, C., 2014. Eosinophil deficiency compromises lung defense against *Aspergillus fumigatus*. Infection and Immunity 82 (3), 1315–1325. Available at https://doi.org/10.1128/IAI.01172-13, http://iai.asm.org/content/82/3/1315.full.pdf.

Luong, A.U., Chua, A., Alim, B.M., Olsson, P., Javer, A., 2022. Allergic fungal rhinosinusitis: the role and expectations of biologics. Journal of Allergy and Clinical Immunology: In Practice 10 (12), 3156–3162. Available at https://doi.org/10.1016/j.jaip.2022.08.021, http://www.elsevier.com/journals/the-journal-of-allergy-and-clinical-immunology-in-practice/2213-2198.

Lupetti, A., van Dissel, J.T., Brouwer, C.P.J.M., Nibbering, P.H., 2008. Human antimicrobial peptides' antifungal activity against *Aspergillus fumigatus*. European Journal of Clinical Microbiology & Infectious Diseases 27 (11), 1125–1129. Available at https://doi.org/10.1007/s10096-008-0553-z.

Macleod, T., Ainscough, J.S., Hesse, C., Konzok, S., Braun, A., Buhl, A.-L., et al., 2020. The Proinflammatory cytokine IL-36γ is a global discriminator of harmless microbes and invasive pathogens within epithelial tissues. Cell Reports 33 (11), 108515. Available at https://doi.org/10.1016/j.celrep.2020.108515.

Mak, G., Porter, P.C., Bandi, V., Kheradmand, F., Corry, D.B., 2013. Tracheobronchial mycosis in a retrospective case-series study of five status asthmaticus patients. Clinical Immunology 146 (2), 77–83. Available at https://doi.org/10.1016/j.clim.2012.11.005, http://www.elsevier.com/inca/publications/store/6/2/2/8/0/6/index.htt.

Manning, S.C., Schaefer, S.D., Close, L.G., Vuitch, F., 1991. Culture-positive allergic fungal sinusitis. Archives of Otolaryngology - Head and Neck Surgery 117 (2), 174–178. Available at https://doi.org/10.1001/archotol.1991.01870140062007.

McAleer, J.P., Kolls, J.K., 2011. Mechanisms controlling Th17 cytokine expression and host defense. Journal of Leukocyte Biology 90 (2), 263–270. Available at https://doi.org/10.1189/jlb.0211099, http://www.jleukbio.org/content/90/2/263.full.pdf+html.

McGuckin, M.A., Lindén, S.K., Sutton, P., Florin, T.H., 2011. Mucin dynamics and enteric pathogens. Nature Reviews. Microbiology 9 (4), 265–278. Available at https://doi.org/10.1038/nrmicro2538.

Mehlhop, P.D., van de Rijn, M., Goldberg, A.B., Brewer, J.P., Kurup, V.P., Martin, T.R., et al., 1997. Allergen-induced bronchial hyperreactivity and eosinophilic inflammation occur in the absence of IgE in a mouse model of asthma. Proceedings of the National Academy of Sciences 94 (4), 1344–1349. Available at https://doi.org/10.1073/pnas.94.4.1344.

Millien, V.O., Lu, W., Shaw, J., Yuan, X., Mak, G., Roberts, L., et al., 2013. Cleavage of fibrinogen by proteinases elicits allergic responses through toll-like receptor 4. Science (New York, N.Y.) 341 (6147), 792–796. Available at https://doi.org/10.1126/science.1240342, http://www.sciencemag.org/content/341/6147/792.full.pdf.

Moss, R.B., 2023. Severe fungal asthma: a role for biologics and inhaled antifungals. MDPI, United States Journal of Fungi 9 (1). Available at https://doi.org/10.3390/jof9010085, www.mdpi.com/journal/jof.

Moyes, D.L., Wilson, D., Richardson, J.P., Mogavero, S., Tang, S.X., Wernecke, J., et al., 2016. Candidalysin is a fungal peptide toxin critical for mucosal infection. Nature 532 (7597), 64–68. Available at https://doi.org/10.1038/nature17625, http://www.nature.com/nature/index.html.

Murai, H., Qi, H., Choudhury, B., Wild, J., Dharajiya, N., Vaidya, S., et al., 2012. Alternaria-induced release of IL-18 from damaged airway epithelial cells: an NF-κB dependent mechanism of Th2 differentiation? PLoS One 7 (2), e30280. Available at https://doi.org/10.1371/journal.pone.0030280.

Murali, P.S., Dai, G., Kumar, A., Fink, J.N., Kurup, V.P., 1992. Aspergillus antigen-induced eosinophil differentiation in a murine model. Infection and Immunity 60 (5), 1952–1956. Available at https://doi.org/10.1128/iai.60.5.1952-1956.1992.

Newcomb, D.C., Sajjan, U.S., Nagarkar, D.R., Wang, Q., Nanua, S., Zhou, Y., et al., 2008. Human rhinovirus 1B exposure induces phosphatidylinositol 3-kinase-dependent airway inflammation in mice. American Journal of Respiratory and Critical Care Medicine 177 (10), 1111–1121. Available at https://doi.org/10.1164/rccm.200708-1243OC, http://ajrccm.atsjournals.org/cgi/reprint/177/10/1111.

Ohashi, Y., Motojima, S., Fukuda, T., Makino, S., 1992. Airway hyperresponsiveness, increased intracellular spaces of bronchial epithelium, and increased infiltration of eosinophils and lymphocytes in bronchial mucosa in asthma. American Review of Respiratory Disease 145 (6), 1469–1476. Available at https://doi.org/10.1164/ajrccm/145.6.1469.

O'Hollaren, M.T., Yunginger, J.W., Offord, K.P., Somers, M.J., O'Connell, E.J., Ballard, D.J., et al., 1991. Exposure to an aeroallergen as a possible precipitating factor in respiratory arrest in young patients with asthma. The New England Journal of Medicine 324 (6), 359–363.

Oppenheim, F.G., Helmerhorst, E.J., Lendenmann, U., Offner, G.D., 2012. Anti-candidal activity of genetically engineered histatin variants with multiple functional domains.

PLoS One 7 (12). Available at https://doi.org/10.1371/journal.pone.0051479, http://www.plosone.org/article/fetchObjectAttachment.action?uri=info%3Adoi%2F10.1371%2Fjournal.pone.0051479&representation=PDF.

Oshikata, C., Watanabe, M., Saito, A., Ishida, M., Kobayashi, S., Konuma, R., et al., 2017. Allergic bronchopulmonary mycosis due to exposure to *Eurotium herbariorum* after the great east Japan earthquake. Prehospital and Disaster Medicine 32 (6), 688–690. Available at https://doi.org/10.1017/s1049023x17006914.

Pashley, C.H., Fairs, A., Morley, J.P., Tailor, S., Agbetile, J., Bafadhel, M., et al., 2012. Routine processing procedures for isolating filamentous fungi from respiratory sputum samples may underestimate fungal prevalence. Medical Mycology 50 (4), 433–438. Available at https://doi.org/10.3109/13693786.2011.615762.

Patel, N.N., Triantafillou, V., Maina, I.W., Workman, A.D., Tong, C.C.L., Kuan, E.C., et al., 2019. Fungal extracts stimulate solitary chemosensory cell expansion in noninvasive fungal rhinosinusitis. International Forum of Allergy and Rhinology 9 (7), 730–737. Available at https://doi.org/10.1002/alr.22334, http://onlinelibrary.wiley.com/journal/10.1002/(ISSN)2042-6984.

Patro, S.K., Verma, R.K., Panda, N.K., Chakrabarti, A., Singh, P., 2015. Efficacy of preoperative itraconazole in allergic fungal rhinosinusitis. American Journal of Rhinology and Allergy 29 (4), 299–304. Available at https://doi.org/10.2500/ajra.2015.29.4187, http://www.ingentaconnect.com/content/ocean/ajra/2015/00000029/00000004/art00018.

Pericolini, E., Gabrielli, E., Amacker, M., Kasper, L., Roselletti, E., Luciano, E., et al., 2015. Secretory aspartyl proteinases cause vaginitis and can mediate vaginitis caused by *Candida albicans* in Mice. mBio 6 (3). Available at https://doi.org/10.1128/mbio.00724-15.

Porter, P., Susarla, S.C., Polikepahad, S., Qian, Y., Hampton, J., Kiss, A., et al., 2009. Link between allergic asthma and airway mucosal infection suggested by proteinase-secreting household fungi. Mucosal Immunology 2 (6), 504–517. Available at https://doi.org/10.1038/mi.2009.102.

Porter, P.C., Lim, D.J., Maskatia, Z.K., Mak, G., Tsai, C.L., Citardi, M.J., et al., 2014. Airway surface mycosis in chronic TH2-associated airway disease. Journal of Allergy and Clinical Immunology 134 (2), 325. Available at https://doi.org/10.1016/j.jaci.2014.04.028, http://www.elsevier.com/inca/publications/store/6/2/3/3/6/8/index.htt.

Porter, P.C., Roberts, L., Fields, A., Knight, M., Qian, Y., Delclos, G.L., et al., 2011. Necessary and sufficient role for T helper cells to prevent fungal dissemination in allergic lung disease. Infection and Immunity 79 (11), 4459–4471. Available at https://doi.org/10.1128/IAI.05209-11.

Pulimood, T.B., Corden, J.M., Bryden, C., Sharples, L., Nasser, S.M., 2007. Epidemic asthma and the role of the fungal mold *Alternaria alternata*. Journal of Allergy and Clinical Immunology 120 (3), 610–617. Available at https://doi.org/10.1016/j.jaci.2007.04.045.

Quansah, R., Jaakkola, M.S., Hugg, T.T., Heikkinen, S.A.M., Jaakkola, J.J.K., Behrens, T., 2012. Residential dampness and molds and the risk of developing asthma: a systematic review and meta-analysis. PLoS One 7 (11), e47526. Available at https://doi.org/10.1371/journal.pone.0047526.

Rains, B.M., Mineck, C.W., 2003. Treatment of allergic fungal sinusitis with high-dose intraconazole. American Journal of Rhinology 17 (1), 1–8. Available at https://doi.org/10.1177/194589240301700101, http://www.ingentaconnect.com/content/ocean/ajr.

Ramirez, G.A., Yacoub, M.R., Ripa, M., Mannina, D., Cariddi, A., Saporiti, N., et al., 2018. Eosinophils from physiology to disease: a comprehensive review. BioMed Research International 2018. Available at https://doi.org/10.1155/2018/9095275, http://www.hindawi.com/journals/biomed/.

Richmond, B.W., Brucker, R.M., Han, W., Du, R.H., Zhang, Y., Cheng, D.S., et al., 2016. Airway bacteria drive a progressive COPD-like phenotype in mice with polymeric immunoglobulin receptor deficiency. Nature Communications 7. Available at https://doi.org/10.1038/ncomms11240, http://www.nature.com/ncomms/index.html.

Roy, M.G., Livraghi-Butrico, A., Fletcher, A.A., McElwee, M.M., Evans, S.E., Boerner, R.M., et al., 2014. Muc5b is required for airway defence. Nature 505 (7483), 412–416. Available at https://doi.org/10.1038/nature12807.

Samant, M., Krings, J.G., Lew, D., Goss, C.W., Koch, T., McGregor, M.C., et al., 2024. Use of quantitative CT imaging to identify bronchial thermoplasty responders. CHEST 165 (4), 775–784. Available at https://doi.org/10.1016/j.chest.2023.12.015.

Sandhu, R.S., Mehta, S.K., Khan, Z.U., Singh, M.M., 1979. Role of *Aspergillus* and *Candida* species in allergic bronchopulmonary mycoses. A comparative study. Scandinavian Journal of Respiratory Diseases 60 (5), 235–242.

Seshasayee, D., Lee, W.P., Zhou, M., Shu, J., Suto, E., Zhang, J., et al., 2007. In vivo blockade of OX40 ligand inhibits thymic stromal lymphopoietin driven atopic inflammation. Journal of Clinical Investigation 117 (12), 3868–3878. Available at https://doi.org/10.1172/jci33559.

Shaw, J.L., Fakhri, S., Citardi, M.J., Porter, P.C., Corry, D.B., Kheradmand, F., et al., 2013. IL-33-responsive innate lymphoid cells are an important source of IL-13 in chronic rhinosinusitis with nasal polyps. American Journal of Respiratory and Critical Care Medicine 188 (4), 432–439. Available at https://doi.org/10.1164/rccm.201212-2227OC, http://www.atsjournals.org/doi/pdf/10.1164/rccm.201212-2227OC.

Sheng, Y.H., Hasnain, S.Z., 2022. Mucus and mucins: the underappreciated host defence system. Frontiers in Cellular and Infection Microbiology 12. Available at https://doi.org/10.3389/fcimb.2022.856962, http://www.frontiersin.org/Cellular_and_Infection_Microbiology/archive.

Shin, S.H., Kim, Y.H., Jin, H.S., Kang, S.H., 2016. Alternaria induces production of thymic stromal lymphopoietin in nasal fibroblasts through toll-like receptor 2. Allergy, Asthma and Immunology Research 8 (1), 63–68. Available at https://doi.org/10.4168/aair.2016.8.1.63, http://www.e-aair.org/Synapse/Data/PDFData/9999AAIR/aair-8-63.pdf.

Silva, J.D.C., Thompson-Souza, G.D.A., Barroso, M.V., Neves, J.S., Figueiredo, R.T., 2021. Neutrophil and eosinophil DNA extracellular trap formation: lessons from pathogenic fungi. Frontiers in Microbiology 12. Available at https://doi.org/10.3389/fmicb.2021.634043, https://www.frontiersin.org/journals/microbiology#.

Srisomboon, Y., Squillace, D.L., Maniak, P.J., Kita, H., O'Grady, S.M., 2020. Fungal allergen-induced IL-33 secretion involves cholesterol-dependent, VDAC-1-mediated ATP release from the airway epithelium. Journal of Physiology 598 (10), 1829–1845. Available at https://doi.org/10.1113/JP279379, http://onlinelibrary.wiley.com/journal/10.1111/(ISSN)1469-7793.

Stevens, W.W., Kato, A., 2021. Group 2 innate lymphoid cells in nasal polyposis. Annals of Allergy, Asthma and Immunology 126 (2), 110–117. Available at https://doi.org/10.1016/j.anai.2020.08.001, http://www.elsevier.com/wps/find/journaldescription.reviewers/722283/description#description.

Stevens, W.W., Peters, A.T., Tan, B.K., Klingler, A.I., Poposki, J.A., Hulse, K.E., et al., 2019. Associations between inflammatory endotypes and clinical presentations in chronic rhinosinusitis. Journal of Allergy and Clinical Immunology: In Practice 7 (8), 2812. Available at https://doi.org/10.1016/j.jaip.2019.05.009, http://www.elsevier.com/journals/the-journal-of-allergy-and-clinical-immunology-in-practice/2213-2198.

Sun, H., Damania, A., Mair, M.L., Otukoya, E., Li, Y.-D., Polsky, K., et al., 2022. Induced eosinophilic chronic rhinosinusitis and asthma, a model of unified airway disease. Frontiers in Immunology 13. Available at https://doi.org/10.3389/fimmu.2022.818017.

Sun, H., Knight, J.M., Li, Y.-D., Ashoori, F., Citardi, M.J., et al., 2024. Allergic fungal rhinosinusitis linked to other hyper-IgE syndromes through defective TH17 responses. Journal of Allergy and Clinical Immunology 154 (5), 1169–1179. Available at https://doi.org/10.1016/j.jaci.2024.06.022.

Sun, N., Ogulur, I., Mitamura, Y., Yazici, D., Pat, Y., Bu, X., et al., 2024. The epithelial barrier theory and its associated diseases. Allergy 79 (12), 3192–3237. Available at https://doi.org/10.1111/all.16318.

Sweerus, K., Lachowicz-Scroggins, M., Gordon, E., LaFemina, M., Huang, X., Parikh, M., et al., 2017. Claudin-18 deficiency is associated with airway epithelial barrier dysfunction and asthma. Journal of Allergy and Clinical Immunology 139 (1), 72. Available at https://doi.org/10.1016/j.jaci.2016.02.035.

Tangye, S.G., Puel, A., 2023. The Th17/IL-17 axis and host defense against fungal infections. Journal of Allergy and Clinical Immunology: In Practice 11 (6), 1624–1634. Available at https://doi.org/10.1016/j.jaip.2023.04.015, http://www.elsevier.com/journals/the-journal-of-allergy-and-clinical-immunology-in-practice/2213-2198.

Tyler, M.A., Lam, K., Marino, M.J., Yao, W.C., Schmale, I., Citardi, M.J., et al., 2021. Revisiting the controversy: the role of fungi in chronic rhinosinusitis. International Forum of Allergy and Rhinology 11 (11), 1577–1587. Available at https://doi.org/10.1002/alr.22826, http://onlinelibrary.wiley.com/journal/10.1002/(ISSN)2042-6984.

Viksne, R.J., Sumeraga, G., Pilmane, M., 2023. Antimicrobial and defense proteins in chronic rhinosinusitis with nasal polyps. Medicina 59 (7), 1259. Available at https://doi.org/10.3390/medicina59071259.

Wan, H., Winton, H.L., Soeller, C., Tovey, E.R., Gruenert, D.C., Thompson, P.J., et al., 1999. Der p 1 facilitates transepithelial allergen delivery by disruption of tight junctions. Journal of Clinical Investigation 104 (1), 123–133. Available at https://doi.org/10.1172/jci5844.

Wark, P., Hussaini, S., Holder, C., Powell, H., Gibson, P., Oldmeadow, C., 2020. Omalizumab is an effective intervention in severe asthma with fungal sensitization. The Journal of Allergy and Clinical Immunology: In Practice 8 (10), 3428. Available at https://doi.org/10.1016/j.jaip.2020.05.055.

Weatherhead, J.E., Porter, P., Coffey, A., Haydel, D., Versteeg, L., Zhan, B., et al., 2018. Ascaris larval infection and lung invasion directly induce severe allergic airway disease in mice. Infection and Immunity 86 (12). Available at https://doi.org/10.1128/IAI.00533-18, http://iai.asm.org/content/by/year.

Weschta, M., Rimek, D., Formanek, M., Podbielski, A., Riechelmann, H., 2006. Effect of nasal antifungal therapy on nasal cell activation markers in chronic rhinosinusitis. Archives of Otolaryngology - Head and Neck Surgery 132 (7), 743–747. Available at https://doi.org/10.1001/archotol.132.7.743Germany, http://archotol.ama-assn.org/cgi/reprint/132/7/743.

Weschta, M., Rimek, D., Formanek, M., Polzehl, D., Podbielski, A., Riechelmann, H., 2004. Topical antifungal treatment of chronic rhinosinusitis with nasal polyps: a randomized, double-blind clinical trial. Journal of Allergy and Clinical Immunology 113 (6), 1122–1128. Available at https://doi.org/10.1016/j.jaci.2004.03.038.

Wu, Y., Zeng, Z., Guo, Y., Song, L., Weatherhead, J.E., Huang, X., et al., 2021. *Candida albicans* elicits protective allergic responses via platelet mediated T helper 2 and T helper 17 cell polarization. Immunity 54 (11), 2595. Available at https://doi.org/10.1016/j.immuni.2021.08.009.

Xiao, C., Puddicombe, S.M., Field, S., Haywood, J., Broughton-Head, V., Puxeddu, I., et al., 2011. Defective epithelial barrier function in asthma. The Journal of Allergy and Clinical Immunology 128 (3). Available at https://doi.org/10.1016/j.jaci.2011.05.038.

Yoo, J.K., Kim, T.S., Hufford, M.M., Braciale, T.J., 2013. Viral infection of the lung: Host response and sequelae. Journal of Allergy and Clinical Immunology 132 (6), 1263–1276. Available at https://doi.org/10.1016/j.jaci.2013.06.006, http://www.elsevier.com/inca/publications/store/6/2/3/3/6/8/index.htt.

Yoon, J., Ponikau, J.U., Lawrence, C.B., Kita, H., 2008. Innate antifungal immunity of human eosinophils mediated by a β2 integrin, CD11b. Journal of Immunology 181 (4), 2907–2915. Available at https://doi.org/10.4049/jimmunol.181.4.2907, http://www.jimmunol.org/cgi/reprint/181/4/2907.

Zhang, Z., Biagini Myers, J.M., Brandt, E.B., Ryan, P.H., Lindsey, M., Mintz-Cole, R.A., et al., 2017. β-Glucan exacerbates allergic asthma independent of fungal sensitization and promotes steroid-resistant TH2/TH17 responses. Journal of Allergy and Clinical Immunology 139 (1). Available at https://doi.org/10.1016/j.jaci.2016.02.031.

CHAPTER

7

Histoplasmosis: current and future perspectives in host responses, diagnosis, and treatment

Alessandro F. Valdez[1], Taiane Nascimento de Souza[2], Clara Pralon[1], Daniel Zamith-Miranda[3], Leonardo Nimrichter[1] and Joshua D. Nosanchuk[3]

[1]*Paulo de Góes Microbiology Institute, Federal University of Rio de Janeiro, UFRJ, Rio de Janeiro, RJ, Brazil,*

[2]*Department of Microbiology and Immunology, Albert Einstein College of Medicine, Bronx, NY, United States,*

[3]*Departments of Medicine (Division of Infectious Diseases) and Microbiology and Immunology, Albert Einstein College of Medicine, Bronx, NY, United States*

Introduction

Histoplasmosis is a cosmopolitan disease caused by the dimorphic ascomycete *Histoplasma capsulatum* (Valdez et al., 2022). In short, infection is initiated when microconidia or mycelial fragments are inhaled by an individual. In the lung, temperature triggers the morphological shift to the yeast form, which replicates in the host with various degrees of success depending on factors such as immune status, age, and inoculum size (Valdez et al., 2022). *H. capsulatum* was initially divided into three different subspecies (Ajello, 1968), but further studies revealed at least eight genetic clusters within *Histoplasma* (Kasuga et al., 2003). More recently, the implementation of genome sequencing allowed the differentiation of seven of those clades into phylogenetic species: *Histoplasma ohiense*, *Histoplasma mississippiense*, *H. capsulatum sensu stricto*, *Histoplasma suramericanum,* and three still unnamed *Histoplasma* lineages from continental Africa, southern Brazil, and India (Sepúlveda et al., 2014; Sepúlveda et al., 2017; Almeida-Silva et al., 2021; Jofre et al., 2022). Regardless, no systematic assessment has been done to determine the degree of phenotypic differences between these phylogenetic species, and although future differentiation may be clinically relevant, for now, we refer to *H. capsulatum* as the causative agent of histoplasmosis in humans.

The disease is endemic in the United States, where most cases used to be associated with the Ohio and Mississippi River Valleys (Kauffman, 2007), although this scenario has changed because of global warming, as the phenomenon is currently expanding geographical areas where *H. capsulatum* and other dimorphic

Immunological Insights and Emerging Therapeutics in Medical Mycology. DOI: https://doi.org/10.1016/B978-0-443-23636-5.00011-3

fungi can thrive (Seidel et al., 2024). Histoplasmosis is also endemic in Brazil and has largely disseminated throughout South America, with cases reported in Ecuador, Argentina, and Uruguay among other countries (Colombo et al., 2011). In the United States and South America, histoplasmosis is often misdiagnosed as tuberculosis (Adenis et al., 2014; Nacher et al., 2014). Histoplasmosis is increasingly reported in China (Pan et al., 2013), whereas the disease is infrequently reported in Australia, Israel, Zimbabwe, South Africa, Uganda, and Tanzania (Lofgren et al., 2012; McLeod et al., 2011; Cottle et al., 2013; Gumbo et al., 2001; Elias et al., 2018). Additionally, some autochthonous cases of histoplasmosis have been reported in Italy, France, and Spain, but most European cases are still associated with travel to endemic areas (Farina et al., 2000; Antinori et al., 2021; Ashbee et al., 2008; Calvopiña et al., 2023).

There is a broad range of presentations for histoplasmosis, and although *H. capsulatum* is one of the few fungal organisms that meet all the requirements to be considered a primary pathogen (Köhler et al., 2014; Köhler et al., 2017), infection in immunocompetent individuals is usually restricted to the lungs, while it can more readily cause disseminated disease in immunocompromised individuals (Valdez et al., 2022; Azar et al., 2020). Pulmonary acute histoplasmosis is usually asymptomatic, and symptoms such as cough, dyspnea, fever, chills, and other milder respiratory symptoms are often misdiagnosed as bacterial pneumonia or viral respiratory diseases (Azar and Hage, 2017). In addition to these symptoms, weight loss, night sweats, and shortness of breath are usually present in chronic pulmonary histoplasmosis, mimicking tuberculosis symptoms and often resulting in empirical antituberculosis therapy and a delayed diagnosis of histoplasmosis (Kauffman, 2007). Disseminated disease is associated with lymphadenopathy, hepatomegaly, splenomegaly, occasional skin and mucosal lesions (and even endovascular lesions), central nervous system (CNS), and gastrointestinal symptoms (Wheat et al., 2016) that, being nonspecific, can lead to misdiagnosis.

Like other fungal infections, histoplasmosis is severely misdiagnosed and/or underreported, either due to low awareness or the lack of species-specific symptoms. Recently, the World Health Organization (WHO) created the Fungal Priority Pathogen List to prioritize fungal pathogens of public health importance and raise awareness, and *Histoplasma* was placed in the "high priority" group (*WHO fungal priority pathogens list to guide research, development, and public health action.*, 2025; Beardsley, 2024; Fisher and Denning, 2023). Antifungal therapies vary according to the degree of disease and the immunological status of the patient, but are usually not recommended in mild cases. In the event of persistent symptoms or immunosuppression, the treatment ranges from itraconazole to the administration of liposomal amphotericin B (Limper et al., 2011; Azar et al., 2020; Wheat et al., 2007). In addition, antifungal therapies are associated with a series of limitations and with increasing drug resistance, so optimal clinical results often depend on early and proper treatment, which also depends on accurate diagnosis (Valdez et al., 2023; Nett and Andes, 2016; Voltan et al., 2016). Taken together, delayed diagnosis, misdiagnosis, and lack of adequate treatment increase the death toll, especially in the setting of disseminated histoplasmosis in immunocompromised patients, where mortality rates reach up to 80% (Denning, 2016; Toscanini et al., 2021; Denning, 2024).

In this chapter, we will review and discuss the overall interaction of *H. capsulatum* with the host, current alternatives regarding diagnosis and treatment, as well as future perspectives for the management of histoplasmosis.

Host-pathogen interaction

Recognition and internalization of *Histoplasma capsulatum* yeast by innate immune cells

After transformation from the hyphal form, *H. capsulatum* yeast cells typically reach the alveoli, where they first encounter alveolar macrophages (AMs), which correspond to 90% of the resident phagocyte population (Morales-Nebreda et al., 2015). These sentinel cells act as the first line of defense against inhaled pathogens and particles entering the lungs, where they recognize microbial products, phagocytose and destroy microorganisms, and secrete mediators to recruit other leukocytes (Crameri and Blaser, 2002). Fungal recognition by AMs is mediated by pattern recognition receptors (PRRs), a class of receptors that recognize microbe-associated molecular patterns (MAMPs) exposed on the surface of microbes. The major PRR involved in the recognition/phagocytosis of *H. capsulatum* is the complement receptor (CR), which is expressed on alveolar and interstitial macrophages as well as neutrophils (PMNs), and dendritic cells (DCs) (Bullock and Wright, 1987; Newman et al., 1990; Long et al., 2003; Guimarães et al., 2019; Vandendriessche et al., 2021). In macrophages, CR3 (CD11b/CD18), CR4 (CD11c/CD18), and LFA-1 (CD11a/CD18) are receptors associated with the phagocytosis of *H. capsulatum*, and blocking the common β-chain (CD18) prevents both attachment and phagocytosis of *H. capsulatum* by macrophages by 50%–90% (Bullock and Wright, 1987; Newman et al., 1990). CR3 is the main receptor used by *H. capsulatum* to enter macrophages. This receptor recognizes the heat-shock protein-60 (Hsp60) on the *H. capsulatum* surface, and the pretreatment of macrophages with recombinant Hsp60 (rHsp60) inhibits attachment of *H. capsulatum* yeasts to macrophages. Furthermore, the expression of CR3 in CHO cells is sufficient to promote the internalization of *H. capsulatum* cells (Long et al., 2003).

Hsp60 is distributed on the yeast's surface in discrete clusters, and it is upregulated in response to the elevation in temperature, facilitating phagocytosis by AMs (Long et al., 2003; Guimarães et al., 2011). Once *H. capsulatum* has been phagocytosed by AMs, it proliferates in aggregates in the perinuclear area, inducing DNA damage and apoptosis in the host cells (Pitangui et al., 2016). Apoptotic AMs as well as soluble factors can modulate the course of the infection (Allen and Deepe, 2005). Yeasts released by apoptotic cells are subsequently internalized by other phagocytes (AMs, PMNs, and DCs), leading to their activation (Deepe et al., 2008). Observations in a murine model of histoplasmosis show an influx of inflammatory cells, including monocytes, PMNs, and DCs, to the lung during early stage infection (Deepe et al., 2008; Baughman et al., 1986).

As part of the early immune events in response to infection by *H. capsulatum*, PMNs recruited to the alveoli phagocytose opsonized and nonopsonized *H. capsulatum* yeasts via FcγRIII (CD16) and CRs, CR1 and CR3 (Newman, Gootee and Gabay, 1993). These leukocytes have important antifungal activities against *H. capsulatum* through the release of their granule contents (defensins, cathepsin G, and bactericidal-permeability-increasing protein) into the phagolysosomes (Newman et al., 1993; Newman et al., 2000). Additionally, the binding of extracellular *H. capsulatum* yeast to the CD18 integrin triggers the release of neutrophil extracellular traps, which are structures composed of DNA-histone complexes and proteins that trap and destroy the fungus (Thompson-Souza et al., 2020).

DCs are also phagocytes that interact with *H. capsulatum*, and they play an important role in connecting innate and adaptive immunity. DCs represent a heterogeneous population in the alveoli and can arise from precursor cells and circulating monocytes (Ardain et al., 2020). DCs infiltrate the lung in the first week of *H. capsulatum* infection in mice (Deepe et al., 2008). DCs phagocytose *H. capsulatum* mainly through the recognition of the fungal protein cyclophilin A by the host receptor very late antigen-5, as opposed to AMs (Gomez et al., 2008). Once phagocytosed, the fungus is processed in the phagolysosome system, and the generated peptides are exposed on the cell surface bound to MHCII. MHCII/peptide-expressing DCs migrate to draining lymph nodes, where they present antigens to T cells (Ardain et al., 2020). DCs can phagocytose apoptotic infected macrophages and process the antigen into the MHCI pathway to activate $CD8^+$ cells (cross-presentation) (Hsieh et al., 2011). Additionally, activated DCs secrete inflammatory cytokines such as IL-12 and TNF-α (Zhou et al., 2001). IL-12 is responsible for inducing the production of interferons (IFN)-γ by Th1 and natural killer (NK) cells, which are important components of the immune response to *H. capsulatum* (Zhou et al., 2001; Allendoerfer et al., 1997; Zhou et al., 1995).

NK cells are important innate lymphoid cells, often found as tissue-resident in the alveolar interstitium but also recruited during infection (Ardain et al., 2020). During *H. capsulatum* infection, NK cells are recruited to the lung at an early stage of the infection and are activated by IL-12 produced by DCs (Cain and Deepe, 1998; Cohen et al., 2011). These cells not only contribute to innate immunity through their direct cytotoxicity, but also through the differentiation of IFN-γ-producing Th1 cells (Zhou et al., 2001). IFN-γ plays a pivotal role during *H. capsulatum* infection, by activating the fungicidal response in macrophages (Brummer et al., 1991; Shen et al., 2018; Newman et al., 2006; Prado et al., 2020).

The cellular component of innate immunity extends beyond phagocytes and NK cells. Alveolar epithelial cells (AECs) also play an important role against fungi, functioning as a physical barrier preventing their access to the blood capillaries, as well as producing antimicrobial peptides that kill the fungus when it is in the alveolar lumen (Whitsett and Alenghat, 2015). The alveoli are covered by type I and type II AECs. The internalization of *H. capsulatum* by tracheal epithelial cells from hamsters decreases the virulence of the internalized yeast, although by an unclear mechanism (Eissenberg et al., 1997). Type II AECs play an antifungal role, by producing surfactant protein (SP)-A and SP-D that increase the permeability of extracellular yeasts, reducing their viability (McCormack et al., 2003). Furthermore, type II AECs produce IL-8 (CXCL8) in response to *H. capsulatum* (Alcantara et al., 2020), recruiting the first wave of leukocytes (PMNs) to the alveolar space (Marshall et al., 2001).

H. capsulatum releases extracellular vesicles (EVs) into the extracellular milieu (Albuquerque et al., 2008). EVs are nanosized compartments that transport a variety of bioactive molecules, including proteins, lipids, RNAs, metabolites, and glycans (A. F. Valdez et al., 2023; Piffer et al., 2021). Emerging evidence suggests that fungal EVs interact with host cells and modulate their activity, potentially influencing the outcome of infection (Baltazar et al., 2016; Honorato et al., 2024, 2022; Baltazar et al., 2018). For example, short-term incubation (1 hour) of macrophages with *H. capsulatum* EVs reduces the ability of these cells to internalize the fungus (Baltazar et al., 2018). Additionally, *H. capsulatum* EVs carry active enzymes such as laccase and urease, which are associated with fungal virulence (Baltazar et al., 2016). Although the specific EV components recognized by host cells remain unidentified, the presence of Hsp60 suggests that EVs may interact with CR3 on macrophages.

Role of host pattern recognition receptors

A wide range of PRRs, including toll-like receptors (TLRs), C-type lectin receptors (CLRs), and notch receptors (NRs), have been associated with the immune response against *H. capsulatum* (Wang et al., 2014; Lin et al., 2010). With the exception of CLRs, none of these receptors are used by macrophages and DCs for the phagocytosis of *H. capsulatum* yeasts (Lin et al., 2010). However, they play pivotal roles in inducing the production of cytokines such as IL-12, IFN-γ, granulocyte-macrophage colony-stimulating factor (GM-CSF), and TNF-α by these cells, which are important in connecting the innate and adaptive immune responses during *H. capsulatum* infection (Kroetz and Deepe, 2012).

The *H. capsulatum* cell wall is the main interface for interaction with PRRs (Valdez et al., 2022). It is composed of a diversity of polysaccharides, such as chitin, β-glucans [β-(1,3)- and β-(1, 6)-linked], and α-(1,3)-glucan, mannans, galactomannans, as well as important proteins, such as Hsp60 (Guimarães et al., 2011; Valdez et al., 2022). However, only a few of these molecules have been identified as ligands for the PRRs mentioned above. Among these components, β-(1,3)-glucan is the most studied and well-characterized ligand of the dectin-1 receptor on the phagocyte surface (Wang et al., 2014; Valdez et al., 2022; Lin et al., 2010).

Dectin-1 is part of the CLRs family and is necessary for protective immunity to many fungal species, but the role of this receptor during *H. capsulatum* infection remains controversial (Drummond and Brown, 2011; Gringhuis et al., 2022). On the surface of virulent strains of *H. capsulatum,* β-(1,3)-glucan is masked, avoiding its recognition by dectin-1 (Rappleye et al., 2007; Rappleye et al., 2004; Garfoot et al., 2016, 2017). Nevertheless, dectin-1 induces the production of TNF-α by macrophages in response to either live or heat-killed *H. capsulatum* (Hsieh et al., 2011). Furthermore, the response triggered by dectin-1 is important for the vaccine-induced immunity against *H. capsulatum* in mice. Dectin-2, another CLR, is associated with the development of antifungal Th17 response, following vaccination and infection (Wang et al., 2014). Both receptors signal through the Syk-CARD9 pathway, but dectin-2 recognizes α-mannan structures on the fungal surface. Additionally, both receptors induce IL-1β production in DCs, an important cytokine for the development of Th17 cells (Chang et al., 2017).

This functional redundancy of dectin-1 with other receptors has led to the hypothesis that these receptors may work collaboratively on the surface of specific cells, enhancing the cytokine response triggered by *H. capsulatum* (Souza et al., 2021). The receptors dectin-1, CD18, and TLR2 are similarly associated with the formation of lipid bodies and the generation of lipid mediators in macrophages stimulated with *H. capsulatum* or β-glucan (Sorgi et al., 2009), suggesting a synergistic role for these receptors in modulating immune responses to fungal pathogens.

Both CR3 and TLR2 are associated with lipid microdomains, dynamic regions of the plasma membrane enriched in cholesterol that dock different PRRs (Hellwing et al., 2018; Guimarães et al., 2019; Lin et al., 2010). Evidence suggests cooperative signaling between CR3 and dectin-1, triggering the secretion of inflammatory cytokines, such as TNF-α and IL-6, in macrophages through integrated signaling at the Syk kinase pathway (Lin et al., 2010; Souza et al., 2021; Huang et al., 2015). However, these findings were demonstrated using heat-killed *H. capsulatum*, which shows increased β-glucan exposure at the cell surface (Wheeler and Fink, 2006). The role of TLR2 during *H. capsulatum* infection in macrophages and DCs remains poorly understood. However, the *H. capsulatum* yeast protein Yps3p has been identified as a ligand for TLR2 in microglia, suggesting the activation of this receptor on phagocytes during *H. capsulatum* infection (Aravalli et al., 2008).

TLRs are a large family of PRRs composed of cell surface and endosomal receptors expressed in a variety of immune and nonimmune cells (Kawai et al., 2024). Except for TLR3, TLRs interact with the adaptor proteins myeloid differentiation factor 88 (MyD88) for the activation of the transcription factors NF-κB and AP-1 to induce cytokine synthesis (Coady et al., 2015). The activation of MyD88 is required for the early innate immune response to *H. capsulatum*, inducing the production of IL-6, TNF-α, IL-1β, IL-12, and also CCL2 and KC during *H. capsulatum* infection in mice. Supporting the importance of TLRs in experimental histoplasmosis, the MyD88 signaling pathway is associated with the recruitment of monocytes, PMNs, and DCs to the lung of infected mice (Coady et al., 2015).

The effective immune response to *H. capsulatum* requires the coordinated participation of multiple PRRs (Souza et al., 2021). Certain PRRs, especially the endosomal ones (TLR7 and TLR9), are activated only following phagocytosis, triggering the innate immune responses from within phagosomes (Kawai et al., 2024). They induce the production of type I interferons (IFN-I) by $CD103^+$ DCs in the lungs during *H. capsulatum* infection (Van Prooyen et al., 2016). The IFN-I production is correlated with the restriction of the fungal growth in DCs. Additionally, activation of TLR7/9 in DCs is important for inducing IFN-γ production by primed $CD4^+$ T cells (Van Prooyen et al., 2016).

NRs are also activated in DCs after phagocytosis of *H. capsulatum* yeasts (Huang and Deepe, 2022). NRs are involved in cell-cell communication, affecting the differentiation and functional state of immune cells, such as phagocytes, T and B cells (Zhou et al., 2022). The levels of Notch 1 and Notch 2, as well as their ligands Jagged 2 and DDL4, are higher in infected DCs with *H. capsulatum* compared to uninfected (Huang and Deepe, 2022). Notch signaling triggered by *H. capsulatum* promotes activation of infected DCs, upregulating the costimulatory molecules CD80 and CD86, and promoting the clearance of yeasts by these cells (Huang and Deepe, 2022).

The fate of internalized *Histoplasma capsulatum*

The elimination of *H. capsulatum* begins with the recognition of MAMPs by PRRs from phagocytes, inducing the internalization of the fungus. After fusing with lysosomes, phagosomes become phagolysosomes, where ingested microorganisms are degraded. While *H. capsulatum* yeasts can survive and replicate within macrophages, ultimately leading to host-cell lysis, PMNs and DCs have fungistatic and fungicidal activity, respectively (Newman et al., 1993; Newman et al., 2000; Eissenberg et al., 1988; Newman et al., 1994; Strasser et al., 1999; Gildea et al., 2005).

Even though phagolysosomes from macrophages feature distinct microbicidal mechanisms, including acidic pH (ranging from 4.5 to 5.0), reactive oxygen species (ROS), nitric oxide (NO), and proteolytic enzymes, *H. capsulatum* is able to survive in this environment (Valdez et al., 2022; Eissenberg et al., 1988; Newman et al., 1994; Strasser et al., 1999; Eissenberg et al., 1993; Holbrook et al., 2013; Youseff et al., 2012). To detoxify ROS, *H. capsulatum* secretes catalase and superoxide dismutase that counteract the effects of hydrogen peroxide (H_2O_2) and superoxide ion ($O_2^{\bullet -}$), respectively. The catalases, CatB and CatP, and superoxide dismutase 3 (SOD3), protect *H. capsulatum* from killing by PMNs and macrophages (Holbrook et al., 2013). Furthermore, yeast mutants lacking SOD3 expression exhibit reduced infectivity in murine models of *H. capsulatum* infection (Holbrook et al., 2013; Youseff et al., 2012).

To escape from the acidic phagolysosome environment, *H. capsulatum* maintains the phagolysosome pH at 6.5 in murine macrophages (Eissenberg, et al., 1988; Eissenberg et al., 1993). At this pH, lysosomal hydrolases are inactivated, but transferrin remains functional, allowing the yeast to acquire iron, an essential nutrient for its survival, within the phagolysosome (Newman et al., 1994; Strasser et al., 1999; Gildea et al., 2005). *H. capsulatum* controls the pH within the phagolysosome of these macrophages by inhibiting the accumulation of the V-ATPase in the phagolysosome membrane, an ATP-dependent proton pump responsible for generating and maintaining phagolysosomal pH (Strasser et al., 1999). In human macrophages, phagosome acidification is not required to mediate fungistatic/fungicidal activity. However, yeasts can still survive and prevent the fusion between phagosomes and lysosomes (Gildea et al., 2005).

H. capsulatum-infected DCs also exhibited marked formation of phagolysosomes. However, unlike in macrophages, this process inhibits the intracellular growth of the yeast (Gildea et al., 2005). The killing of *H. capsulatum* within the phagolysosome of DCs has been associated with proteolytic enzymes belonging to the hydrolase class, whose activity is not dependent on acidification. Furthermore, ROS and NO production, which are critical for the microbicidal function of macrophages, appear to have little to no effect on fungal death by DCs, as inhibitors of $O_2\bullet^-$, H_2O_2, and NO production do not impair the ability of DCs to control the intracellular growth of *H. capsulatum* (Gildea et al., 2005).

DCs are inherently resistant to the virulence mechanisms employed by *H. capsulatum*. This is associated with the type of signaling pathway activated during the phagocytosis of *H. capsulatum*. It is hypothesized that the phagocytosis mediated by CR3 in macrophages is advantageous to the fungus because CR3 signaling alone, without cytokine costimuli and cooperation with other PRRs, such as dectin-1, does not promote ROS production (Ehlers, 2000). To effectively kill the invading fungus, macrophages require activation by IFN-γ produced by Th1 lymphocytes. IFN-γ stimulates increased NO production in macrophages and restricts the entry of iron and copper into the phagolysosome, which are essential for the growth of *H. capsulatum* in this environment (Nakamura et al., 1994; Lane et al., 1994; Cain and Deepe, 1998; Shen et al., 2018; Prado et al., 2020; Lane et al., 1991). GM-CSF also increases the fungicidal activity and ROS production of macrophages against *H. capsulatum* (Subramanian Vignesh et al., 2013; Deepe and Gibbons, 2000). Part of the fungicidal effect of GM-CSF occurs through zinc deprivation (Subramanian Vignesh et al., 2013). At low zinc concentrations, *H. capsulatum* is more sensitive to the effects of ROS, while at normal zinc concentrations the yeast is more resistant to ROS (Subramanian Vignesh et al., 2013). These findings suggest that nutrient deprivation within the *H. capsulatum*-containing phagosome may be a key mechanism by which macrophages activated during the adaptive immune response control fungal infection.

Adaptive immunity to *Histoplasma capsulatum*

The innate immune response may be insufficient to eliminate *H. capsulatum* infection, necessitating the activation of adaptive immunity to control and clear the infection. For example, *H. capsulatum* within the phagolysosome of macrophages may not be completely cleared by the adaptive response, leading to granuloma formation in the lungs. Granulomas isolate the fungus and protect surrounding healthy tissue from the inflammatory response. Inside the granulomas, yeasts may persist in a dormant state. If local immunity wanes, yeasts can resume replication and, ultimately, disseminate beyond the lungs, affecting other organs, such as the skin, bone marrow, CNS, gastrointestinal tract, and adrenal glands (Valdez et al., 2022; Heninger et al., 2006).

Most of the host response to histoplasmosis is primarily driven by cell-mediated immunity (CMI) (Valdez et al., 2022). The protective role of the humoral immune response, however, remains less clear. In the lungs of mice infected with *H. capsulatum*, an increased number of B cells appears in the first week after infection, and remains elevated until the end of the second week (Cain and Deepe, 1998). In an acute infection model of histoplasmosis, the absence of B cells does not alter the clearance of *H. capsulatum* in the lungs and spleen of infected mice (Allendoerfer, Boivin and Deepe, 1997). Nevertheless, in a reactivation model of histoplasmosis, induced by blocking $CD4^+$ and $CD8^+$ T cells in mice 6 weeks after infection, the absence of B cells reduced the survival of mice and fungal clearance in the lungs and spleen (Allendoerfer et al., 1997; Allen and Deepe, 2006). These findings suggest that B cells may contribute to long-term immune protection through antibody responses.

Increased levels of IgM and IgA antibodies are observed in the serum of patients with acute histoplasmosis within the first 2 weeks of symptoms, followed by IgG antibodies after the first month (Chandler et al., 1969; Nosanchuk et al., 2012). Additionally, the protective effect of passive immunization by monoclonal antibodies (mAbs) has been demonstrated (Nosanchuk et al., 2012). The use of mAbs to fungal cell surface antigens, such as histone-like protein and Hsp60, can trigger a protective immune response with reduced fungal burden and organ damage in murine experimental *H. capsulatum* infection (Nosanchuk et al., 2003; Guimarães et al., 2009). Protective mAbs increased phagocytosis of *H. capsulatum* by macrophages, and phagolysosomal fusion, and consequently intracellular fungal survival in vitro (Nosanchuk et al., 2003; Guimarães et al., 2009; Shi et al., 2008). Additionally, treatment of *H. capsulatum* with Hsp60-binding mAbs in vitro can modulate EV cargo and enzymatic activity of laccase and phosphatase, known virulence factors, in a mechanism that appears to participate in the protective immune response mediated by mAbs (Baltazar et al., 2016).

The protective role of T cells in histoplasmosis is well-established (Wüthrich et al., 2003; Allendoerfer et al., 1997; Allen and Deepe, 2006). DCs activate $CD4^+$ and $CD8^+$ T cell responses through direct antigen presentation and cross-presentation, respectively (Gildea et al., 2001; Lin et al., 2005). Depletion of $CD4^+$ T cells leads to the death of mice with a sublethal infection of *H. capsulatum* yeast, a phenotype not observed with the depletion of $CD8^+$ T cells (Allendoerfer et al., 1997). However, similar to B cells, $CD8^+$ T cells appear to be essential for long-term immune protection against histoplasmosis (Allen and Deepe, 2006). The protective immune response to *H. capsulatum* elicited by vaccination, when $CD4^+$ T cell support is lacking, is dependent on $CD8^+$ T cells (Wüthrich et al., 2003). Similarly, in a reactivation model of histoplasmosis, depletion of both $CD4^+$ and $CD8^+$ cells 6 weeks after infection exhibits increased fungal loads in the lungs and spleen (Allen and Deepe, 2006). For both $CD4^+$ and $CD8^+$ T cell responses, the protective effect is mediated by the secretion of cytokines IFN-γ and TNF-α, while the secretion of IL-10 exacerbates the infection (Wüthrich et al., 2003; Allendoerfer et al., 1997; Allen and Deepe, 2006).

Overall, the $CD4^+$ T cell responses that confer antifungal activity are Th1 and Th17, while the Th2 and regulatory T cells (Treg) responses exacerbate fungal infection (Valdez et al., 2022; Horwath et al., 2015). The development of these responses is stimulated by cytokines produced in response to microorganisms. The secretion of IL-12 by macrophages and DCs promotes the differentiation of Th1 cells, while the production of IL-6, IL-1β, TGF-β, and IL-23 promotes the differentiation of Th17 cells. The Th1 response is characterized by the secretion of inflammatory cytokines such as IFN-γ, TNF-α, and GM-CSF, and promotes the classical activation of macrophages, as mentioned previously (Kroetz and Deepe, 2012).

TNF-α is a multifunctional cytokine that is critically important in host defenses to *H. capsulatum* yeast (Allendoerfer and Deepe, 1998). A case study of three patients undergoing treatment with the TNF-α inhibitor infliximab showed a direct correlation between the absence of this cytokine and the reactivation of *H. capsulatum* (Wood et al., 2003). Infliximab reduced the human AM-induced proliferation of lymphocytes and the production of IFN-γ (Wood et al., 2003). TNF-α also regulates the population of Treg cells responsible for increased susceptibility to histoplasmosis. Treatment with anti-TNF-α induces the recruitment of intestinal DCs ($CD11b^+$ $CD103^+$) to the lungs during *H. capsulatum* infection, which induces a tolerogenic response of Treg cells through the secretion of retinoic acid (Tweedle and Deepe, 2018).

The protective role of the Th17 response in *H. capsulatum* yeast infection remains unclear (Wang et al., 2014; Deepe and Gibbons, 2009; Puerta-Arias et al., 2020). IL-23 induces the differentiation of naive $CD4^+$ T cells into Th17, which produce IL-17A, IL-17F, IL-6, and TNF-α in mice, but not IFN-γ and IL-4 (Korn et al., 2009). Levels of IL-23 and IL-17A peak during the first week in the lungs of mice infected with *H. capsulatum* (Deepe and Gibbons, 2009). Neutralization of IL-17A by antibodies reduces fungal clearance, decreases recruitment of inflammatory cells, and increases IL-10 production (antiinflammatory cytokine) (Deepe and Gibbons, 2009). Furthermore, neutralizing IL-17A, in the absence of IL-12 and TNF-α, increases mice susceptibility to *H. capsulatum* infection (Deepe and Gibbons, 2009). Mice immunized with inactivated *H. capsulatum* develop a protective Th1 and Th17 response after infection, characterized by the increased production of IFN-γ and IL-17A, respectively (Wang et al., 2014). The induction of this response by DCs has been associated with the stimulation of dectin-1 and dectin-2 (Wang et al., 2014).

The imbalance between Th1 and Th17 responses due to cytokines produced by Th2 cells compromises host defense. The cytokine IL-4 is a central mediator of the Th2 response and induces alternatively activated macrophages, a phenotype that facilitates *H. capsulatum* yeast infection (Kroetz and Deepe, 2012). This cytokine inhibits the production of NO and increases the release of IL-10 by macrophages (Fecher et al., 2016; Kroetz and Deepe, 2012). When infected with *H. capsulatum*, mice genetically deficient for IL-10 present better fungal clearance than wild-type mice, which can be reversed by blocking TNF-α, reinforcing the importance of this cytokine for the control of histoplasmosis (Deepe and Gibbons, 2003).

The dynamic relationship between *H. capsulatum* yeasts and major receptors from different phagocytes can be observed in Fig. 7.1.

Diagnosis and treatment

Current strategies for diagnosis

For fungal diseases in general, definitive diagnosis depends on either histopathological or culture confirmation, and a probable diagnosis is based on clinical presentations, predisposing conditions, and evidence of mycosis, such as the presence of antigens in the urine (antigenuria) (Azar and Hage, 2017; De Pauw et al., 2008). According to the European Confederation of Medical Mycology (ECMM), management of histoplasmosis and other endemic mycosis requires a thorough understanding of epidemiology, diagnostic methods, risk factors and overall disease development in different patient populations (Thompson et al., 2021), thus requiring an all-round approach, including epidemiological and laboratorial evidence of the disease (Azar and Hage, 2017; Valdez et al., 2022).

The gold standard is the isolation and culture of *H. capsulatum* from either fluids or tissue samples, followed by observation by microscopy. The ECMM guidelines state that all biopsied tissues should be submitted to either periodic acid-Schiff or Grocott-Gomori's methenamine silver staining. Unlike other medical important yeasts, such as *Candida sp.* and *Cryptococcus sp.*, *H. capsulatum* stains poorly with Gram stain, being rarely detected this way. The sensitivity of both histopathology- and culture-based diagnosis will highly depend on the immune status, fungal burden, and specimen chosen (Hage et al., 2011; Barros, Wheat and Hage, 2023).

Enzyme immunoassays (EIA) specific for *H. capsulatum* polysaccharide in both urine and serum, such as the Clarus *Histoplasma* GM Enzyme Immunoassay (Immunomycologics) and MiraVista *Histoplasma* Urine Antigen LFA (Miravista), have been FDA-approved and show excellent performance in multicenter studies (Azar and Hage, 2017; Barros et al., 2023; Martínez-Gamboa et al., 2021). Overall, studies show that the sensitivity of antigen testing is higher in samples from immunocompromised patients, and the performance varies depending on the severity of the disease (Hage et al., 2011; Barros, Wheat and Hage, 2023;

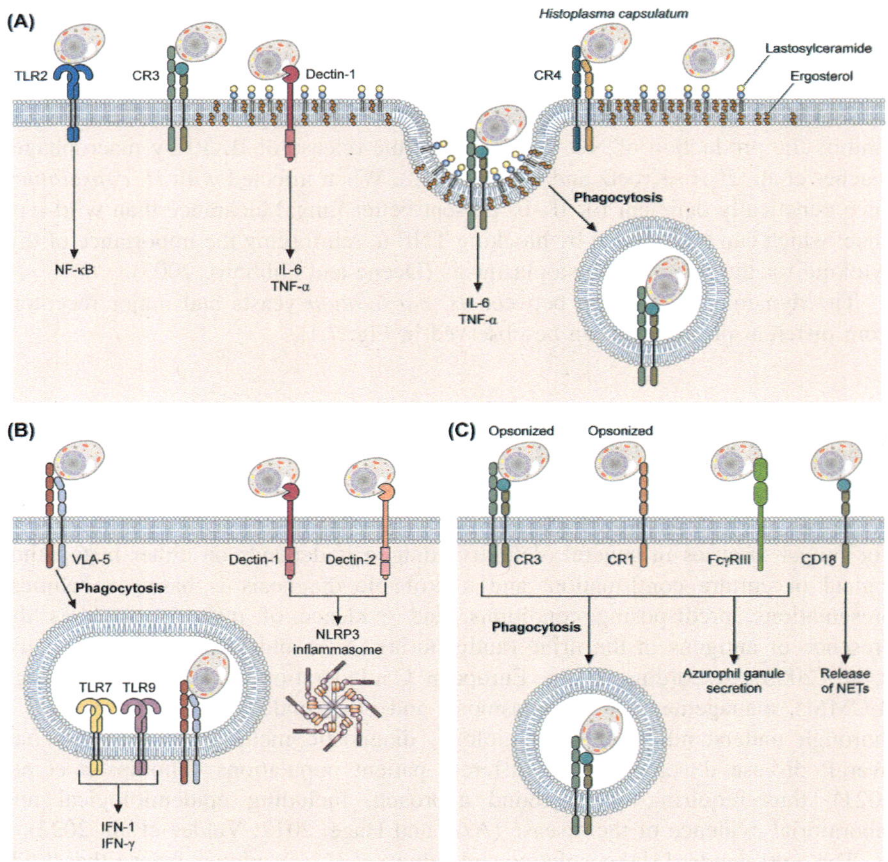

FIGURE 7.1 Major receptors involved with *Histoplasma capsulatum* recognition by phagocytes.

Association of *H. capsulatum* with phagocytes. (A) TLR2, CR3, CR4, dectin-1, and lactosylceramide participate in the recognition of yeasts of *H. capsulatum* by macrophages. TLR2 and dectin-1 are involved with the activation of NF-kB and production of cytokines IL-6 and TNF-α, respectively. During *H. capsulatum* adhesion and internalization, CR3 is recruited to lipid microdomains. (B) Dendritic cells interact with *H. capsulatum* using plasma membrane receptors very late antigen-5 (VLA-5), CR3, dectin-1, and dectin-2. VLA-5 is the main receptor involved in phagocytosis of *H. capsulatum* yeasts, CR3 is involved with fungal phagocytosis, and dectin-1 and dectin-2 with the activation of NLRP3 inflammasome. Intracellular receptors TLR7 and TLR9 are involved with the production of type I interferons (IFN-1). (C) In neutrophils, the major receptors for ic3b-opsonized *H. capsulatum* are CR1 and CR3, while nonopsonized yeasts are recognized by FcγRIII. Neutrophil extracellular trap (NET) release is dependent on CD18.

This figure is a reproduction from Valdez et al., 2022, originally published in Virulence volume 13, 2022, issue 1.

Martínez-Gamboa et al., 2021). Nonetheless, antigen detection in body fluids is considered one of the most sensitive and time-saving options to diagnose histoplasmosis (Azar and Hage, 2017). Although antigen detection can be performed with different specimen types (Bloch et al., 2018; Barros, Wheat, and Hage, 2023; Hage et al., 2010), combined detection in urine and serum appears to provide the best performance, even though there are some small differences between FDA-cleared tests (Azar and Hage, 2017; Torres-González et al., 2018; Theel et al., 2013; Fandiño-Devia et al., 2016; Buitrago and Martín-Gómez, 2020). Complete cross-reactivity occurs between histoplasmosis and blastomycosis, as the same galactomannan that has (1→6)-α-d-galactofuranosyl side chains is detected in both diseases (Buitrago and Martín-Gómez, 2020; Connolly et al., 2007). Additionally, low-level cross-reactivity with other invasive fungal pathogens such as *Coccidioides* spp., *Aspergillus* spp., *Paracoccidioides* spp., *Sporothrix schenckii,* and *Talaromyces marneffei* occurs, but this is generally differentiated when correlated with other clinical aspects in the setting of a low-positive *Histoplasma* antigen result to suggest an etiology other than histoplasmosis (Wheat et al., 1997; Hage et al., 2011; Kuberski et al., 2007; Assi, Lakkis, and Wheat, 2011; Ghorra et al., 2022; Hage et al., 2015). Notably, despite its shortcomings, histoplasma antigen testing is now included in the WHO Essential Diagnostics List (Toscanini et al., 2021).

Antibody testing can also be used for the diagnosis of histoplasmosis, but this approach is severely limited as certain immunocompromised patients do not produce detectable antibody levels, and the time required for antibody detection ranges from 4 to 8 weeks after infection (Wheat et al., 1982). Among the options, three methodologies are more commonly utilized: immunodiffusion (ID), complement fixation (CF), and immunoglobulin G and M EIA. ID can detect antibodies against antigens M and H: the M antigen is present in up to 80% of patients, but will remain positive for years, making it impossible to assess whether the patient has acute disease or if the detection is resulting from a prior resolved exposure. In contrast, the H antigen remains positive for approximately 6 months, indicating acute infection, but is present in only 25% of patients (Wheat et al., 1982; Wheat, 1992; Eichenberger et al., 2025). CF utilizes histoplasmin, a crude antigenic extract, and a fourfold increase in the antibody titer to histoplasmin obtained 2 weeks apart is diagnostic of acute infection, whereas a single titer of 32-fold or greater is suggestive of infection but not considered diagnostic (Kauffman, 2007; Richer et al., 2016). EIA-based antibody testing for IgG and IgM offers higher sensitivity than both CF and ID (Richer et al., 2016). In addition to the already mentioned shortcomings, false-positive serologies have been reported related to other fungi, such as *Blastomyces* and *Coccidioides*, but also in diseases manifesting with lymphadenopathy and pulmonary nodules, such as lymphoma, sarcoidosis, and tuberculosis (Kauffman, 2007; Eichenberger, et al., 2025). Nevertheless, combining antigen and antibody EIA testing provides an enhanced method for the diagnosis of acute pulmonary and CNS histoplasmosis (Bloch et al., 2018; Barros, Wheat, and Hage, 2023; Richer et al., 2016).

Molecular-based diagnosis is another option. Although polymerase chain reactions methods for identifying histoplasmosis have been described, none of them are FDA-approved for clinical specimens (Tang et al., 2006; Simon et al., 2010). However, antigen detection tests are often not available in nonendemic regions, making molecular techniques a valuable alternative for these cases (Buitrago and Martín-Gómez, 2020). Although data are limited on histoplasmosis, next-generation sequencing can assist with the diagnosis of a broad range of fungal infections. A notable example is the Karius test, which relies on the detection of cell-free DNA in blood specimens and is able to detect over 400 different fungi, including *Histoplasma* (Tsang et al., 2021; Chang et al., 2022).

Future perspectives for diagnosis

Several groups are advancing novel approaches for the diagnosis of histoplasmosis. Puerta-Arias et al. (2023) developed a novel in silico strategy to identify *H. capsulatum*-specific antigens that could be potential candidates for diagnostic methods. In short, using a computational analysis model that included the application of bioinformatic tools and the analysis of experimental data from transcriptomics and proteomics, the authors identified two antigens (*Hc670_Ag* and *Hc212_Ag*) and produced polyclonal antibodies (PAbs) against them. Although more validation and research are needed, the PAbs serve as proof of concept, as they were reactive against purified *H. capsulatum* antigens, culture extracts, and fluid samples from patients with histoplasmosis, showing the potential of the in silico method to identify targets not only for histoplasmosis but also for other difficult-to-diagnose fungal infections (Puerta-Arias et al., 2023). Additionally, Laboccetta et al. (2023) performed a comparative analysis of several novel antigen candidates. Among the antigens, the *H. capsulatum* 100 kDa protein (Hcp100) was the most promising candidate, with high sensitivity and specificity as well as the least cross-reactions. As highlighted by the authors, an anti-Hcp100 antibody detection ELISA would particularly benefit low-resourced countries where histoplasmosis is endemic due to its low estimated cost in comparison to currently available commercial kits (Laboccetta et al., 2023).

In a different approach, Rubio-Carrasquilla et al. (2019) developed an IFN-γ release assay (IGRA) to detect latent *H. capsulatum* infection in asymptomatic individuals, since latent infections may occur and currently there is no laboratory test capable of detecting subclinical or latent histoplasmosis. IGRA tests are based on the stimulation of the CMI by certain microorganisms, causing the development of memory T cells or a specific effector response. When restimulated in vitro with the same specific antigens, lymphocytes will release IFN-γ, which can be easily quantified with an immunoassay (Whitworth et al., 2013). Although IGRA has developed for a broad range of pathogens, the authors were the first to explore an IGRA test to detect *H. capsulatum* (Rubio-Carrasquilla et al., 2019). Using crude culture filtrates from both mycelium and yeast morphologies that contain a variety of common antigens, including glycoproteins M and H (Deepe and Durose, 1995), the authors were able to induce a highly specific IFN-γ response that allowed differentiation between most proven histoplasmosis cases and individuals not exposed to the fungus with high sensitivity and specificity, comparable to commercially available IGRAs for other diseases (Rubio-Carrasquilla et al., 2019). Additionally, the comparison of serological responses with IGRA showed that cellular immune memory to *H. capsulatum* lasts considerably longer than humoral memory, since serological responses tended to fade with time while the cellular immune response was detected in all patients with proven histoplasmosis, regardless of the time elapsed since the primary infection (Rubio-Carrasquilla et al., 2019). Similarly, Datta et al. (2022) developed another IGRA, the histoSPOT assay, an enzyme-linked immunospot assay that detects antigens from a yeast cell lysate. The assay performance is 78% sensitivity and 100% specificity for diagnosis in patients with active disease (Datta et al., 2022). However, the authors highlight some limitations, such as the use of a crude antigen extract, which can result in sensitivity and specificity differences across endemic areas, because different *H. capsulatum* strains have different glucan compositions and gene expression patterns (Datta et al., 2022). Taken together, IGRAs offer a powerful alternative for the diagnosis of histoplasmosis. Even though optimization of antigen preparation and studies comprising larger populations from multiple endemic areas are needed, the further development of IGRA assays will allow their use either as an auxiliary tool for diagnosis in combination with serology and confirmation by other methods or even as a stand-alone methodology.

Treatment—standard and novel tools

Standard treatment for histoplasmosis consists of itraconazole therapy for mild-to-moderate cases. For severe histoplasmosis or immunocompromised hosts, the disease is tackled with liposomal amphotericin B induction therapy, which is the therapy of choice over deoxycholate amphotericin B because of its improved safety, tolerance, and efficacy, especially in immunocompromised hosts (Saullo and Miller, 2022; Johnson et al., 2002). Individuals receiving itraconazole should have blood levels of the drug monitored to validate the drug dosing (Arnold et al., 2025). Prophylaxis for histoplasmosis with itraconazole is recommended only for people living with HIV with a low $CD4^{+}$ count (less than 150 cells/mm^3 (Kasuga et al., 2003)), but only in areas of hyperendemicity (Wheat et al., 2007).

Treatment duration is also highly variable and depends on the severity of illness and response to treatment. While mild-to-moderate histoplasmosis is generally treated for 6–12 weeks, 12 to over 18 months of treatment is recommended for cavitary disease. Patients with more severe disease often receive 1–2 weeks of liposomal amphotericin B, followed by a year of itraconazole therapy. Secondary prophylaxis may be necessary, especially in the setting of ongoing immunosuppression. Urine and blood antigen levels should be monitored to demonstrate a therapeutic response (Arnold et al., 2025). Notably, the decision process regarding treatment of pregnant women should include a balanced consideration of the potential benefits and harms, and, if treatment is necessary, azoles should be avoided in the first trimester in favor of amphotericin B (Arnold et al., 2025).

Tri-azoles such as voriconazole have been explored in a CNS histoplasmosis setting. Voriconazole has an enhanced CNS penetration when compared to itraconazole, making it suitable for the treatment of histoplasmosis at this site (Eichenberger et al., 2025). There are, however, conflicting reports on mortality rates of patients receiving voriconazole compared to itraconazole, with a retrospective study indicating significantly higher mortality associated with voriconazole (Freifeld et al., 2009) and a systematic review of CNS histoplasmosis indicating no difference between both therapies (de Oliveira et al., 2023). Posoconazole and isavuconazole have also been explored in limited settings, in in vitro studies and in reports of treatment of very few patients (Restrepo et al., 2007; Schwartz et al., 2021; Spec et al., 2018; Thompson et al., 2016).

Recently, a multicenter randomized comparative trial performed by Spec et al. (2024) compared efficacy, safety, and pharmacokinetics of a novel antifungal agent, superbioavailability itraconazole (SUBA-itraconazole), against conventional itraconazole over several endemic fungal infections, such as histoplasmosis, blastomycosis, coccidioidomycosis, and sporotrichosis. The study concluded that SUBA-itraconazole is effective and performed with fewer adverse events than itraconazole, even at one-third of its dose, corroborating an overall better cost-effect relationship between efficacy and safety (Spec et al., 2024). The current recommended dosage of SUBA-itraconazole in adults by the Infectious Diseases Society of America is 130 mg three times a day for 3 days, then 130 mg twice a day for 6–12 weeks (Arnold et al., 2025). Off-label use may be considered for children (based on weight) who meet criteria for antifungal treatment (Arnold et al., 2025).

Concluding remarks

H. capsulatum is a complex pathogen that poses a serious threat to people globally, and there are a series of challenges posed by histoplasmosis that need to be tackled in order to mitigate the effects of this WHO high-priority threat. The information reviewed in this chapter discusses how the host immune response perceives and defends against *H. capsulatum* yeasts. Although the T cell response can activate an effective response to the fungus, yeasts employ diverse survival mechanisms within hosts. The production and release of potent virulence factors facilitate disease in immunocompetent and immunocompromised individuals. *H. capsulatum* tolerates different environments, and its ability to transition from a free-living environmental organism to an intracellular parasite in macrophages highlights its dynamic resilience. Notably, interactions of the fungus with environmental predators, such as amoebae that have similarities with host phagocytes, may have enabled this microbe's capacity to mask itself from the human immune response and enable progressive infection. Further identification and characterization of these multiple interactions between the pathogen and its surroundings, including soil predators and host immune components that facilitate intracellular growth, will be useful for the development of novel therapeutic strategies against histoplasmosis, as well as other fungal diseases. Conventional treatment for histoplasmosis, like many fungal diseases, faces a broad range of limitations and a general lack of investment in novel drug development, a scenario that needs to be improved. Similarly, diagnosis needs to be enhanced, particularly with a more cost-effective test for under-resourced nations, while maintaining the already existing high sensitivity and specificity of the existing lab tests. It is also important to note that global warming has accelerated the geographic expansion of the endemic areas of histoplasmosis, putting more people at risk for disease. Consequently, as with other critically important neglected mycoses, it is now, more than ever, necessary to raise efforts in research and awareness about histoplasmosis among physicians, clinical microbiologists, and the public in order to better prevent, diagnose, and treat the disease.

References

Adenis, A., Nacher, M., Hanf, M., Basurko, C., Dufour, J., Huber, F., et al., 2014. Tuberculosis and histoplasmosis among human immunodeficiency virus-infected patients: a comparative study. The American Journal of Tropical Medicine and Hygiene 90 (2), 216–223. Available at https://doi.org/10.4269/ajtmh.13-0084.

Ajello, L., 1968. Comparative morphology and immunology of members of the genus histoplasma. Mycoses 11 (7), 507–514. Available at https://doi.org/10.1111/j.1439-0507.1968.tb03370.x.

Albuquerque, P.C., Nakayasu, E.S., Rodrigues, M.L., Frases, S., Casadevall, A., Zancope-Oliveira, R.M., et al., 2008. Vesicular transport in *Histoplasma capsulatum*: an effective mechanism for trans-cell wall transfer of proteins and lipids in ascomycetes. Cellular Microbiology 10 (8), 1695–1710. Available at https://doi.org/10.1111/j.1462-5822.2008.01160.x.

Alcantara, C., Almeida, B.R., Barros, B.C.S.C., Orikaza, C.M., Toledo, M.S., Suzuki, E., 2020. *Histoplasma capsulatum* chemotypes I and II induce IL-8 secretion in lung epithelial cells in distinct manners. Medical Mycology 58 (8), 1169–1177. Available at https://doi.org/10.1093/mmy/myaa006.

Allendoerfer, R., Boivin, G.P., Deepe, G.S., 1997. Modulation of immune responses in murine pulmonary histoplasmosis. Journal of Infectious Diseases 175 (4), 905–914. Available at https://doi.org/10.1086/513989, http://jid.oxfordjournals.org/content/current.

Allendoerfer, R., Deepe, G.S., 1998. Blockade of endogenous TNF-α exacerbates primary and secondary pulmonary histoplasmosis by differential mechanisms. Journal of Immunology 160 (12), 6072–6082. Available at https://doi.org/10.4049/jimmunol.160.12.6072, http://www.jimmunol.org/.

Allen, H.L., Deepe, G.S., 2005. Apoptosis modulates protective immunity to the pathogenic fungus *Histoplasma capsulatum*. Journal of Clinical Investigation 115 (10), 2875–2885. Available at https://doi.org/10.1172/JCI25365.

Allen, H.L., Deepe, G.S., 2006. B cells and CD4-CD8- T cells are key regulators of the severity of reactivation histoplasmosis. Journal of Immunology 177 (3), 1763–1771. Available at https://doi.org/10.4049/jimmunol.177.3.1763, http://www.jimmunol.org/.

Almeida-Silva, F., de Melo Teixeira, M., Matute, D.R., de Faria Ferreira, M., Barker, B.M., Almeida-Paes, R., et al., 2021. Genomic diversity analysis reveals a strong population structure in *Histoplasma capsulatum* LAmA (*Histoplasma suramericanum*). Journal of Fungi 7 (10), 865. Available at https://doi.org/10.3390/jof7100865.

Antinori, S., Giacomelli, A., Corbellino, M., Torre, A., Schiuma, M., Casalini, G., et al., 2021. Histoplasmosis diagnosed in Europe and Israel: a case report and systematic review of the literature from 2005 to 2020. Journal of Fungi 7 (6), 481. Available at https://doi.org/10.3390/jof7060481.

Aravalli, R.N., Hu, S., Woods, J.P., Lokensgard, J.R., 2008. Histoplasma capsulatum yeast phase-specific protein Yps3p induces Toll-like receptor 2 signaling. Journal of neuroinflammation 5. Available at https://doi.org/10.1186/1742-2094-5-30.

Ardain, A., Marakalala, M.J., Leslie, A., 2020. Tissue-resident innate immunity in the lung. Immunology 159 (3), 245–256. Available at https://doi.org/10.1111/imm.13143, http://onlinelibrary.wiley.com/journal/10.1111/(ISSN)1365-2567.

Arnold, S.R., Spec, A., Baddley, J.W., Pappas, P., Lentz, R.J., Wolf, J., et al., 2025. 2025 Clinical practice guideline update by the infectious diseases society of america on histoplasmosis: treatment of asymptomatic histoplasma pulmonary nodules (*Histoplasmomas*) and mild or moderate acute pulmonary histoplasmosis in adults, children, and pregnant people. Clinical Infectious Diseases 81. Available at https://doi.org/10.1093/cid/ciaf256.

Ashbee, H.R., Evans, E.G.V., Ashbee, H.R., Evans, E.G.V., Viviani, M.A., Dupont, B., et al., 2008. Histoplasmosis in Europe: report on an epidemiological survey from the European confederation of medical mycology working group. Medical Mycology 46 (1), 57–65. Available at https://doi.org/10.1080/13693780701591481.

Assi, M., Lakkis, I.E., Wheat, L.J., 2011. Cross-reactivity in the Histoplasma antigen enzyme immunoassay caused by sporotrichosis. Clinical and Vaccine Immunology 18 (10), 1781–1782. Available at https://doi.org/10.1128/CVI.05017-11, http://cvi.asm.org/cgi/reprint/18/10/1781.

Azar, M.M., Hage, C.A., 2017. Laboratory diagnostics for histoplasmosis. Journal of Clinical Microbiology 55 (6), 1612–1620. Available at https://doi.org/10.1128/JCM.02430-16, http://jcm.asm.org/content/55/6/1612.full.pdf.

Azar, M.M., Loyd, J.L., Relich, R.F., Wheat, L.J., Hage, C.A., 2020. Current concepts in the epidemiology, diagnosis, and management of histoplasmosis syndromes. Seminars in respiratory and critical care medicine 41 (1), 13–30. Available at https://doi.org/10.1055/s-0039-1698429, http://www.thieme-connect.com/ejournals/toc/srccm.

Baltazar, L.M., Nakayasu, E.S., Sobreir, T.J.P., Choi, H., Casadevall, A., Nimrichter, L., et al., 2016. Antibody binding alters the characteristics and contents of extracellular vesicles released by *Histoplasma capsulatum*. mSphere 1 (2). Available at https://doi.org/10.1128/mSphere.00085-15, http://msphere.asm.org/content/msph/1/2/e00085-15.full.pdf.

Baltazar, L.M., Zamith-Miranda, D., Burnet, M.C., Choi, H., Nimrichter, L., Nakayasu, E.S., et al., 2018. Concentration-dependent protein loading of extracellular vesicles released by Histoplasma capsulatum after antibody treatment and its modulatory action upon macrophages. Scientific Reports 8 (1). Available at https://doi.org/10.1038/s41598-018-25665-5, www.nature.com/srep/index.html.

Barros, N., Wheat, J.L., Hage, C., 2023. Pulmonary histoplasmosis: a clinical update. Journal of Fungi. 9 (2). Available at https://doi.org/10.3390/jof9020236, www.mdpi.com/journal/jof.

Baughman, R.P., Kim, C.K., Vinegar, A., Hendricks, D.E., Schmidt, D.J., Bullock, W.E., 1986. The pathogenesis of experimental pulmonary histoplasmosis: correlative studies of histopathology, bronchoalveolar lavage, and respiratory function. American Review of Respiratory Disease 134 (4), 771–776.

Beardsley, J., 2024. Pathogens of importance in lung disease—implications of the WHO fungal priority pathogen list. Respirology 29 (1), 21–23. Available at https://doi.org/10.1111/resp.14623.

Bloch, K.C., Myint, T., Raymond-Guillen, L., Hage, C.A., Davis, T.E., Wright, P.W., et al., 2018. Improvement in diagnosis of histoplasma meningitis by combined testing for histoplasma antigen and immunoglobulin G and immunoglobulin M anti-histoplasma antibody in cerebrospinal fluid. Clinical Infectious Diseases 66 (1), 89–94. Available at https://doi.org/10.1093/cid/cix706, http://cid.oxfordjournals.org/content/by/year.

Brummer, Kurita, Yoshida, Nishimura, Miyaji, 1991. Killing of *Histoplasma capsulatum* by γ-interferon-activated human monocyte-derived macrophages: evidence for a superoxide anion-dependent mechanism. Journal of Medical Microbiology 35 (1), 29–34. Available at https://doi.org/10.1099/00222615-35-1-29.

Buitrago, M.J., Martín-Gómez, M.T., 2020. Timely diagnosis of histoplasmosis in non-endemic countries: a laboratory challenge. Frontiers in Microbiology 11. Available at https://doi.org/10.3389/fmicb.2020.00467, https://www.frontiersin.org/journals/microbiology#.

Bullock, W.E., Wright, S.D., 1987. Role of the adherence-promoting receptors, CR3, LFA-1, and p150,95, in binding of histoplasma capsulatum by human macrophages. Journal of Experimental Medicine 165 (1), 195–210. Available at https://doi.org/10.1084/jem.165.1.195.

Cain, J.A., Deepe, G.S., 1998. Evolution of the primary immune response to *Histoplasma capsulatum* in murine lung. Infection and Immunity 66 (4), 1473–1481. Available at https://doi.org/10.1128/iai.66.4.1473-1481.1998, http://iai.asm.org/content/by/year.

Calvopiña, M., Toro, M., Bastidas-Caldes, C., Vasco-Julio, D., Muñoz, G., 2023. A fatal case of disseminated histoplasmosis by *Histoplasma capsulatum* var. capsulatum misdiagnosed as visceral leishmaniasis—molecular diagnosis and identification. Pathogens 12 (9), 1112. Available at https://doi.org/10.3390/pathogens12091112.

Chandler, J.W., Smith, T.K., Newberry, W.M., Chin, T.D., Kirkpatrick, C.H., 1969. Immology of the mycoses. II. Characterization of the immunoglobulin and antibody responses in histoplasmosis. The Journal of Infectious Diseases 119 (3), 247–254.

Chang, T.-H., Huang, J.-H., Lin, H.-C., Chen, W.-Y., Lee, Y.-H., Hsu, L.-C., et al., 2017. Dectin-2 is a primary receptor for NLRP3 inflammasome activation in dendritic cell response to *Histoplasma capsulatum*. PLoS Pathogens 13 (7), e1006485. Available at https://doi.org/10.1371/journal.ppat.1006485.

Chang, B., Saleh, T., Wales, C., Kuklinski, L., Malla, P., Yang, S., et al., 2022. Case report: disseminated histoplasmosis in a renal transplant recipient from a non-endemic region. Frontiers in Pediatrics 10. Available at https://doi.org/10.3389/fped.2022.985475.

Coady, A., Sil, A., Deepe, G.S., 2015. MyD88-dependent signaling drives host survival and early cytokine production during *Histoplasma capsulatum* infection. Infection and Immunity 83 (4), 1265–1275. Available at https://doi.org/10.1128/iai.02619-14.

Cohen, N.R., Tatituri, R.V.V., Rivera, A., Watts, G.F.M., Kim, E.Y., Chiba, A., et al., 2011. Innate recognition of cell wall β-Glucans drives invariant natural killer T cell responses against fungi. Cell Host and Microbe 10 (5), 437–450. Available at https://doi.org/10.1016/j.chom.2011.09.011.

Colombo, A.L., Tobn, A., Restrepo, A., Queiroz-Telles, F., Nucci, M., 2011. Epidemiology of endemic systemic fungal infections in Latin America. Medical Mycology 49 (8), 785–798. Available at https://doi.org/10.3109/13693786.2011.577821.

Connolly, P.A., Durkin, M.M., LeMonte, A.M., Hackett, E.J., Wheat, L.J., 2007. Detection of Histoplasma antigen by a quantitative enzyme immunoassay. Clinical and Vaccine Immunology 14 (12), 1587–1591. Available at https://doi.org/10.1128/CVI.00071-07.

Cottle, L.E., Gkrania-Klotsas, E., Williams, H.J., Brindle, H.E., Carmichael, A.J., Fry, G., et al., 2013. A multinational outbreak of histoplasmosis following a biology field trip in the Ugandan rainforest. Journal of Travel Medicine 20 (2), 83–87. Available at https://doi.org/10.1111/jtm.12012.

Crameri, R., Blaser, K., 2002. Allergy and immunity to fungal infections and colonization. European Respiratory Journal 19 (1), 151–157. Available at https://doi.org/10.1183/09031936.02.00229102.

Datta, K., LaRue, R., Permpalung, N., Das, S., Zhang, S., Steinke, S.M., et al., 2022. Development of an interferon-gamma release assay (IGRA) to aid diagnosis of histoplasmosis. Journal of Clinical Microbiology 60 (10). Available at https://doi.org/10.1128/jcm.01128-22.

Deepe, G.S., Durose, G.G., 1995. Immunobiological activity of recombinant H antigen from Histoplasma capsulatum. Infection and Immunity 63 (8), 3151–3157. Available at https://doi.org/10.1128/iai.63.8.3151-3157.1995.

Deepe, G.S., Gibbons, R., 2000. Recombinant murine granulocyte-macrophage colony-stimulating factor modulates the course of pulmonary histoplasmosis in immunocompetent and immunodeficient mice. Antimicrobial Agents and Chemotherapy 44 (12), 3328–3336. Available at https://doi.org/10.1128/aac.44.12.3328-3336.2000.

Deepe, G.S., Gibbons, R.S., 2009. Interleukins 17 and 23 influence the host response to Histoplasma capsulatum. Journal of Infectious Diseases 200 (1), 142–151. Available at https://doi.org/10.1086/599333.

Deepe, G.S., Gibbons, R.S., 2003. Protective and memory immunity to *Histoplasma capsulatum* in the absence of IL-10. Journal of Immunology 171 (10), 5353–5362. Available at https://doi.org/10.4049/jimmunol.171.10.5353, http://www.jimmunol.org/.

Deepe Jr., G.S., Gibbons, R.S., Smulian, A.G., 2008. *Histoplasma capsulatum* manifests preferential invasion of phagocytic subpopulations in murine lungs. Journal of Leukocyte Biology 84 (3), 669–678. Available at https://doi.org/10.1189/jlb.0308154, http://www.jleukbio.org/cgi/reprint/84/3/669.

Denning, D.W., 2024. Global incidence and mortality of severe fungal disease. The Lancet Infectious Diseases 24 (7), e428. Available at https://doi.org/10.1016/S1473-3099(23)00692-8, https://www.sciencedirect.com/science/journal/14733099.

Denning, D.W., 2016. Minimizing fungal disease deaths will allow the UNAIDS target of reducing annual AIDS deaths below 500 000 by 2020 to be realized. Philosophical Transactions of the Royal Society B: Biological Sciences 371 (1709), 20150468. Available at https://doi.org/10.1098/rstb.2015.0468.

Drummond, R.A., Brown, G.D., 2011. The role of Dectin-1 in the host defence against fungal infections. Current Opinion in Microbiology 14 (4), 392–399. Available at https://doi.org/10.1016/j.mib.2011.07.001.

Ehlers, M.R.W., 2000. CR3: a general purpose adhesion-recognition receptor essential for innate immunity. Microbes and Infection 2 (3), 289–294. Available at https://doi.org/10.1016/s1286-4579(00)00299-9.

Eichenberger, E.M., Little, J.S., Baddley, J.W., 2025. Histoplasmosis. Infectious Disease Clinics of North America 39 (1), 145–161. Available at https://doi.org/10.1016/j.idc.2024.11.009, https://www.sciencedirect.com/science/journal/08915520.

Eissenberg, L.G., Goldman, W.E., Schlesinger, P.H., 1993. *Histoplasma capsulatum* modulates the acidification of phagolysosomes. Journal of Experimental Medicine 177 (6), 1605–1611. Available at rupress.org/jem.

Eissenberg, L.G., Moser, S.A., Goldman, W.E., 1997. Alterations to the cell wall of *Histoplasma capsulatum* yeasts during infection of macrophases or epithelial cells. Journal of Infectious Diseases 175 (6), 1538–1544. Available at https://doi.org/10.1086/516496, http://jid.oxfordjournals.org/content/current.

Eissenberg, L.G., Schlesinger, P.H., Goldman, W.E., 1988. Phagosome-lysosome fusion in P388D1 macrophages infected with histoplasma capsulatum. Journal of Leukocyte Biology 43 (6), 483–491. Available at https://doi.org/10.1002/jlb.43.6.483.

Elias, A., Saleh, K.A., Faranesh, N., Dalal, R., Geffen, Y., Fisher, Y., et al., 2018. Case report: histoplasmosis: first autochthonous case from Israel. The American Journal of Tropical Medicine and Hygiene 98 (1), 278–280. Available at https://doi.org/10.4269/ajtmh.17-0603.

Fandiño-Devia, E., Rodríguez-Echeverri, C., Cardona-Arias, J., Gonzalez, A., 2016. Antigen detection in the diagnosis of histoplasmosis: a meta-analysis of diagnostic performance. Mycopathologia 181 (3-4), 197–205. Available at https://doi.org/10.1007/s11046-015-9965-3.

Farina, Gnecchi, Michetti, Parma, Cavanna, Nasta, 2000. Imported and autochthonous histoplasmosis in Bergamo Province, Northern Italy. Scandinavian Journal of Infectious Diseases 32 (3), 271–274. Available at https://doi.org/10.1080/00365540050165901, http://www.tandf.co.uk/journals/titles/00365548.asp.

Fecher, R.A., Horwath, M.C., Friedrich, D., Rupp, J., Deepe, G.S., 2016. Inverse correlation between IL-10 and HIF-1a in macrophages infected with histoplasma capsulatum. Journal of Immunology 197 (2), 565–579. Available at https://doi.org/10.4049/jimmunol.1600342, http://www.jimmunol.org/content/197/2/565.full.pdf.

Fisher, M.C., Denning, D.W., 2023. The WHO fungal priority pathogens list as a game-changer. Nature Reviews. Microbiology 21 (4), 211–212. Available at https://doi.org/10.1038/s41579-023-00861-x, https://www.nature.com/nrmicro/.

Freifeld, A., Proia, L., Andes, D., Baddour, L.M., Blair, J., Spellberg, B., et al., 2009. Voriconazole use for endemic fungal infections. Antimicrobial Agents and Chemotherapy 53 (4), 1648–1651. Available at https://doi.org/10.1128/aac.01148-07.

Garfoot, A.L., Dearing, K.L., VanSchoiack, A.D., Wysocki, V.H., Rappleye, C.A., 2017. Eng1 and Exg8 are the major β-glucanases secreted by the fungal pathogen *Histoplasma capsulatum*. Journal of Biological Chemistry 292 (12), 4801–4810. Available at https://doi.org/10.1074/jbc.M116.762104, http://www.jbc.org/content/292/12/4801.full.pdf.

Garfoot, A.L., Shen, Q., Wüthrich, M., Klein, B.S., Rappleye, C.A., 2016. The eng1 β-glucanase enhances *Histoplasma* virulence by reducing β-glucan exposure. mBio 7 (2). Available at https://doi.org/10.1128/mBio.01388-15, http://mbio.asm.org/content/7/2/e01388-15.full.pdf.

Ghorra, N., Goushchi, A., Konopnicki, D., Libois, A., Lagrou, K., Wind, A.D., et al., 2022. Disseminated histoplasmosis diagnosed by cross-reactivity with the *Aspergillus galactomannan* antigen in an HIV-positive patient. Journal of Medical Mycology 32 (2), 101244. Available at https://doi.org/10.1016/j.mycmed.2022.101244.

Gildea, L.A., Ciraolo, G.M., Morris, R.E., Newman, S.L., 2005. Human dendritic cell activity against *Histoplasma capsulatum* is mediated via phagolysosomal fusion. Infection and Immunity 73 (10), 6803–6811. Available at https://doi.org/10.1128/IAI.73.10.6803-6811.2005.

Gildea, Morris, Newman, 2001. *Histoplasma capsulatum* yeasts are phagocytosed via very late antigen-5, killed, and processed for antigen presentation by human dendritic cells. Journal of Immunology 166 (2), 1049–1056. Available at https://doi.org/10.4049/jimmunol.166.2.1049.

Gomez, F.J., Pilcher-Roberts, R., Alborzi, A., Newman, S.L., 2008. *Histoplasma capsulatum* cyclophilin A mediates attachment to dendritic cell VLA-5. Journal of Immunology 181 (10), 7106–7114. Available at https://doi.org/10.4049/jimmunol.181.10.7106, http://www.jimmunol.org/cgi/reprint/181/10/7106.

Gringhuis, S.I., Kaptein, T.M., Remmerswaal, E.B.M., Drewniak, A., Wevers, B.A., Theelen, B., et al., 2022. Fungal sensing by dectin-1 directs the non-pathogenic polarization of TH17 cells through balanced type I IFN responses in human DCs. Nature Immunology 23 (12), 1735–1748. Available at https://doi.org/10.1038/s41590-022-01348-2, https://www.nature.com/ni.

Guimarães, A.J., Cerqueira, M.D.de, Nosanchuk, J.D., 2011. Surface architecture of *Histoplasma capsulatum*. Frontiers in Microbiology 2. Available at https://doi.org/10.3389/fmicb.2011.00225, http://www.frontiersin.org/Journal/DownloadFile.ashx?pdf=1&FileId=2130&articleId=15430&Version=1&ContentTypeId=21&FileName=fmicb-02-00225.pdf.

Guimarães, A.J., de Cerqueira, M.D., Zamith-Miranda, D., Lopez, P.H., Rodrigues, M.L., Pontes, B., et al., 2019. Host membrane glycosphingolipids and lipid microdomains facilitate *Histoplasma capsulatum* internalisation by macrophages. Cellular Microbiology 21 (3). Available at https://doi.org/10.1111/cmi.12976, http://onlinelibrary.wiley.com/journal/10.1111/(ISSN)1462-5822.

Guimarães, A.J., Frases, S., Gomez, F.J., Zancopé-Oliveira, R.M., Nosanchuk, J.D., 2009. Monoclonal antibodies to heat shock protein 60 alter the pathogenesis of *Histoplasma capsulatum*. Infection and Immunity 77 (4), 1357–1367. Available at https://doi.org/10.1128/iai.01443-08.

Guimarães, A.J., Nakayasu, E.S., Sobreira, T.J.P., Cordero, R.J.B., Nimrichter, L., Almeida, I.C., et al., 2011. *Histoplasma capsulatum* heat-shock 60 orchestrates the adaptation of the fungus to temperature stress. PLoS ONE 6 (2), e14660. Available at https://doi.org/10.1371/journal.pone.0014660.

Gumbo, T., Just-Nübling, G., Robertson, V., Latif, A.S., Borok, M.Z., Hohle, R., 2001. Clinicopathological features of cutaneous histoplasmosis in human immunodeficiency virus-infected patients in Zimbabwe. Transactions of the Royal Society of Tropical Medicine and Hygiene 95 (6), 635–636. Available at https://doi.org/10.1016/S0035-9203(01)90103-8.

Hage, C.A., Azar, M.M., Bahr, N., Loyd, J., Wheat, L.J., 2015. Histoplasmosis: up-to-date evidence-based approach to diagnosis and management. Seminars in respiratory and critical care medicine 36 (5), 729–745. Available at https://doi.org/10.1055/s-0035-1562899, http://www.thieme-connect.com/ejournals/toc/srccm.

Hage, C.A., Davis, T.E., Fuller, D., Egan, L., Witt, J.R., Wheat, L.J., et al., 2010. Diagnosis of histoplasmosis by antigen detection in BAL fluid. Chest 137 (3),

623–628. Available at https://doi.org/10.1378/chest.09-1702, http://chestjournal.chestpubs.org/content/137/3/623.full.pdf+html.

Hage, C.A., Ribes, J.A., Wengenack, N.L., Baddour, L.M., Assi, M., McKinsey, D.S., et al., 2011. A multicenter evaluation of tests for diagnosis of histoplasmosis. Clinical Infectious Diseases: An Official Publication of the Infectious Diseases Society of America 53 (5), 448–454. Available at https://doi.org/10.1093/cid/cir435.

Hellwing, C., Schoeniger, A., Roessler, C., Leimert, A., Schumann, J., 2018. Lipid raft localization of TLR2 and its co-receptors is independent of membrane lipid composition. PeerJ 6, e4212. Available at https://doi.org/10.7717/peerj.4212.

Heninger, E., Hogan, L.H., Karman, J., Macvilay, S., Hill, B., Woods, J.P., et al., 2006. Characterization of the *Histoplasma capsulatum* -induced granuloma. The Journal of Immunology 177 (5), 3303–3313. Available at https://doi.org/10.4049/jimmunol.177.5.3303.

Holbrook, E.D., Smolnycki, K.A., Youseff, B.H., Rappleye, C.A., 2013. Redundant catalases detoxify phagocyte reactive oxygen and facilitate *Histoplasma capsulatum* pathogenesis. Infection and Immunity 81 (7), 2334–2346. Available at https://doi.org/10.1128/IAI.00173-13, http://iai.asm.org/content/81/7/2334.full.pdf.

Honorato, L., Bonilla, J.J.A., Valdez, A.F., Frases, S., Araújo, G.R.de S., Sabino, A.L.R.do N., et al., 2024. Toll-like receptor 4 (TLR4) is the major pattern recognition receptor triggering the protective effect of a *Candida albicans* extracellular vesicle-based vaccine prototype in murine systemic candidiasis. mSphere 9 (8). Available at https://doi.org/10.1128/msphere.00467-24.

Honorato, L., de Araujo, J.F.D., Ellis, C.C., Piffer, A.C., Pereira, Y., Frases, S., et al., 2022. Extracellular vesicles regulate biofilm formation and yeast-to-hypha differentiation in *Candida albicans*. mBio 13 (3). Available at https://doi.org/10.1128/mbio.00301-22.

Horwath, M.C., Fecher, R.A., Deepe, G.S., 2015. *Histoplasma capsulatum*, lung infection and immunity. Future Microbiology 10 (6), 967–975. Available at https://doi.org/10.2217/fmb.15.25, http://www.futuremedicine.com/loi/fmb.

Hsieh, S.H., Lin, J.S., Huang, J.H., Wu, S.Y., Chu, C.L., Kung, J.T., et al., 2011. Immunization with apoptotic phagocytes containing *Histoplasma capsulatum* activates functional CD^{8+} T cells to protect against histoplasmosis. Infection and Immunity 79 (11), 4493–4502. Available at https://doi.org/10.1128/IAI.05350-11Taiwan, http://iai.asm.org/content/79/11/4493.full.pdf.

Huang, S., Deepe, G.S., 2022. Notch regulates *Histoplasma capsulatum* clearance in mouse lungs during innate and adaptive immune response phases in primary infection. Journal of Leukocyte Biology 112 (5), 1137–1154. Available at https://doi.org/10.1002/JLB.4A1221-743R, http://jlb.onlinelibrary.wiley.com/hub/journal/10.1002/(ISSN)1938-3673/.

Huang, J.-H., Lin, C.-Y., Wu, S.-Y., Chen, W.-Y., Chu, C.-L., Brown, G.D., et al., 2015. CR3 and Dectin-1 collaborate in macrophage cytokine response through association on lipid rafts and activation of Syk-JNK-AP-1 pathway. PLoS Pathogens 11 (7), e1004985. Available at https://doi.org/10.1371/journal.ppat.1004985.

Jofre, G.I., Singh, A., Mavengere, H., Sundar, G., D'Agostino, E., Chowdhary, A., et al., 2022. An Indian lineage of *Histoplasma* with strong signatures of differentiation and selection. Fungal Genetics and Biology 158, 103654. Available at https://doi.org/10.1016/j.fgb.2021.103654.

Johnson, P.C., Wheat, L.J., Cloud, G.A., Goldman, M., Lancaster, D., Bamberger, D.M., et al., 2002. Safety and efficacy of liposomal amphotericin B compared with conventional amphotericin B for induction therapy of histoplasmosis in patients with AIDS. Annals of Internal Medicine 137 (2), 105–109. Available at https://doi.org/10.7326/0003-4819-137-2-200207160-00008, http://annals.org/issues.aspx.

Kasuga, T., White, T.J., Koenig, G., Mcewen, J., Restrepo, A., Castañeda, E., et al., 2003. Phylogeography of the fungal pathogen *Histoplasma capsulatum*. Molecular Ecology 12 (12), 3383–3401. Available at https://doi.org/10.1046/j.1365-294x.2003.01995.x.

Kauffman, C.A., 2007. Histoplasmosis: a clinical and laboratory update. Clinical Microbiology Reviews 20 (1), 115–132. Available at https://doi.org/10.1128/CMR.00027-06.

Kawai, T., Ikegawa, M., Ori, D., Akira, S., 2024. Decoding toll-like receptors: recent insights and perspectives in innate immunity. Immunity 57 (4), 649–673. Available at https://doi.org/10.1016/j.immuni.2024.03.004.

Korn, T., Bettelli, E., Oukka, M., Kuchroo, V.K., 2009. IL-17 and Th17 cells. Annual Review of Immunology 27, 485–517. Available at https://doi.org/10.1146/annurev.immunol.021908.132710Germany, http://arjournals.annualreviews.org/doi/pdf/10.1146/annurev.immunol.021908.132710.

Kroetz, D.N., Deepe, G.S., 2012. The role of cytokines and chemokines in *Histoplasma capsulatum* infection. Cytokine 58 (1), 112–117. Available at https://doi.org/10.1016/j.cyto.2011.07.430.

Kuberski, T., Myers, R., Wheat, L.J., Durkin, M., Connolly, P., Kubak, B.M., et al., 2007. Diagnosis of coccidioidomycosis by antigen detection using cross-reaction with a *Histoplasma antigen*. Clinical Infectious Diseases: An Official Publication of the Infectious Diseases Society of America 44 (5). Available at https://doi.org/10.1086/511684.

Köhler, J.R., Casadevall, A., Perfect, J., 2014. The spectrum of fungi that infects humans. Cold Spring Harbor Perspectives in Medicine 5 (1). Available at https://doi.org/10.1101/cshperspect.a019273.

Köhler, J.R., Hube, B., Puccia, R., Casadevall, A., Perfect, J.R., 2017. Fungi that infect humans. Microbiology Spectrum 5 (3). Available at https://doi.org/10.1128/microbiolspec.FUNK-0014-2016, http://www.asmscience.org/docserver/fulltext/microbiolspec/5/3/FUNK-0014-2016.pdf?expires=1497002495&id=id&accname=45052&checksum=D5D7DC99D96F69B7DFC14A9ED3BDE168.

Laboccetta, C.R., Toscanini, M.A., Garrido, A.V., Posse, G.B., Capece, P., Valdez, R.M., et al., 2023. Evaluation of the *Histoplasma capsulatum* 100-kilodalton antigen dot blot for the rapid diagnosis of progressive histoplasmosis in HIV/AIDS patients. Diagnostic Microbiology and Infectious Disease 107 (4), 116060. Available at https://doi.org/10.1016/j.diagmicrobio.2023.116060.

Lane, T.E., Wu-Hsieh, B.A., Howard, D.H., 1991. Iron limitation and the gamma interferon-mediated antihistoplasma state of murine macrophages. Infection and Immunity 59 (7), 2274–2278. Available at https://doi.org/10.1128/iai.59.7.2274-2278.1991.

Lane, T.E., Wu-Hsieh, B.A., Howard, D.H., 1994. Antihistoplasma effect of activated mouse splenic macrophages involves production of reactive nitrogen intermediates. Infection and Immunity 62 (5), 1940–1945.

Limper, A.H., Knox, K.S., Sarosi, G.A., Ampel, N.M., Bennett, J.E., Catanzaro, A., et al., 2011. An official American Thoracic Society statement: treatment of fungal infections in adult pulmonary and critical care patients. American Journal of Respiratory and Critical Care Medicine 183 (1), 96–128. Available at https://doi.org/10.1164/rccm.2008-740STundefined, http://ajrccm.atsjournals.org/cgi/reprint/183/1/96.

Lin, S., Huang, J.H., Hung, L.Y., Wu, S.Y., Wu-Hsieh, B.A., 2010. Distinct roles of complement receptor 3, Dectin-1, and sialic acids in murine macrophage interaction with Histoplasma yeast. Journal of Leukocyte Biology 88 (1), 95–106. Available at https://doi.org/10.1189/jlb.1109717Taiwan, http://www.jleukbio.org/cgi/reprint/88/1/95.

Lin, J.S., Yang, C.W., Wang, D.W., Wu-Hsieh, B.A., 2005. Dendritic cells cross-present exogenous fungal antigens to stimulate a protective CD8 T cell response in infection by *Histoplasma capsulatum*. Journal of Immunology 174 (10), 6282–6291. Available at https://doi.org/10.4049/jimmunol.174.10.6282, http://www.jimmunol.org/.

Lofgren, S.M., Kirsch, E.J., Maro, V.P., Morrissey, A.B., Msuya, L.J., Kinabo, G.D., et al., 2012. Histoplasmosis among hospitalized febrile patients in northern Tanzania. Transactions of the Royal Society of Tropical Medicine and Hygiene 106 (8), 504–507. Available at https://doi.org/10.1016/j.trstmh.2012.05.009.

Long, K.H., Gomez, F.J., Morris, R.E., Newman, S.L., 2003. Identification of heat shock protein 60 as the ligand on *Histoplasma capsulatum* that mediates binding to CD18 receptors on human macrophages. Journal of Immunology 170 (1), 487–494. Available at https://doi.org/10.4049/jimmunol.170.1.487, http://www.jimmunol.org/.

Marshall, L.J., Perks, B., Ferkol, T., Shute, J.K., 2001. IL-8 released constitutively by primary bronchial epithelial cells in culture forms an inactive complex with secretory component. Journal of Immunology 167 (5), 2816–2823. Available at https://doi.org/10.4049/jimmunol.167.5.2816, http://www.jimmunol.org/.

Martínez-Gamboa, A., Niembro-Ortega, M.D., Torres-González, P., Santiago-Cruz, J., Velázquez-Zavala, N.G., Rangel-Cordero, A., et al., 2021. Diagnostic accuracy of antigen detection in urine and molecular assays testing in different clinical samples for the diagnosis of progressive disseminated histoplasmosis in patients living with HIV/AIDS: a prospective multicenter study in Mexico. PLoS neglected tropical diseases 15 (3), e0009215. Available at https://doi.org/10.1371/journal.pntd.0009215.

McCormack, F.X., Gibbons, R., Ward, S.R., Kuzmenko, A., Wu, H., Deepe, G.S., 2003. Macrophage-independent fungicidal action of the pulmonary collectins. Journal of Biological Chemistry 278 (38), 36250–36256. Available at https://doi.org/10.1074/jbc.M303086200.

McLeod, D.S.A., Mortimer, R.H., Perry-Keene, D.A., Allworth, A., Woods, M.L., Perry-Keene, J., et al., 2011. Histoplasmosis in Australia: report of 16 cases and literature review. Medicine 90 (1), 61–68. Available at https://doi.org/10.1097/MD.0b013e318206e499.

Morales-Nebreda, L., Misharin, A.V., Perlman, H., Budinger, G.R.S., 2015. The heterogeneity of lung macrophages in the susceptibility to disease. European Respiratory Review 24 (137), 505–509. Available at https://doi.org/10.1183/16000617.0031-2015.

Nacher, M., Adenis, A., Sambourg, E., Huber, F., Abboud, P., Epelboin, L., et al., 2014. Histoplasmosis or tuberculosis in HIV-infected patients in the Amazon: what should be treated first. PLoS neglected tropical diseases 8 (12), e3290. Available at https://doi.org/10.1371/journal.pntd.0003290.

Nakamura, L.T., Wu-Hsieh, B.A., Howard, D.H., 1994. Recombinant murine gamma interferon stimulates macrophages of the RAW cell line to inhibit intracellular growth of *Histoplasma capsulatum*. Infection and Immunity 62 (2), 680–684.

Nett, J.E., Andes, D.R., 2016. Antifungal agents: spectrum of activity, pharmacology, and clinical indications. Infectious Disease Clinics of North America 30 (1), 51–83. Available at https://doi.org/10.1016/j.idc.2015.10.012, http://www.elsevier.com/inca/publications/store/6/2/3/3/0/2/index.htt.

Newman, S.L., Bucher, C., Rhodes, J., Bullock, W.E., 1990. Phagocytosis of *Histoplasma capsulatum* yeasts and microconidia by human cultured macrophages and alveolar macrophages. Cellular cytoskeleton requirement for attachment and ingestion. Journal of Clinical Investigation 85 (1), 223–230. Available at https://doi.org/10.1172/JCI114416.

Newman, S.L., Gootee, L., Brunner, G., Deepe, G.S., 1994. Chloroquine induces human macrophage killing of *Histoplasma capsulatum* by limiting the availability of intracellular iron and is therapeutic in a murine model of histoplasmosis. Journal of Clinical Investigation 93 (4), 1422–1429. Available at https://doi.org/10.1172/JCI117119, http://www.jci.org.

Newman, S.L., Gootee, L., Gabay, J.E., Selsted, M.E., 2000. Identification of constituents of human neutrophil azurophil granules that mediate fungistasis against *Histoplasma capsulatum*. Infection and Immunity 68 (10), 5668–5672. Available at https://doi.org/10.1128/IAI.68.10.5668-5672.2000.

Newman, S.L., Gootee, L., Gabay, J.E., 1993. Human neutrophil-mediated fungistasis against *Histoplasma capsulatum*: localization of fungistatic activity to the azurophil granules. Journal of Clinical Investigation 92 (2), 624–631. Available at http://www.jci.org.

Newman, S.L., Gootee, L., Hilty, J., Morris, R.E., 2006. Human macrophages do not require phagosome acidification to mediate fungistatic/fungicidal activity against *Histoplasma* capsulation. Journal of Immunology 176 (3), 1806–1813. Available at https://doi.org/10.4049/jimmunol.176.3.1806, http://www.jimmunol.org/.

Nosanchuk, J.D., Steenbergen, J.N., Shi, L., Deepe, G.S., Casadevall, A., 2003. Antibodies to a cell surface histone-like protein protect against *Histoplasma capsulatum*. Journal of Clinical Investigation 112 (8), 1164–1175. Available at https://doi.org/10.1172/JCI19361, http://www.jci.org.

Nosanchuk, J.D., Zancopé-Oliveira, R.M., Hamilton, A.J., Guimarães, A.J., 2012. Antibody therapy for histoplasmosis. Frontiers in Microbiology 3. Available at https://doi.org/10.3389/fmicb.2012.00021, http://www.frontiersin.org/Journal/DownloadFile.ashxpdf=1&FileId=3251&articleId=19022&Version=1&ContentTypeId=21&FileName=fmicb-03-00021.pdf.

de Oliveira, V.F., Kruschewsky, W.L.L., Sekiguchi, W.K., Costa, S.F., Levin, A.S., Magri, M.M.C., et al., 2023. Clinical, radiological and laboratory characteristics of central nervous system histoplasmosis: a systematic review of a severe disease. Mycoses 66 (8), 659–670. Available at https://doi.org/10.1111/myc.13600, http://onlinelibrary.wiley.com/journal/10.1111/(ISSN)1439-0507.

Pan, B., Chen, M., Pan, W., Liao, W., 2013. Histoplasmosis: a new endemic fungal infection in China? Review and analysis of cases. Mycoses 56 (3), 212–221. Available at https://doi.org/10.1111/myc.12029.

De Pauw, B., Walsh, T.J., Donnelly, J.P., Stevens, D.A., Edwards, J.E., Calandra, T., et al., 2008. Revised definitions of invasive fungal disease from the European Organization for Research and Treatment of Cancer/Invasive Fungal Infections Cooperative Group and the National Institute of Allergy and Infectious Diseases Mycoses Study Group (EORTC/MSG) Consensus Group. Clinical Infectious Diseases 46 (12), 1813–1821. Available at https://doi.org/10.1086/588660.

Piffer, A.C., Kuczera, D., Rodrigues, M.L., Nimrichter, L., 2021. The paradoxical and still obscure properties of fungal extracellular vesicles. Molecular Immunology 135, 137–146. Available at https://doi.org/10.1016/j.molimm.2021.04.009, www.elsevier.com/locate/molimm.

Pitangui, N.de S., Sardi, J.de C.O., Voltan, A.R., dos Santos, C.T., da Silva, J.de F., da Silva, R.A.M., et al., 2016. An intracellular arrangement of *Histoplasma capsulatum* yeast-aggregates generates nuclear damage to the cultured murine alveolar macrophages. Frontiers in Microbiology 6. Available at https://doi.org/10.3389/fmicb.2015.01526.

Prado, M.K.B., Fontanari, C., Souza, C.O.S., Gardinassi, L.G., Zoccal, K.F., de Paula-Silva, F.W.G., et al., 2020. IL-22 promotes IFN-γ-mediated immunity against histoplasma capsulatum infection. Biomolecules 10 (6), 1–18. Available at https://doi.org/10.3390/biom10060865, https://www.mdpi.com/2218-273X/10/6/865/pdf.

Van Prooyen, N., Henderson, C.A., Hocking Murray, D., Sil, A., 2016. CD103+ conventional dendritic cells are critical for TLR7/9-dependent host defense against *Histoplasma capsulatum*, an endemic fungal pathogen of humans. PLoS pathogens 12 (7), e1005749. Available at https://doi.org/10.1371/journal.ppat.1005749.

Puerta-Arias, J.D., Mejía, S.P., González, A., 2020. The role of the interleukin-17 axis and neutrophils in the pathogenesis of endemic and systemic mycoses. Frontiers in Cellular and Infection Microbiology 10. Available at https://doi.org/10.3389/fcimb.2020.595301, http://www.frontiersin.org/Cellular_and_Infection_Microbiology/archive.

Puerta-Arias, J.D., Pablo, J., Agudelo, I., Williams Naranjo Preciado, T., Joshua, J., 2023. Obar, Identification and production of novel potential pathogen-specific biomarkers for diagnosis of histoplasmosis. Microbiology Spectrum 11 (6). Available at https://doi.org/10.1128/spectrum.00939-23.

Rappleye, C.A., Eissenberg, L.G., Goldman, W.E., 2007. *Histoplasma capsulatum* α-(1,3)-glucan blocks innate immune recognition by the β-glucan receptor. Proceedings of the National Academy of Sciences of the United States of America 104 (4), 1366–1370. Available at https://doi.org/10.1073/pnas.0609848104.

Rappleye, C.A., Engle, J.T., Goldman, W.E., 2004. RNA interference in *Histoplasma capsulatum* demonstrates a role for α-(1,3)-glucan in virulence. Molecular Microbiology 53 (1), 153–165. Available at https://doi.org/10.1111/j.1365-2958.2004.04131.x.

Restrepo, A., Tobón, A., Clark, B., Graham, D.R., Corcoran, G., Bradsher, R.W., et al., 2007. Salvage treatment of histoplasmosis with posaconazole. Journal of Infection 54 (4), 319–327. Available at https://doi.org/10.1016/j.jinf.2006.05.006.

Richer, S.M., Smedema, M.L., Durkin, M.M., Herman, K.M., Hage, C.A., Fuller, D., et al., 2016. Improved diagnosis of acute pulmonary histoplasmosis by combining antigen and antibody detection. Clinical Infectious Diseases 62 (7), 896–902. Available at https://doi.org/10.1093/cid/ciw007, http://cid.oxfordjournals.org/content/by/year.

Rubio-Carrasquilla, M., Santa, C.D., Rendón, J.P., Botero-Garcés, J., Guimarães, A.J., Moreno, E., et al., 2019. An interferon gamma release assay specific for *Histoplasma capsulatum* to detect asymptomatic infected individuals: a proof of concept study. Medical Mycology 57 (6), 724–732. Available at https://doi.org/10.1093/mmy/myy131.

Saullo, J.L., Miller, R.A., 2022. Updates on histoplasmosis in solid organ transplantation. Current Fungal Infection Reports 16 (4), 165–178. Available at https://doi.org/10.1007/s12281-022-00441-1, https://www.springer.com/journal/12281.

Schwartz, S., Cornely, O.A., Hamed, K., Marty, F.M., Maertens, J., Rahav, G., et al., 2021. Isavuconazole for the treatment of patients with invasive fungal diseases involving the central nervous system. Medical Mycology 58 (4), 417–424. Available at https://doi.org/10.1093/mmy/myz103.

Seidel, D., Wurster, S., Jenks, J.D., Sati, H., Gangneux, J.-P., Egger, M., et al., 2024. Impact of climate change and natural disasters on fungal infections. The Lancet Microbe 5 (6), e594. Available at https://doi.org/10.1016/s2666-5247(24)00039-9.

Sepúlveda, V.E., Márquez, R., Turissini, D.A., Goldman, W.E., Matute, D.R., 2017. Genome sequences reveal cryptic speciation in the human pathogen *Histoplasma capsulatum*. mBio 8 (6). Available at https://doi.org/10.1128/mBio.01339-17, http://mbio.asm.org/content/8/6/e01339-17.full.pdf.

Sepúlveda, V.E., Williams, C.L., Goldman, W.E., 2014. Comparison of phylogenetically distinct *Histoplasma* strains reveals evolutionarily divergent virulence strategies. mBio 5 (4). Available at https://doi.org/10.1128/mBio.01376-14, http://mbio.asm.org/content/5/4/e01376-14.full.pdf+html.

Shen, Q., Beucler, M.J., Ray, S.C., Rappleye, C.A., 2018. Macrophage activation by IFN-γ triggers restriction of phagosomal copper from intracellular pathogens. PLoS pathogens 14 (11). Available at https://doi.org/10.1371/journal.ppat.1007444, https://journals.plos.org/plospathogens/.

Shi, L., Albuquerque, P.C., Lazar-Molnar, E., Wang, X., Santambrogio, L., Gácser, A., et al., 2008. A monoclonal antibody to *Histoplasma capsulatum* alters the intracellular fate of the fungus in murine macrophages. Eukaryotic Cell 7 (7), 1109–1117. Available at https://doi.org/10.1128/ec.00036-08.

Simon, S., Veron, V., Boukhari, R., Blanchet, D., Aznar, C., 2010. Detection of *Histoplasma capsulatum* DNA in human samples by real-time polymerase chain reaction. Diagnostic Microbiology and Infectious Disease 66 (3), 268–273. Available at https://doi.org/10.1016/j.diagmicrobio.2009.10.010.

Sorgi, C.A., Secatto, A., Fontanari, C., Turato, W.M., Belangér, C., De Medeiros, A.I., et al., 2009. *Histoplasma capsulatu*m cell wall β-glucan induces lipid body formation through CD18, TLR2, and dectin-1 receptors: correlation with leukotriene B 4 generation and role in HIV-1 infection. Journal of Immunology 182 (7), 4025–4035. Available at https://doi.org/10.4049/jimmunol.0801795Brazil, http://www.jimmunol.org/cgi/reprint/182/7/4025.

Souza, T.N., Valdez, A.F., Rizzo, J., Zamith-Miranda, D., Guimarães, A.J., Nosanchuk, J.D., et al., 2021. Host cell membrane microdomains and fungal infection. Cellular Microbiology 23 (12). Available at https://doi.org/10.1111/cmi.13385, http://onlinelibrary.wiley.com/journal/10.1111/(ISSN)1462-5822.

Spec, A., Connolly, P., Montejano, R., Wheat, L.J., 2018. In vitro activity of isavuconazole against fluconazole-resistant isolates of *Histoplasma capsulatum*. Medical Mycology 56 (7), 834–837. Available at https://doi.org/10.1093/mmy/myx130, https://mmy.oxfordjournals.org/.

Spec, A., Thompson, G.R., Miceli, M.H., Hayes, J., Proia, L., McKinsey, D., et al., 2024. MSG-15: super-bioavailability itraconazole versus conventional itraconazole in the treatment of endemic mycoses - a multicenter, open-label, randomized comparative trial. Open Forum Infectious Diseases 11 (3). Available at https://doi.org/10.1093/ofid/ofae010.

Strasser, J.E., Newman, S.L., Ciraolo, G.M., Morris, R.E., Howell, M.L., Dean, G.E., 1999. Regulation of the macrophage vacuolar ATPase and phagosome-lysosome fusion by *Histoplasma capsulatum*. Journal of Immunology 162 (10), 6148–6154. Available at https://doi.org/10.4049/jimmunol.162.10.6148, http://www.jimmunol.org/.

Subramanian Vignesh, K., Landero Figueroa, J.A., Porollo, A., Caruso, J.A., Deepe, G.S., 2013. Granulocyte macrophage-colony stimulating factor induced Zn sequestration enhances macrophage superoxide and limits intracellular pathogen survival. Immunity 39 (4), 697–710.

Tang, Y.-W., Li, H., Durkin, M.M., Sefers, S.E., Meng, S., Connolly, P.A., et al., 2006. Urine polymerase chain reaction is not as sensitive as urine antigen for the diagnosis of disseminated histoplasmosis. Diagnostic Microbiology and Infectious Disease 54 (4), 283–287. Available at https://doi.org/10.1016/j.diagmicrobio.2005.10.008.

Theel, E.S., Jespersen, D.J., Harring, J., Mandrekar, J., Binnicker, M.J., 2013. Evaluation of an enzyme immunoassay for detection of *Histoplasma capsulatum* antigen from urine specimens. Journal of Clinical Microbiology 51 (11), 3555–3559. Available at https://doi.org/10.1128/JCM.01868-13, http://jcm.asm.org/content/51/11/3555.full.pdf+html.

Thompson-Souza, G.A., Santos, G.M.P., Silva, J.C., Muniz, V.S., Braga, Y.A.V., Figueiredo, R.T., et al., 2020. *Histoplasma capsulatum*-induced extracellular DNA trap release in human neutrophils. Cellular Microbiology 22 (7). Available at https://doi.org/10.1111/cmi.13195, http://onlinelibrary.wiley.com/journal/10.1111/(ISSN)1462-5822.

Thompson, G.R., Le, T., Chindamporn, A., Kauffman, C.A., Alastruey-Izquierdo, A., Ampel, N.M., et al., 2021. Global guideline for the diagnosis and management of the endemic mycoses: an initiative of the European Confederation of Medical Mycology in cooperation with the International Society for Human and Animal Mycology. The Lancet Infectious Diseases 21 (12), e364. Available at https://doi.org/10.1016/S1473-3099(21)00191-2, http://www.journals.elsevier.com/the-lancet-infectious-diseases.

Thompson, G.R., Rendon, A., Ribeiro Dos Santos, R., Queiroz-Telles, F., Ostrosky-Zeichner, L., Azie, N., et al., 2016. Isavuconazole treatment of cryptococcosis and dimorphic mycoses. Clinical Infectious Diseases 63 (3), 356–362. Available at https://doi.org/10.1093/cid/ciw305, http://cid.oxfordjournals.org/content/by/year.

Torres-González, P., Niembro-Ortega, M.D., Martínez-Gamboa, A., Ahumada-Topete, V.H., Andrade-Villanueva, J., Araujo-Meléndez, J., et al., 2018. Diagnostic accuracy cohort study and clinical value of the Histoplasma urine antigen (ALPHA Histoplasma EIA) for disseminated histoplasmosis among HIV infected patients: a multicenter study. PLoS neglected tropical diseases 12 (11), e0006872. Available at https://doi.org/10.1371/journal.pntd.0006872.

Toscanini, M.A., Nusblat, A.D., Cuestas, M.L., 2021. Diagnosis of histoplasmosis: current status and perspectives. Applied Microbiology and Biotechnology 105 (5), 1837–1859. Available at https://doi.org/10.1007/s00253-021-11170-9, http://link.springer.de/link/service/journals/00253/index.htm.

Tsang, C.C., Teng, J.L.L., Lau, S.K.P., Woo, P.C.Y., 2021. Rapid genomic diagnosis of fungal infections in the age of next-generation sequencing. Journal of Fungi 7 (8). Available at https://doi.org/10.3390/jof7080636, https://www.mdpi.com/2309-608X/7/8/636/pdf.

Tweedle, J.L., Deepe, G.S., 2018. Tumor necrosis factor alpha antagonism reveals a gut/ lung axis that amplifies regulatory T cells in a pulmonary fungal infection. Infection and Immunity 86 (6). Available at https://doi.org/10.1128/IAI.00109-18, http://iai.asm.org/content/86/6/e00109-18.full.pdf#page=1&view=FitH.

Valdez, A.F., de Souza, T.N., Bonilla, J.J.A., Zamith-Miranda, D., Piffer, A.C., Araujo, G.R.S., et al., 2023. Traversing the cell wall: the chitinolytic activity of *Histoplasma capsulatum* extracellular vesicles facilitates their release. Journal of Fungi 9 (11), 1052. Available at https://doi.org/10.3390/jof9111052.

Valdez, A.F., Miranda, D.Z., Guimarães, A.J., Nimrichter, L., Nosanchuk, J.D., 2022. Pathogenicity & virulence of *Histoplasma capsulatum* - a multifaceted organism adapted to intracellular environments. Virulence 13 (1), 1900–1919. Available at https://doi.org/10.1080/21505594.2022.2137987, http://www.tandfonline.com/loi/kvir20.

Valdez, A.F., Zamith-Miranda, D., Nimrichter, L., Nosanchuk, J.D., 2023. Micro- and nanoparticles as platforms for the treatment of fungal infections: present and future perspectives. Future microbiology 18 (15), 1007–1011. Available at https://doi.org/10.2217/fmb-2023-0079, http://www.futuremedicine.com/loi/fmb.

Vandendriessche, S., Cambier, S., Proost, P., Marques, P.E., 2021. Complement receptors and their role in leukocyte recruitment and phagocytosis. Frontiers in Cell and Developmental Biology 9. Available at https://doi.org/10.3389/fcell.2021.624025, https://www.frontiersin.org/journals/cell-and-developmental-biology#.

Voltan, A.R., Quindós, G., Alarcón, K.P.M., Fusco-Almeida, A.M., Mendes-Giannini, M.J.S., Chorilli, M., 2016. Fungal diseases: could nanostructured drug delivery systems be a novel paradigm for therapy? International journal of nanomedicine 11, 3715–3730. Available at https://doi.org/10.2147/IJN.S93105, https://www.dovepress.com/getfile.php?fileID=31770.

Wang, H., LeBert, V., Hung, C.Y., Galles, K., Saijo, S., Lin, X., et al., 2014. C-type lectin receptors differentially induce th17 cells and vaccine immunity to the endemic mycosis of north america. Journal of Immunology 192 (3), 1107–1119. Available at https://doi.org/10.4049/jimmunol.1302314.

Wheat, L.J., Azar, M.M., Bahr, N.C., Spec, A., Relich, R.F., Hage, C., 2016. Histoplasmosis. Infectious Disease Clinics of North America 30 (1), 207–227.

Wheat, L.J., Freifeld, A.G., Kleiman, M.B., Baddley, J.W., McKinsey, D.S., Loyd, J.E., et al., 2007. Clinical practice guidelines for the management of patients with histoplasmosis: 2007 update by the Infectious Diseases Society of America. Clinical Infectious Diseases 45 (7), 807–825. Available at https://doi.org/10.1086/521259.

Wheat, French, Kohler, Zimmerman, Smith, Norton, et al., 1982. The diagnostic laboratory tests for histoplasmosis. Analysis of experience in a large urban outbreak. Annals of Internal Medicine 97 (5), 680–685. Available at https://doi.org/10.7326/0003-4819-97-5-680.

Wheat, J., Wheat, Connolly, Kleiman, Supparatpinyo, Nelson, Bradsher, Restrepo, 1997. Cross-reactivity in *Histoplasma capsulatum* variety capsulatum antigen assays of urine samples from patients with endemic mycoses. Clinical Infectious Diseases 24 (6), 1169–1171. Available at https://doi.org/10.1086/513647.

Wheat, L.J., 1992. Histoplasmosis in indianapolis. Clinical Infectious Diseases: An Official Publication of the Infectious Diseases Society of America 14 (Suppl 1).

Wheeler, R.T., Fink, G.R., 2006. A drug-sensitive genetic network masks fungi from the immune system. PLoS Pathogens 2 (4), 328–339. Available at https://doi.org/10.1371/journal.ppat.0020035, http://pathogens.plosjournals.org/archive/1553-7374/2/4/pdf/10.1371_journal.ppat.0020035-L.pdf.

Whitsett, J.A., Alenghat, T., 2015. Respiratory epithelial cells orchestrate pulmonary innate immunity. Nature Immunology 16 (1), 27–35. Available at https://doi.org/10.1038/ni.3045, http://www.nature.com/ni.

Whitworth, H.S., Scott, M., Connell, D.W., Dongés, B., Lalvani, A., 2013. IGRAs - The gateway to T cell based TB diagnosis. Methods 61 (1), 52–62. Available at https://doi.org/10.1016/j.ymeth.2012.12.012.

WHO fungal priority pathogens list to guide research, development and public health action, 2025. Available at https://www.who.int/publications/i/item/9789240060241.

Wood, K.L., Hage, C.A., Knox, K.S., Kleiman, M.B., Sannuti, A., Day, R.B., et al., 2003. Histoplasmosis after treatment with anti-tumor necrosis factor-α therapy. American Journal of Respiratory and Critical Care Medicine 167 (9), 1279–1282. Available at https://doi.org/10.1164/rccm.200206-563OC.

Wüthrich, M., Filutowicz, H.I., Warner, T., Deepe Jr., G.S., Klein, B.S., 2003. Vaccine immunity to pathogenic fungi overcomes the requirement for CD4 help in exogenous antigen presentation to CD8+ T cells: implications for vaccine development in immune-deficient hosts. Journal of Experimental Medicine 197 (11), 1405–1416. Available at https://doi.org/10.1084/jem.20030109.

Youseff, B.H., Holbrook, E.D., Smolnycki, K.A., Rappleye, C.A., 2012. Extracellular superoxide dismutase protects Histoplasma yeast cells from host-derived oxidative stress. PLoS Pathogens 8 (5). Available at https://doi.org/10.1371/journal.ppat.1002713, http://www.plospathogens.org/article/fetchObjectAttachment.action?uri=info%3Adoi%2F10.1371%2Fjournal.ppat.1002713&representation=PDF.

Zhou, P., Freidag, B.L., Caldwell, C.C., Seder, R.A., 2001. Perforin is required for primary immunity to *Histoplasma capsulatum*. Journal of Immunology 166 (3), 1968–1974. Available at https://doi.org/10.4049/jimmunol.166.3.1968, http://www.jimmunol.org/.

Zhou, B., Lin, W., Long, Y., Yang, Y., Zhang, H., Wu, K., et al., 2022. Notch signaling pathway: architecture, disease, and therapeutics. Signal Transduction and Targeted Therapy 7 (1). Available at https://doi.org/10.1038/s41392-022-00934-y.

Zhou, P., Sieve, M.C., Bennett, J., Kwon-Chung, K.J., Tewari, R.P., Gazzinelli, R.T., et al., 1995. IL-12 prevents mortality in mice infected with *Histoplasma capsulatum* through induction of IFN-γ The Journal of Immunology 155 (2), 785–795. Available at https://doi.org/10.4049/jimmunol.155.2.785.

CHAPTER

Tumor necrosis factor-alpha antagonists and susceptibility to histoplasmosis

8

Bradford Leonard Crowther[1,2] and George Samuel Deepe[2]

[1]*Department of Molecular and Cellular Biosciences, University of Cincinnati College of Medicine, Cincinnati, OH, United States,*

[2]*Division of Infectious Diseases, Department of Internal Medicine, University of Cincinnati College of Medicine, Cincinnati, OH, United States*

Histoplasma capsulatum: pathogenesis and epidemiology

H. capsulatum is a thermally dimorphic fungal pathogen that exists as spores in soil containing bat or bird droppings. Once inhaled, these fungal elements convert to pathogenic intracellular yeasts in the mammalian lung. Human infection with *H. capsulatum* is the result of accidental inhalation of spores that become airborne upon disruption of the soil (Deepe Jr, 2020). Once inside the lungs, spores that are ingested by resident lung macrophages, but not dendritic cells (DCs), and transform into yeast cells (Newman et al., 2011). The change from ambient temperature to body temperature (37°C) triggers a series of genetic changes that transform spores into yeast cells (Gilmore et al., 2015; Sil, 2019; Webster and Sil, 2008). It is this morphotype that causes nearly all the manifestations associated with histoplasmosis. Yeast cells replicate principally within macrophages present in the lung and draining lymph nodes. Subsequently, they are transported within these phagocytes to remote tissues, including, but not limited to, secondary lymphoid organs, the spleen, and the liver. Fungal growth continues until activation of T-cell-mediated immunity terminates it.

H. capsulatum is found worldwide but is endemic to the Ohio and Mississippi River Valley regions in the United States and to many countries in South America (Ashraf et al., 2020). Exposures are common in the American Midwest and Southeast, with an incidence rate of up to 80% (Deepe Jr, 2020; Horwath et al., 2015). Once considered to be endemic only to the Midwestern and Southeastern United States, the epidemiology of this fungus has undergone a reassessment with the discovery of cases in areas previously considered to be nonendemic (Nett et al., 2015). The cause of this northern and westward march is likely multifactorial, but climate change is one of the key elements (Laux et al., 2023; van Rhijn and

Immunological Insights and Emerging Therapeutics in Medical Mycology. DOI: https://doi.org/10.1016/B978-0-443-23636-5.00001-0

Bromley, 2021). In addition to changes in the epidemiology, recent studies have uncovered a more complex genetic composition with the discovery of four cryptic species (Sepúlveda et al., 2017). This finding may have implications for disease severity in humans.

Overview of the immune response

Host immunity to *H. capsulatum* develops in two distinct phases: initially, the innate immune response, comprised of macrophages, DCs, and neutrophils (PMNs), deploys several fungistatic and fungicidal mechanisms in an attempt to contain invasion by this pathogen (Newman et al., 2011; Newman et al., 1993; Wu-Hsieh et al., 1998; Wu-Hsieh and Howard, 1987; Wu-Hsieh et al., 1992). Despite their vast armamentarium, the fungus continues to replicate, but only in macrophages. DCs kill yeast cells, and PMNs exert a fungistatic effect (Newman et al., 1993; Gildea et al., 2005). Subsequently, activation of adaptive immunity, particularly T-cell-mediated immunity, ensues; when this occurs, yeast cells are eliminated from tissues (Cain and Deepe, 1998). Although both $CD4^+$ and $CD8^+$ T cells are engaged, it is the former that is required for elimination of the fungus (Gomez et al., 1988; Allendoerfer et al., 1999). The pivotal role that $CD4^+$ T cells exert in host immunity is exemplified by the susceptibility of AIDS patients to disseminated histoplasmosis. The principal mechanism by which $CD4^+$ T cells halt fungal replication is by delivery of granulocyte-macrophage colony-stimulating factor (GM-CSF) and interferon-gamma (IFN-γ) to macrophages to promote their capacity to kill *H. capsulatum* (Deepe et al., 1999; Kroetz and Deepe, 2012). If just one element of immunity does not properly function, immunity to *H. capsulatum* will fail.

The lung is the portal of entry; therefore the first encounter that *Histoplasma* has with host immune cells is with lung macrophages. These cells recognize yeast cells through the integrin CD11/CD18 (CR3), which binds to the *H. capsulatum* ligand heat shock protein 60 (Long et al., 2003). β-Glucan is expressed on multiple isolates of this fungus and attaches to dectin-1. This cell surface molecule is dispensable for ingestion but is key in promoting proinflammatory cytokines by macrophages (Ray and Rappleye, 2019; Garfoot and Rappleye, 2016; Lin et al., 2010). Macrophages are a replicative niche for yeast cells but exhibit several mechanisms to inhibit intracellular growth of yeasts, including metal sequestration, nitric oxide generation, and lysosomal hydrolases. These traits require exposure to external cytokine stimulation (Seider et al., 2010; Winters et al., 2010; Subramanian Vignesh et al., 2013; Newman et al., 1992; Eissenberg et al., 1993; Nittler et al., 2005). Nitric oxide is one of the more controversial mediators of fungal killing. Although mouse macrophages generate this gas upon exposure to cytokines such as IFN-γ, it has been difficult to demonstrate that human macrophages manufacture this cytocidal gas (Newman and Gootee, 1992).

Two distinct resident macrophage populations exist in the lung: alveolar macrophages (AMs) and interstitial macrophages (IMs), and these are commonly differentiated by their transcriptome and expression of cell surface markers (Shi et al., 2021). AMs exist in the airway and thus are likely the first cells to contact the inhaled fungal elements (Malainou et al., 2023; Allard et al., 2018; Guth et al., 2009). IMs reside in the interstitium, and contact with yeast cells might follow that of AMs (Schyns et al., 2018). IMs and AMs perform complementary functions, with the major exception that the former bear major histocompatibility class II molecules and therefore may serve as a means to activate $CD4^+$ T cells.

DCs are another major phagocytic population in the lung that is crucial for immunity to *H. capsulatum*. Lung DCs are located in the epithelium, submucosa, and parenchyma (Mellman, 2013; Plantinga et al., 2010). In contrast to macrophages, yeast cells bind to the very late antigen-5 (VLA-5) molecule, a fibronectin receptor. The ligand for this interaction is cyclophilin A on the yeast surface (Gildea et al., 2005; Gomez et al., 2008; Thind et al., 2015). Once ingested, yeast cells are quickly eliminated intracellularly by massive phagolysosomal fusion. Since this event is not observed in macrophages, it raises the possibility that operating through the VLA-5 receptor pathway triggers a different trafficking pathway that culminates in the death of the fungus (Gildea et al., 2005).

Clinical manifestations of histoplasmosis

Symptoms of infection vary depending on the competency of the host immune response. Many cases manifest no signs or symptoms and require little to no treatment. A smaller proportion of patients with infection limited to the lung may exhibit a flu-like illness. Shortness of breath, chest pain, and dyspnea are observed in those with more extensive lung disease. There is a chronic cavitary form of the infection that was primarily observed in male smokers years ago (Goodwin et al., 1976). More recently, this manifestation has been observed in younger nonsmoking patients (Kennedy and Limper, 2007). In contrast, patients who are prescribed corticosteroids or tumor necrosis factor-alpha (TNF-α) inhibitors, or those with AIDS, the infection presents in the disseminated form with involvement of multiple organs, including the liver, spleen, bone marrow, adrenals, and central nervous system (Deepe Jr, 2020). Fever, malaise, and chills are common findings. Physical findings include lymphadenopathy, hepatosplenomegaly, weight loss, and rales in the lungs. This form of infection may be life-threatening if not promptly diagnosed and treated. There is a subacute form of disseminated histoplasmosis in which the course of infection is slower and not abrupt. Fever and weight loss are relatively common. Physical findings include hepatosplenomegaly and oral ulcerations that are frequently mistaken for oral malignancy.

Tumor necrosis factor-α as a functional unit of immunity

TNF-α is a member of the TNF superfamily of proteins with pleiotropic effects on numerous immune functions (Beutler and Cerami, 1989). TNF-α is generated in a soluble form by immune and nonimmune cells to induce the production of inflammatory molecules upon recognition by its receptors (van Loo and Bertrand, 2023; Kalliolias and Ivashkiv, 2016; Tracey and Cerami, 1994). TNF-α signals through two receptors, TNF receptor type 1 (TNFR1), a ubiquitous protein that triggers signaling cascades through the TNF receptor-associated death domain (TRADD), and TNF receptor type 2 (TNFR2), found primarily on B and T cells, that signals through the TNF receptor-associated factor (Vandenabeele et al., 1995; Locksley et al., 2001; Gough and Myles, 2020; Medler et al., 2022) (see Fig. 8.1). Though TNF-α is generated by cells in a soluble form, a transmembrane form exists and is converted to the soluble form once it is processed by the disintegrin metalloproteinase TNF-α-converting enzyme (Horiuchi et al., 2010; Ramana, 2010) (see Fig. 8.2). The cytokine becomes biologically active when it is properly folded into a homotrimeric structure (Hlodan and Pain, 1995).

Upon TNF-α recognition by its receptors, downstream receptor-mediated signaling stimulates a wide variety of functions. TRADD recruitment following

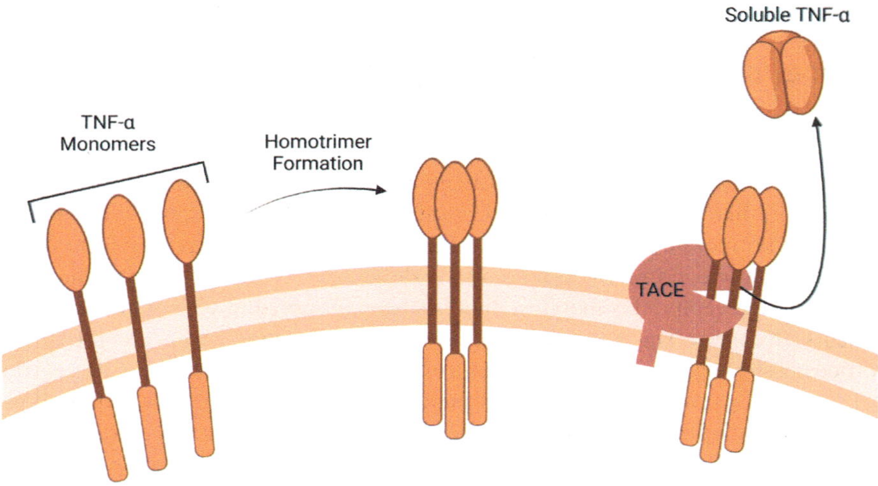

FIGURE 8.1 Tumor necrosis factor-alpha (TNF-α) homotrimers and soluble cytokine.

TNF-α is produced by multiple cell populations. The principal ones are phagocytes, including macrophages and dendritic cells. T cells also release this cytokine. Functional TNF-α is a homotrimer formed from three TNF-α monomers on the cell membrane. The transmembrane form of TNF-α is converted to a soluble form after cleavage by the TNF-α-converting enzyme and released to be recognized by TNF receptors.

Image created in BioRender.

cytokine recognition by TNFR1 leads to the formation of one of four unique signaling complexes (Jang et al., 2021; Wajant and Siegmund, 2019). Complex I stimulates NF-κB and mitogen-activated protein kinases (MAPKs) to promote inflammation, host defense, tissue degeneration, cell proliferation, or cell survival (Jang et al., 2021; Wajant and Siegmund, 2019). Complexes IIa and IIb activate caspase 8, which is responsible for apoptosis, and Complex IIc induces necroptosis and inflammation through mixed lineage kinase domain-like protein activation (Jang et al., 2021). Recognition by TNFR2 initiates formation of a complex containing TNF receptor-associated factor 1 (TRAF1), TNF receptor-associated factor 2 (TRAF2), cellular inhibitor of apoptosis cellular inhibitors of apoptosis 1 (cIAP1), and cIAP2 to stimulate NF-κB, MAPKs, and protein kinase B (AKT) to stimulate homeostatic activities such as cell proliferation, cell survival, and tissue regeneration (Jang et al., 2021). TNFR2 is activated by soluble and transmembrane TNF-α (Jang et al., 2021;Wajant and Siegmund, 2019). In this regard, transmembrane TNF-α acts as a receptor, binds antibodies to this cytokine, and generates reverse signaling. The consequence of reverse signaling can be stimulatory or inhibitory (Eissner et al.,et al., 2004).

Tumor necrosis factor-α antagonism: a double-edged sword

Unequivocally, TNF-α is one of the most vital components of host defenses to the fungal pathogen *H. capsulatum* (Vergidis et al., 2015; Lee et al., 2002; Wood et al., 2003; Allendoerfer and Deepe, 1998; Zhou et al., 1998). This cytokine regulates multiple functions of innate and adaptive immunity (Beutler and Cerami, 1989; Beyer et al., 2016; Brown et al., 2003; Chan et al., 2000; Mehrad et al., 1999; Roach et al., 2002; Sundquist and Wick, 2005), and interference with its activity produces an overly aggressive infection in animal models. Naive or immune mice given an anti-TNF-α fail to survive an otherwise sublethal infection (Wu-Hsieh et al., 1992; Allendoerfer and Deepe, 1998; Zhou et al., 1998; Smith et al., 1990). The lack of TNF-α in mice produces marked differences in several cytokines, including IFN-γ, interleukins (IL)-12, -4, -10, and GM-CSF, that are known to dampen or enhance immunity to *H. capsulatum*. Of particular interest is that blockade of TNF-α does not diminish but rather enhances the production of IFN-γ in the lungs of infected mice. This is perplexing since IFN-γ is necessary for protective immunity in both mice and humans (Wu-Hsieh and Howard, 1987; Zhou et al., 1998; Allendoerfer and Deepe, 1997; Merkhofer and Klein, 2020). This raises the hypothesis that the protective function of IFN-γ depends on the presence TNF-α.

Although TNF-α choreographs many facets of immunity, excessive generation of this cytokine may result in hyperinflammation that accompanies inflammatory diseases such as rheumatoid arthritis and Crohn's disease (Beutler and Cerami, 1989; Levin et al., 2016; Choy and Panayi, 2001). To mitigate the deleterious effects of this cytokine on inflammation, TNF-α antagonists are used to neutralize its biological activity. These biologics have emerged as major advances in the treatment of inflammatory disease. They dampen excessive inflammation and are considered disease-modifying drugs. However, neutralization of this cytokine is not without its consequences, as patients are at greater risk of contracting one or more infections (Crawford and Curtis, 2008; Ali et al., 2013). Several different TNF-α blockers are available today. Infliximab, adalimumab, and golimumab are

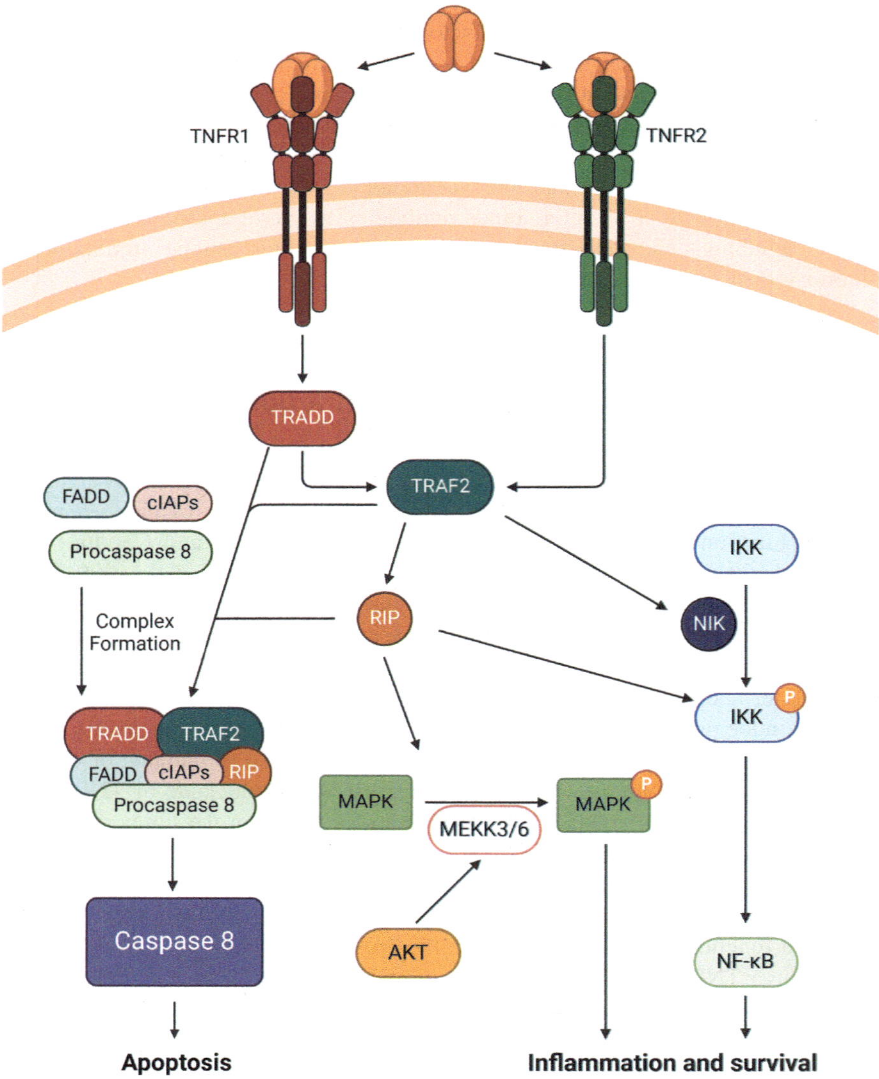

monoclonal antibodies that have affinity for soluble and transmembrane TNF-α to prevent recognition of the cytokine by its receptors at both available ligands (Tsiodras et al., 2008; Vena and Cassano, 2007; Guo et al., 2013). Etanercept is comprised of TNFR2 fused to the Fc portion of IgG1 and bind TNF-α to decrease interactions with its receptors (Hlodan and Pain, 1995; Tsiodras et al., 2008). Certolizumab contains only an anti-TNF-α Fab' fragment that is attached to polyethylene glycol that prolongs its half-life (Goel and Stephens, 2010). Each of the inhibitors mentioned possesses different half-lives, on-off activities, and binding affinities for TNF-α. There are no data to indicate if susceptibility to *H. capsulatum* varies by biologic agent. However, based on studies in patients with tuberculosis, disease develops sooner in recipients of infliximab compared to etanercept, but after two years, the risk is similar between the two pharmaceuticals (Wallis et al., 2005). We would predict similar outcomes in histoplasmosis.

The clinically prescribed TNF-α antagonists have emerged as a major risk factor for the development of life-threatening histoplasmosis (Vergidis et al., 2015; Lee et al., 2002; Smith and Kauffman, 2009; Hage et al., 2010). In this regard, the preclinical studies were prescient. An important consideration is whether these cases represent reactivation or reinfection. In one study, the development of infections, including histoplasmosis, occurred early after treatment initiation with infliximab (Wallis et al., 2004b). The authors interpreted these data to suggest that the TNF-α antagonists cause reactivation of latent infection. While reactivation does occur, the frequency is unknown (Limaye et al., 2000). Reinfection is an equally plausible mechanism, and there is support for this contention. It has long been recognized that recovery of yeast cells from tissues of remotely infected individuals has often been unsuccessful, thus suggesting the organisms, although

FIGURE 8.2 Tumor necrosis factor-alpha (TNF-α) recognition and signaling.

Soluble TNF-α is recognized by TNF receptor type 1 and TNF receptor type 2 to signal through TNF receptor-associated death domain (TRADD) after binding. Through this domain and interaction with TNF receptor-associated factor 2 (TRAF2), the signal leads to one of two outcomes: apoptosis or inflammation and survival. (1) In the apoptosis pathway, TRADD and TRAF2 form a complex with FAS-associated death domain, RIP death domain, and cellular inhibitors of apoptosis (cIAPs). Upon interface with procaspase 8, the endoprotease caspase 8 is activated to induce apoptosis. (2) Alternatively, TRADD, TRAF2, and RIP may initiate inflammatory and survival functions through NF-κB-inducing kinase, which phosphorylates inhibitory κB kinase to activate the transcription factor NF-κB and initiate the transcription and translation of anticaspase proteins associated with cell survival. Another survival pathway involves the TRADD–TRAF2–RIP complex signaling the phosphorylation of mitogen-activated protein kinase (MAPK) by mitogen-activated protein kinase kinase-3 (MEKK-3) and MEKK-6 from AKT to perform similar inflammatory and survival functions.

Image created in BioRender.

apparent on tissue stains, are not viable (Okudaira et al., 1961). This implies that much of the disease in those who receive TNF-α antagonists may represent reinfection rather than reactivation unless the acquisition of disease has been recent.

Risk assessment for developing histoplasmosis in patients on a tumor necrosis factor-α antagonist

One of the impediments to risk reduction in patients living in endemic areas for *H. capsulatum* is the lack of a screening test. In the case of tuberculosis, it is recommended that all patients who will be treated with a TNF-α antagonist be screened for exposure to *M. tuberculosis* either by the PPD skin test or the (IFN-γ) release assay. This approach works well with tuberculosis because of the low incidence in the United States and because well-established laboratory tests are available to identify those who have been infected. Such is not the case with histoplasmosis. In the endemic areas where the proportion of individuals has been infected, a screening test would not be valuable. Therefore the assumption should be that any patient from the endemic region who is about to be treated will be at risk for histoplasmosis. Recognition of signs and symptoms, should the patient become ill, is paramount. Laboratory studies to diagnose histoplasmosis must be initiated promptly and if positive, treatment must be begun as soon as possible.

What are the chances of developing disseminated histoplasmosis while on a TNF-α blocker? Early studies compared the risk in patients receiving infliximab and those receiving etanercept since these were the first two to enter the clinical arena. Patients receiving infliximab appeared to be at higher risk within the first 6 months of treatment (Wallis et al., 2005). The differences were speculated to be a consequence of the degree of inhibition of TNF-α activity between the two drugs (Wallis and Ehlers, 2005). Germane to this analysis, however, is an investigation of the development of tuberculosis during treatment with either of these drugs. In those who received infliximab, cases of tuberculosis were higher early after treatment, but by two years, the incidence was similar (Wallis et al., 2004a). The same may be true for histoplasmosis.

In a recent metaanalysis of 11 studies principally performed in North America, the calculated incidence of histoplasmosis was 33.5/100,000 patients treated with TNF-α inhibitors (Cipolat et al., 2023). This value is far higher than the centers for disease control and prevention estimate of 1.8 cases/100,000 individuals (Smith et al., 2022). Several concerns exist with these data, but the chief one is that reporting cases of histoplasmosis is not mandatory in all states. Thus the true number of cases is unknown. Nevertheless, the data clearly reveal an elevated risk among those receiving a TNF-α antagonist. Moreover, the risk is even higher in those who are administered monoclonal antibodies (~55/100,000) and those with inflammatory bowel disease as compared to rheumatoid disease (Cipolat et al., 2023).

A cohort study was conducted in Brazil in which 54 patients at risk of *H. capsulatum* infection were assessed for development of histoplasmosis using a urine antigen test before and after administration of TNF-α inhibitor therapy (Cipolat et al., 2024). After 6 months of follow-up, none of the 54 developed histoplasmosis. Among the 54 were eight who initially tested positive for urinary antigen. This leads to the conclusion that the positive initial urinary antigen was a false positive, as this small study was likely underpowered to arrive at any meaningful conclusions.

Mechanistic explanations for the effect of tumor necrosis factor-α antagonists

The factors that promote susceptibility to histoplasmosis in the absence of TNF-α are likely multifactorial and not solitary, given the impact of this cytokine on numerous immune and nonimmune cells. One explanation does have experimental evidence to support it and stems from a study conducted with infliximab in patients with rheumatoid arthritis. The efficacy of infliximab in these patients was directly correlated with increased regulatory T cell numbers and suppressive function (Ehrenstein et al., 2004). These T cells are crucial for tempering inflammation and altering pathology, but consequently, they may alter the protective function of inflammatory cells. Thus inflammation is dampened, but the ability of T cells to combat infections is impaired. This finding regarding regulatory T cells prompted our group to examine whether TNF-α neutralization promoted the emergence of this T cell subset in a mouse model of histoplasmosis. Indeed, neutralization of TNF-α increased the number of regulatory T cells in the lungs and their immunosuppressive function. Elimination of these cells restored protective immunity to mice. The suppressive effect of the regulatory T cells was reversed by administration of a monoclonal antibody to IL-10, which is known to inhibit activation of macrophages (Deepe and Gibbons, 2008; Moore et al., 2001). As mentioned earlier, another intriguing possibility is that TNF-α is required for the antifungal activity of IFN-γ on macrophages (see Fig. 8.3).

Management of patients with histoplasmosis

Any patient receiving a TNF-α antagonist who presents with a febrile illness, pneumonitis, or signs of a progressive infection should immediately be evaluated for histoplasmosis. Once diagnosed, treatment should also be prompt. Those who are critically ill should be administered amphotericin B since it is fungicidal and reduces the fungal burden more quickly than azoles. Subsequently, the patient can be switched to an azole. If the illness appears mild, azoles are reasonable to begin with, and the biologic should be discontinued. Duration of treatment should be 12

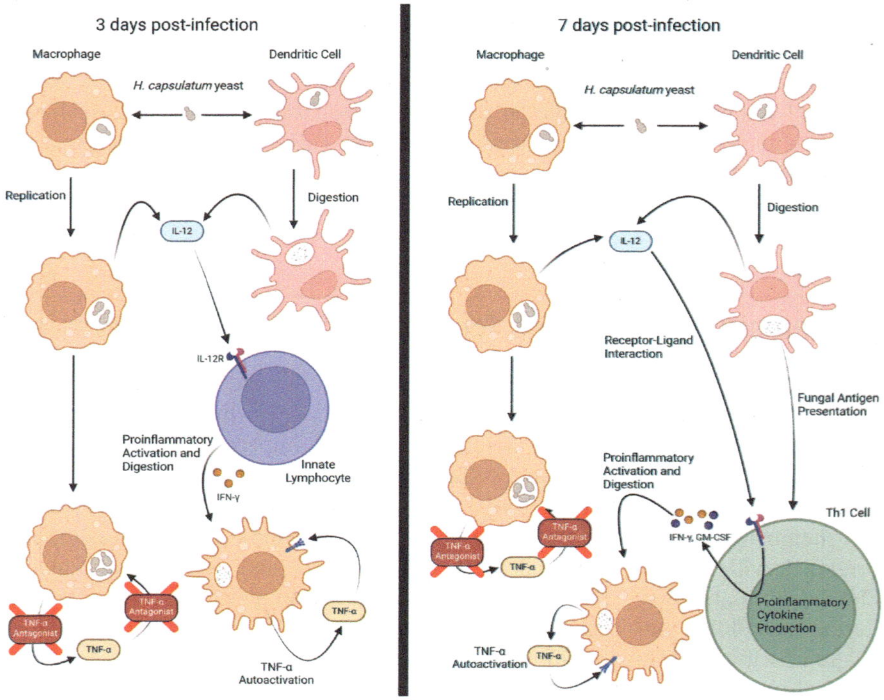

FIGURE 8.3 The intersection of tumor necrosis factor-alpha (TNF-α) and interferon-gamma (IFN-γ) on macrophage handling of *Histoplasma capsulatum*.

Human and mouse macrophages and dendritic cells (DCs) phagocytose *H. capsulatum* yeasts, but the yeasts undergo different fates. In DCs, the yeasts are killed, but in macrophages, they replicate inside phagosomes until the phagocyte has been activated by cytokines (Newman, 2005). We conjecture that before the onset of adaptive immunity in mice (<5 days postinfection), innate lymphoid cells produce IFN-γ in an IL-12-dependent manner to activate macrophages to kill *H. capsulatum* yeasts. This response requires the presence of TNF-α. At 7 days postinfection, infected macrophages and DCs produce IL-12 that enables differentiation of T cells into Th1 cells. These cells, in turn, release IFN-γ that promotes the antifungal activity of macrophages. When TNF-α is absent or blocked by a TNF-α antagonist, the impact of IFN-γ is blunted.

Image created in BioRender.

months, and if the patient remains symptom- and antigenuria-free during this time, it is safe to restart on TNF-α blockers (Vergidis et al., 2015). The risk of recurrence is low, but not zero. Some of that risk may be related to the environment they inhabit. The patient should be encouraged to avoid areas such as barns, renovated homes, and caves to avoid re-exposure.

Conclusion

TNF-α antagonism presents a plethora of challenges in histoplasmosis therapy. If a robust inflammatory response is required for control of *H. capsulatum* infection, it is not surprising that the absence of TNF-α might be deleterious to immunity. Clinicians need to be aware of the possibility of histoplasmosis in their patients, and they need to act quickly to diagnose and, if necessary, treat the infection. Once more is known about the mechanisms that drive susceptibility to histoplasmosis, host-directed therapies may be deployed to hasten resolution of infection.

References

Ali, T., Kaitha, S., Mahmood, S., Ftaisi, A., Stone, J., Bronze, M., 2013. Clinical use of anti-TNF therapy and increased risk of infections. Drug, Healthcare and Patient Safety 5, 79–99. Available at https://doi.org/10.2147/DHPS.S28801.

Allard, B., Panariti, A., Martin, J.G., 2018. Alveolar macrophages in the resolution of inflammation, tissue repair, and tolerance to infection. Frontiers in Immunology 9. Available at https://doi.org/10.3389/fimmu.2018.01777, https://www.frontiersin.org/journals/immunology#.

Allendoerfer, R., Deepe, G.S., 1997. Intrapulmonary response to *Histoplasma capsulatum* in gamma interferon knockout mice. Infection and Immunity 65 (7), 2564–2569. Available at https://doi.org/10.1128/iai.65.7.2564-2569.1997, http://iai.asm.org/content/by/year.

Allendoerfer, R., Deepe, G.S., 1998. Blockade of endogenous TNF-α exacerbates primary and secondary pulmonary histoplasmosis by differential mechanisms. Journal of Immunology 160 (12), 6072–6082.

Allendoerfer, R., Brunner, G.D., Deepe, G.S., 1999. Complex requirements for nascent and memory immunity in pulmonary histoplasmosis. Journal of Immunology 162 (12), 7389–7396.

Ashraf, N., Kubat, R.C., Poplin, V., Adenis, A.A., Denning, D.W., Wright, L., et al., 2020. Re-drawing the maps for endemic mycoses. Mycopathologia 185 (5), 843–865. Available at https://doi.org/10.1007/s11046-020-00431-2, https://rd.springer.com/journal/11046.

Beutler, B., Cerami, A., 1989. The biology of cachectin/TNF - A primary mediator of the host response. Annual Review of Immunology 7, 625–655. Available at https://doi.org/10.1146/annurev.iy.07.040189.003205.

Beyer, M., Abdullah, Z., Chemnitz, J.M., Maisel, D., Sander, J., Lehmann, C., et al., 2016. Tumor-necrosis factor impairs CD4+ T cell-mediated immunological control in chronic viral infection. Nature Immunology 17 (5), 593–603. Available at https://doi.org/10.1038/ni.3399, http://www.nature.com/ni.

Brown, G.R., Lee, E.L., Thiele, D.L., 2003. TNF enhances CD4+ T cell alloproliferation, IFN-γ responses, and intestinal graft-versus-host disease by IL-12-independent mechanisms. Journal of Immunology 170 (10), 5082–5088. Available at https://doi.org/10.4049/jimmunol.170.10.5082, http://www.jimmunol.org/.

Cain, J.A., Deepe, G.S., 1998. Evolution of the primary immune response to *Histoplasma capsulatum* in murine lung. Infection and Immunity 66 (4), 1473–1481. Available at https://doi.org/10.1128/iai.66.4.1473-1481.1998, http://iai.asm.org/content/by/year.

Chan, F.K.M., Siegel, R.M., Lenardo, M.J., 2000. Signaling by the TNF receptor superfamily and T cell homeostasis. Immunity 13 (4), 419–422. Available at https://doi.org/10.1016/S1074-7613(00)00041-8, http://www.immunity.com.

Choy, E.H.S., Panayi, G.S., 2001. Cytokine pathways and joint inflamation in rheumatoid arthritis. New England Journal of Medicine 344 (12), 907–916. Available at https://doi.org/10.1056/NEJM200103223441207.

Cipolat, M.M., Rodrigues, D.R.R., Brenol, C.V., Pasqualotto, A.C., Falci, D.R., 2023. Incidence of histoplasmosis in patients receiving TNF-alpha inhibitors A systematic review and meta-analysis. Medicine (United States) 102 (49), E36450. Available at https://doi.org/10.1097/MD.0000000000036450, https://journals.lww.com/md-journal/pages/default.aspx.

Cipolat, M.M., Rodrigues, D.R.R., Silveira, L.G., Silveira, I.G., Nothaft, M.S.V., Brenol, C.V., et al., 2024. Screening with urine Histoplasma antigen test in asymptomatic patients starting TNF-alpha inhibitor therapy: a cohort study. Therapeutic Advances in Infectious Disease 11. Available at https://doi.org/10.1177/20499361231222134, https://journals.sagepub.com/home/TAI.

Crawford, M., Curtis, J.R., 2008. Tumor necrosis factor inhibitors and infection complications. Current Rheumatology Reports 10 (5), 383–389. Available at https://doi.org/10.1007/s11926-008-0062-1.

Deepe, G.S., Gibbons, R.S., 2008. TNF-α antagonism generates a population of antigen-specific CD4 +CD25+ T cells that inhibit protective immunity in murine histoplasmosis. Journal of Immunology 180 (2), 1088–1097. Available at https://doi.org/10.4049/jimmunol.180.2.1088, http://www.jimmunol.org/cgi/reprint/180/2/1088.

Deepe, G.S., Gibbons, R., Woodward, E., 1999. Neutralization of endogenous granulocyte-macrophage colony-stimulating factor subverts the protective immune response to *Histoplasma capsulatum*. Journal of Immunology 163 (9), 4985–4993.

Deepe Jr, G.S., 2020. Principles and Practices of Infectious Diseases Histoplasma capsulatum. Elsevier, Philadelphia, pp. 3162–3176 2.

Ehrenstein, M.R., Evans, J.G., Singh, A., Moore, S., Warnes, G., Isenberg, D.A., et al., 2004. Compromised function of regulatory T cells in rheumatoid arthritis and reversal by anti-TNFα therapy. Journal of Experimental Medicine 200 (3), 277–285. Available at https://doi.org/10.1084/jem.20040165.

Eissenberg, L.G., Goldman, W.E., Schlesinger, P.H., 1993. *Histoplasma capsulatum* modulates the acidification of phagolysosomes. Journal of Experimental Medicine 177 (6), 1605–1611. Available at http://rupress.org/jem.

Eissner, G., Kolch, W., Scheurich, P., 2004. Ligands working as receptors: reverse signaling by members of the TNF superfamily enhance the plasticity of the immune system. Cytokine and Growth Factor Reviews 15 (5), 353–366. Available at https://doi.org/10.1016/j.cytogfr.2004.03.011.

Garfoot, A.L., Rappleye, C.A., 2016. *Histoplasma capsulatum* surmounts obstacles to intracellular pathogenesis. FEBS Journal 283 (4), 619–633. Available at https://doi.org/10.1111/febs.13389, http://onlinelibrary.wiley.com/journal/10.1111/(ISSN)1742-4658.

Gildea, L.A., Ciraolo, G.M., Morris, R.E., Newman, S.L., 2005. Human dendritic cell activity against *Histoplasma capsulatum* is mediated via phagolysosomal fusion. Infection and Immunity 73 (10), 6803–6811. Available at https://doi.org/10.4049/jimmunol.166.2.1049.

Gilmore, S.A., Voorhies, M., Gebhart, D., Sil, A., 2015. Genome-wide reprogramming of transcript architecture by temperature specifies the developmental states of the human pathogen histoplasma. PLoS Genetics 11 (7), e1005395. Available at https://doi.org/10.1371/journal.pgen.1005395.

Goel, N., Stephens, S., 2010. Certolizumab pegol. mAbs. 2 (2), 137–147. Available at https://doi.org/10.4161/mabs.2.2.11271, http://www.landesbioscience.com/journals/mabs/GoelMABS2-2.pdf.

Gomez, A.M., Bullock, W.E., Taylor, C.L., Deepe, G.S., 1988. Role of L3T4+ T cells in host defense against *Histoplasma capsulatum*. Infection and Immunity 56 (7), 1685–1691.

Gomez, F.J., Pilcher-Roberts, R., Alborzi, A., Newman, S.L., 2008. *Histoplasma capsulatum* cyclophilin A mediates attachment to dendritic cell VLA-5. Journal of Immunology 181 (10), 7106–7114. Available at https://doi.org/10.4049/jimmunol.181.10.7106, http://www.jimmunol.org/cgi/reprint/181/10/7106.

Goodwin, R.A., Owens, F.T., Snell, J.D., Hubbard, W.W., Buchanan, R.D., Terry, R.T., et al., 1976. Chronic pulmonary histoplasmosis. Medicine (United States) 55 (6), 413–452. Available at https://doi.org/10.1097/00005792-197611000-00001.

Gough, P., Myles, I.A., 2020. Tumor necrosis factor receptors: pleiotropic signaling complexes and their differential effects. Frontiers in Immunology 11. Available at https://doi.org/10.3389/fimmu.2020.585880, https://www.frontiersin.org/journals/immunology#.

Guo, Y., Lu, N., Bai, A., 2013. Clinical use and mechanisms of infliximab treatment on inflammatory bowel disease: a recent update. BioMed Research International 2013. Available at https://doi.org/10.1155/2013/581631.

Guth, A.M., Janssen, W.J., Bosio, C.M., Crouch, E.C., Henson, P.M., Dow, S.W., 2009. Lung environment determines unique phenotype of alveolar macrophages. American Journal of Physiology - Lung Cellular and Molecular Physiology 296 (6), L936. Available at https://doi.org/10.1152/ajplung.90625.2008, http://ajplung.physiology.org/cgi/reprint/296/6/L936.

Hage, C.A., Bowyer, S., Tarvin, S.E., Helper, D., Kleiman, M.B., Wheat, L.J., 2010. Recognition, diagnosis, and treatment of histoplasmosis complicating tumor necrosis factor blocker therapy. Clinical Infectious Diseases 50 (1), 85–92. Available at https://doi.org/10.1086/648724.

Hlodan, R., Pain, R.H., 1995. The folding and assembly pathway of tumour necrosis factor TNFα, a globular trimeric protein. European Journal of Biochemistry 231 (2), 381–387. Available at https://doi.org/10.1111/j.1432-1033.1995.tb20710.x.

Horiuchi, T., Mitoma, H., Harashima, S.I., Tsukamoto, H., Shimoda, T., 2010. Transmembrane TNF-α: structure, function and interaction with anti-TNF agents. Rheumatology 49 (7), 1215–1228. Available at https://doi.org/10.1093/rheumatology/keq031.

Horwath, M.C., Fecher, R.A., Deepe, G.S., 2015. *Histoplasma capsulatum*, lung infection and immunity. Future Microbiology 10 (6), 967–975. Available at https://doi.org/10.2217/fmb.15.25, http://www.futuremedicine.com/loi/fmb.

Jang, D.I., Lee, A.H., Shin, H.Y., Song, H.R., Park, J.H., Kang, T.B., et al., 2021. The role of tumor necrosis factor alpha (Tnf-α) in autoimmune disease and current tnf-α inhibitors in therapeutics. International Journal of Molecular Sciences 22 (5), 1–16. Available at https://doi.org/10.3390/ijms22052719, https://www.mdpi.com/1422-0067/22/5/2719/pdf.

Kalliolias, G.D., Ivashkiv, L.B., 2016. TNF biology, pathogenic mechanisms and emerging therapeutic strategies. Nature Reviews Rheumatology 12 (1), 49–62. Available at https://doi.org/10.1038/nrrheum.2015.169, http://www.nature.com/nrrheum/archive/index.html.

Kennedy, C.C., Limper, A.H., 2007. Redefining the clinical spectrum of chronic pulmonary histoplasmosis: a retrospective case series of 46 patients. Medicine 86 (4), 252–258. Available at https://doi.org/10.1097/MD.0b013e318144b1d9.

Kroetz, D.N., Deepe, G.S., 2012. The role of cytokines and chemokines in *Histoplasma capsulatum* infection. Cytokine 58 (1), 112–117. Available at https://doi.org/10.1016/j.cyto.2011.07.430.

Laux, K., Teixeira, M.de M., Barker, B., 2023. Love in the time of climate change: a review of sexual reproduction in the order Onygenales. Fungal Genetics and Biology 167, 103797. Available at https://doi.org/10.1016/j.fgb.2023.103797.

Lee, J.H., Slifman, N.R., Gershon, S.K., Edwards, E.T., Schwieterman, W.D., Siegel, J.N., et al., 2002. Life-threatening histoplasmosis complicating immunotherapy with tumor necrosis factor α antagonists infliximab and etanercept. Arthritis and Rheumatism 46 (10), 2565–2570. Available at https://doi.org/10.1002/art.10583.

Levin, A.D., Wildenberg, M.E., van den Brink, G.R., 2016. Mechanism of action of anti-TNF therapy in inflammatory bowel disease. Journal of Crohn's and Colitis 10 (8), 989–997. Available at https://doi.org/10.1093/ecco-jcc/jjw053, https://academic.oup.com/ecco-jcc/issue.

Limaye, A.P., Connolly, P.A., Sagar, M., Fritsche, T.R., Cookson, B.T., Wheat, L.J., et al., 2000. Transmission of *Histoplasma capsulatum* by organ transplantation. New England Journal of Medicine 343 (16), 1163–1166. Available at https://doi.org/10.1056/nejm200010193431605.

Lin, S., Huang, J.H., Hung, L.Y., Wu, S.Y., Wu-Hsieh, B.A., 2010. Distinct roles of complement receptor 3, Dectin-1, and sialic acids in murine macrophage interaction with Histoplasma yeast. Journal of Leukocyte Biology 88 (1), 95–106. Available at https://doi.org/10.1189/jlb.1109717Taiwan, http://www.jleukbio.org/cgi/reprint/88/1/95.

Locksley, R.M., Killeen, N., Lenardo, M.J., 2001. The TNF and TNF receptor superfamilies: integrating mammalian biology. Cell 104 (4), 487–501. Available at https://doi.org/10.1016/S0092-8674(01)00237-9, http://www.cell.com.

Long, K.H., Gomez, F.J., Morris, R.E., Newman, S.L., 2003. Identification of heat shock protein 60 as the ligand on *Histoplasma capsulatum* that mediates binding to CD18 receptors on human macrophages. Journal of Immunology 170 (1), 487–494. Available at https://doi.org/10.4049/jimmunol.170.1.487, http://www.jimmunol.org/.

Malainou, C., Abdin, S.M., Lachmann, N., Matt, U., Herold, S., 2023. Alveolar macrophages in tissue homeostasis, inflammation, and infection: evolving concepts of therapeutic targeting. The Journal of Clinical Investigation 133 (19).

Medler, J., Kucka, K., Wajant, H., 2022. Tumor necrosis factor receptor 2 (TNFR2): an emerging target in cancer therapy. Cancers 14 (11). Available at https://doi.org/10.3390/cancers14112603, https://www.mdpi.com/2072-6694/14/11/2603/pdf?version=1653465634.

Mehrad, B., Strieter, R.M., Standiford, T.J., 1999. Role of TNF-α in pulmonary host defense in murine invasive aspergillosis. Journal of Immunology 162 (3), 1633–1640.

Mellman, I., 2013. Dendritic cells: master regulators of the immune response. Cancer immunology research 1 (3), 145–149. Available at https://doi.org/10.1158/2326-6066.CIR-13-0102.

Merkhofer, R.M., Klein, B.S., 2020. Advances in understanding human genetic variations that influence innate immunity to fungi. Frontiers in Cellular and Infection Microbiology 10. Available at https://doi.org/10.3389/fcimb.2020.00069, http://www.frontiersin.org/Cellular_and_Infection_Microbiology/archive.

Moore, K.W., De Waal Malefyt, R., Coffman, R.L., O'Garra, A., 2001. Interleukin-10 and the interleukin-10 receptor. Annual Review of Immunology 19, 683–765. Available at https://doi.org/10.1146/annurev.immunol.19.1.683.

Nett, R.J., Skillman, D., Riek, L., Davis, B., Blue, S.R., Sundberg, E.E., et al., 2015. Histoplasmosis in Idaho and Montana, USA, 2012–2013. Emerging Infectious Diseases 21 (6), 1071–1072. Available at https://doi.org/10.3201/eid2106.141367.

Newman, S.L., Gootee, L., 1992. Colony-stimulating factors activate human macrophages to inhibit intracellular growth of *Histoplasma capsulatum* yeasts. Infection and Immunity 60 (11), 4593–4597.

Newman, S.L., Gootee, L., Morris, R., Bullock, W.E., 1992. Digestion of *Histoplasma capsulatum* yeasts by human macrophages. The Journal of Immunology 149 (2), 574–580. Available at https://doi.org/10.4049/jimmunol.149.2.574.

Newman, S.L., Gootee, L., Gabay, J.E., 1993. Human neutrophil-mediated fungistasis against *Histoplasma capsulatum*: localization of fungistatic activity to the azurophil granules. Journal of Clinical Investigation 92 (2), 624–631. Available at http://www.jci.org.

Newman, S.L., Lemen, W., Smulian, A.G., 2011. Dendritic cells restrict the transformation of *Histoplasma capsulatum* conidia into yeasts. Medical Mycology 49 (4), 356–364. Available at https://doi.org/10.3109/13693786.2010.531295.

Newman, S.L., 2005. Interaction of *Histoplasma capsulatum* with human macrophages, dendritic cells, and neutrophils. Methods in Molecular Medicine 118, 181–191.

Nittler, M.P., Hocking-Murray, D., Foo, C.K., Sil, A., 2005. Identification of *Histoplasma capsulatum* transcripts induced in response to reactive nitrogen species. Molecular Biology of the Cell 16 (10), 4792–4813. Available at https://doi.org/10.1091/mbc.E05-05-0434.

Okudaira, M., Straub, M., Schwarz, J., 1961. The etiology of discrete splenic and hepatic calcifications in an endemic area of histoplasmosis. The American Journal of Pathology 39 (5), 599–611.

Plantinga, M., Hammad, H., Lambrecht, B.N., 2010. Origin and functional specializations of DC subsets in the lung. European Journal of Immunology 40 (8), 2112–2118. Available at https://doi.org/10.1002/eji.201040562Belgium, http://onlinelibrary.wiley.com/doi/10.1002/eji.201040562/pdf.

Ramana, K.V., 2010. Tumor necrosis factor-alpha converting enzyme: implications for ocular inflammatory diseases. International Journal of Biochemistry and Cell Biology 42 (7), 1076–1079. Available at https://doi.org/10.1016/j.biocel.2010.03.011.

Ray, S.C., Rappleye, C.A., 2019. Flying under the radar: *Histoplasma capsulatum* avoidance of innate immune recognition. Seminars in Cell and Developmental Biology 89, 91–98. Available at https://doi.org/10.1016/j.semcdb.2018.03.009, http://www.elsevier.com/inca/publications/store/6/2/2/9/4/4/index.htt.

Roach, D.R., Bean, A.G.D., Demangel, C., France, M.P., Briscoe, H., Britton, W.J., 2002. TNF regulates chemokine induction essential for cell recruitment, granuloma formation, and clearance of mycobacterial infection. Journal of Immunology 168 (9), 4620–4627. Available at https://doi.org/10.4049/jimmunol.168.9.4620, http://www.jimmunol.org/.

Schyns, J., Bureau, F., Marichal, T., 2018. Lung interstitial macrophages: past, present, and future. Journal of Immunology Research 2018. Available at https://doi.org/10.1155/2018/5160794, http://www.hindawi.com/journals/jir/.

Seider, K., Heyken, A., Lüttich, A., Miramón, P., Hube, B., 2010. Interaction of pathogenic yeasts with phagocytes: survival, persistence and escape. Current Opinion in Microbiology 13 (4), 392–400. Available at https://doi.org/10.1016/j.mib.2010.05.001.

Sepúlveda, V.E., Márquez, R., Turissini, D.A., Goldman, W.E., Matute, D.R., 2017. Genome sequences reveal cryptic speciation in the human pathogen *Histoplasma capsulatum*. mBio 8 (6). Available at https://doi.org/10.1128/mBio.01339-17, http://mbio.asm.org/content/8/6/e01339-17.full.pdf.

Shi, T., Denney, L., An, H., Ho, L.-P., Zheng, Y., 2021. Alveolar and lung interstitial macrophages: definitions, functions, and roles in lung fibrosis. Journal of Leukocyte Biology 110 (1), 107–114. Available at https://doi.org/10.1002/jlb.3ru0720-418r.

Sil, A., 2019. Molecular regulation of *Histoplasma dimorphism*. Current Opinion in Microbiology 52, 151–157. Available at https://doi.org/10.1016/j.mib.2019.10.011, http://www.elsevier.com/locate/mib.

Smith, D.J., Williams, S.L., Endemic Mycoses State Partners, Benedict, K.M., Jackson, B.R., Toda, M., 2022. Surveillance for coccidioidomycosis, histoplasmosis, and blastomycosis - United States, 2019. Morbidity and mortality weekly report. Surveillance summaries 71 (7), 1–14.

Smith, J.A., Kauffman, C.A., 2009. Endemic fungal infections in patients receiving tumour necrosis factor-α inhibitor therapy. Drugs 69 (11), 1403–1415. Available at https://doi.org/10.2165/00003495-200969110-00002.

Smith, J.G., Magee, D.M., Williams, D.M., Graybill, J.R., 1990. Tumor necrosis factor-alpha plays a role in host defense against *Histoplasma capsulatum*. Journal of Infectious Diseases 162 (6), 1349–1353. Available at https://doi.org/10.1093/infdis/162.6.1349.

Subramanian Vignesh, K., Landero Figueroa, J.A., Porollo, A., Caruso, J.A., Deepe, G.S., 2013. Granulocyte macrophage-colony stimulating factor induced Zn sequestration enhances macrophage superoxide and limits intracellular pathogen survival. Immunity 39 (4), 697–710. Available at https://doi.org/10.1016/j.immuni.2013.09.006.

Sundquist, M., Wick, M.J., 2005. TNF-α-dependent and -independent maturation of dendritic cells and recruited CD11cintCD11b+ cells during oral *Salmonella* infection. Journal of Immunology 175 (5), 3287–3298. Available at https://doi.org/10.4049/jimmunol.175.5.3287, http://www.jimmunol.org/.

Thind, S.K., Taborda, C.P., Nosanchuk, J.D., 2015. Dendritic cell interactions with *Histoplasma* and *Paracoccidioides*. Virulence 6 (5), 424–432. Available at https://doi.org/10.4161/21505594.2014.965586, http://www.tandfonline.com/loi/kvir20.

Tracey, K.J., Cerami, A., 1994. Tumor necrosis factor: a pleiotropic cytokine and therapuetic target. Annual Review of Medicine 45, 491–503. Available at http://www.annualreviews.org/journal/med.

Tsiodras, S., Samonis, G., Boumpas, D.T., Kontoyiannis, D.P., 2008. Fungal infections complicating tumor necrosis factor α blockade therapy. Mayo Clinic Proceedings 83 (2), 181–194. Available at https://doi.org/10.4065/83.2.181, http://www.mayoclinicproceedings.com/pdf%2F8302%2F8302r2%2Epdf.

van Loo, G., Bertrand, M.J.M., 2023. Death by TNF: a road to inflammation. Nature Reviews. Immunology 23 (5), 289–303. Available at https://doi.org/10.1038/s41577-022-00792-3, https://www.nature.com/nri/.

van Rhijn, N., Bromley, M., 2021. The consequences of our changing environment on life threatening and debilitating fungal diseases in humans. Journal of Fungi 7 (5). Available at https://doi.org/10.3390/jof7050367, https://www.mdpi.com/2309-608X/7/5/367/pdf.

Vandenabeele, P., Declercq, W., Beyaert, R., Fiers, W., 1995. Two tumour necrosis factor receptors: structure and function. Trends in Cell Biology 5 (10), 392–399. Available at https://doi.org/10.1016/S0962-8924(00)89088-1.

Vena, G.A., Cassano, N., 2007. Drug focus: Adalimumab in the treatment of moderate to severe psoriasis. Biologics: Targets and Therapy 1 (2), 93–103. Available at https://www.dovepress.com/getfile.php?fileID=1648.

Vergidis, P., Avery, R.K., Wheat, L.J., Dotson, J.L., Assi, M.A., Antoun, S.A., et al., 2015. Histoplasmosis complicating tumor necrosis factor-α blocker therapy: a retrospective analysis of 98 cases. Clinical Infectious Diseases 61 (3), 409–417. Available at https://doi.org/10.1093/cid/civ299, http://cid.oxfordjournals.org/content/by/year.

Wajant, H., Siegmund, D., 2019. TNFR1 and TNFR2 in the control of the life and death balance of macrophages. Frontiers in Cell and Developmental Biology 7 (May). Available at https://doi.org/10.3389/fcell.2019.00091, https://www.frontiersin.org/journals/cell-and-developmental-biology#.

Wallis, R.S., Ehlers, S., 2005. Seminars in arthritis and rheumatism. Tumor necrosis factor and granuloma biology: Explaining the differential infection risk of etanercept and infliximab 34 (5), 34–38. Available at https://doi.org/10.1016/j.semarthrit.2005.01.009, http://www.elsevier.com/inca/publications/store/6/2/3/3/3/2/index.htt.

Wallis, R.S., Broder, M.S., Wong, J.Y., Hanson, M.E., Beenhouwer, D.O., 2004a. Granulomatous infectious diseases associated with tumor necrosis factor antagonists. Clinical Infectious Diseases 38 (9), 1261–1265. Available at https://doi.org/10.1086/383317.

Wallis, R.S., Broder, M., Wong, J., Beenhouwer, D., 2004b. Granulomatous infections due to tumor necrosis factor blockade: correction [4]. Clinical Infectious Diseases 39 (8), 1254–1255. Available at https://doi.org/10.1086/424455.

Wallis, R.S., Broder, M., Wong, J., Lee, A., Hoq, L., 2005. Reactivation of latent granulomatous infections by infliximab. Clinical Infectious Diseases 41 (3), S194. Available at https://doi.org/10.1086/429996.

Webster, R.H., Sil, A., 2008. Conserved factors Ryp2 and Ryp3 control cell morphology and infectious spore formation in the fungal pathogen *Histoplasma capsulatum*. Proceedings of the National Academy of Sciences of the United States of America 105 (38), 14573–14578. Available at https://doi.org/10.1073/pnas.0806221105, http://www.pnas.org/content/105/38/14573.full.pdf.

Winters, M.S., Chan, Q., Caruso, J.A., Deepe, G.S., 2010. Metallomic analysis of macrophages infected with *Histoplasma capsulatum* reveals a fundamental role for zinc in host defenses. Journal of Infectious Diseases 202 (7), 1136–1145. Available at https://doi.org/10.1086/656191, http://www.journals.uchicago.edu/doi/pdf/10.1086/656191.

Wood, K.L., Hage, C.A., Knox, K.S., Kleiman, M.B., Sannuti, A., Day, R.B., et al., 2003. Histoplasmosis after treatment with anti-tumor necrosis factor-α therapy. American Journal of Respiratory and Critical Care Medicine 167 (9), 1279–1282. Available at https://doi.org/10.1164/rccm.200206-563OC.

Wu-Hsieh, B.A., Howard, D.H., 1987. Inhibition of the intracellular growth of *Histoplasma capsulatum* by recombinant murine gamma interferon. Infection and Immunity 55 (4), 1014–1016.

Wu-Hsieh, B.A., Lee, G.S., Franco, M., Hofman, F.M., 1992. Early activation of splenic macrophages by tumor necrosis factor alpha is important in determining the outcome of experimental histoplasmosis in mice. Infection and Immunity 60 (10), 4230–4238.

Wu-Hsieh, B.A., Chen, W., Lee, H.J., 1998. Nitric oxide synthase expression in macrophages of *Histoplasma capsulatum*-infected mice is associated with splenocyte apoptosis and unresponsiveness. Infection and Immunity 66 (11), 5520–5526. Available at https://doi.org/10.1128/iai.66.11.5520-5526.1998, http://iai.asm.org/content/by/year.

Zhou, P., Miller, G., Seder, R.A., 1998. Factors involved in regulating primary and secondary immunity to infection with *Histoplasma capsulatum*: TNF-α plays a critical role in maintaining secondary immunity in the absence of IFN-γ Journal of Immunology 160 (3), 1359–1368.

CHAPTER

Immunogenetics underlying severe coccidioidomycosis

9

Amy P. Hsu

Laboratory of Clinical Immunology and Microbiology, National Institute of Allergy and Infectious Diseases, National Institutes of Health, Bethesda, MD, United States

Coccidioides as a pathogen

Coccidioidomycosis, commonly known as Valley Fever, is caused by the dimorphic fungi, *Coccidioides posadasii* and *Coccidioides immitis*, endemic to the arid and semiarid desert soils of the southwestern United States and Mexico, and within select regions in Central and South America. They are found in the soil, frequently near rodent burrows, as septated hyphae which break apart into single-cell arthroconidia. When the soil is disrupted, the small, 2–5 μm arthroconidia become airborne, allowing inhalation by a mammalian host.

There are an estimated 150,000 *Coccidioides* infections per year in the United States (Galgiani et al., 2023). Mandatory reporting occurs in 28 states plus the District of Columbia (Centers for Disease Control, 2025), and only diagnosed patients are reported; therefore, it is likely the actual incidence is underestimated. In fact, a recent national estimate suggests approximately 273,000 symptomatic cases and 900 deaths per year (Williams et al., 2025). Among infected individuals, the majority will remain asymptomatic, roughly one-third will develop respiratory symptoms such as cough or fever, which resolve over the course of approximately 2 weeks. In a small number of cases, 2%–5%, patients will be unable to clear the infection despite appropriate antifungal therapy and develop a chronic pulmonary disease, while in a fraction of 1% of cases, patients will lose control of the fungus and experience extrapulmonary disseminated coccidioidomycosis (DCM) (Fig. 9.1). Frequent sites of DCM include the skin, bone, and brain, with soft tissue and joint infections also reported.

Data from the CDC demonstrates an increasing incidence of coccidioidomycosis over the past two decades, with more than 95% of United States cases occurring in Arizona and California, followed by the remaining endemic states, Nevada, New Mexico, and Utah. The economic burden has likewise increased. Cases reported in California in 2017 were estimated to have total lifetime costs of $700 million (Wilson et al., 2019). A similar study in Arizona calculated the lifetime cost of the 10,359 cases diagnosed in 2019 to be $736 million (Grizzle et al., 2021). Not surprisingly, in both studies, disseminated disease was associated with the highest financial burden, calculated to be almost $1.4 million in

Immunological Insights and Emerging Therapeutics in Medical Mycology. DOI: https://doi.org/10.1016/B978-0-443-23636-5.00007-1
2027 Published by Elsevier Inc.

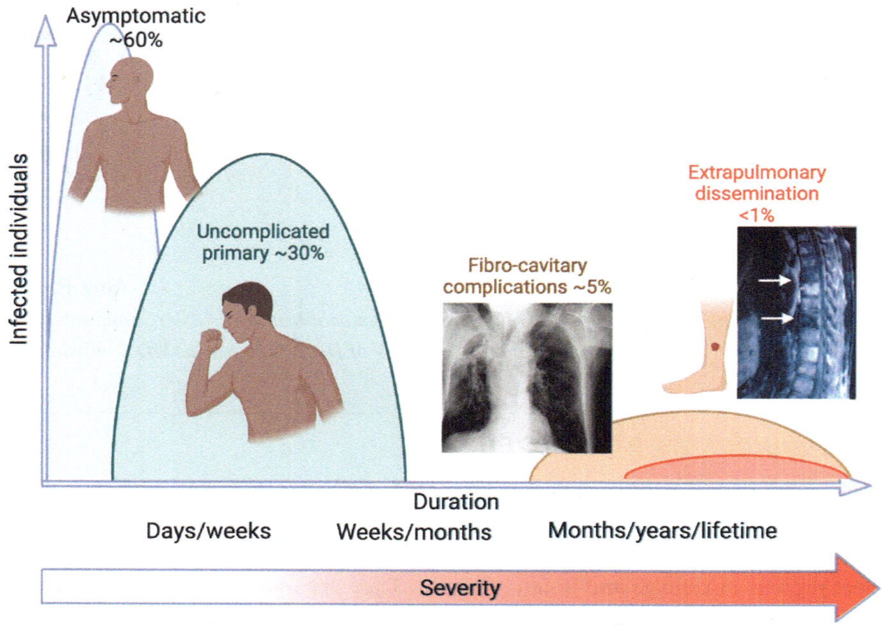

FIGURE 9.1 Spectrum of coccidioidomycosis presentations.

The majority of those infected will remain asymptomatic; approximately 30% of patients have self-resolving respiratory symptoms, possibly requiring medical attention; 2%–5% will develop a chronic pulmonary infection or fibro-cavitary complications requiring prolonged antifungal therapy; and less than 1% will develop extrapulmonary dissemination.

From Hsu AP. J Fungi (Basel). 2024;10(4):256.

direct and indirect costs per person (Grizzle et al., 2021). More recently, *C. immitis* soil colonization in Washington state was demonstrated to be the source of a traumatic inoculation in a patient (Litvintseva et al., 2015). Whole genome sequencing confirmed that the patient and soil isolates were identical (Litvintseva et al., 2015), indicating infection from the soil and not acquired elsewhere. Since 2010, there have been 16 human (Washington Department of Health Coccidioidomycosis Valley Fever, 2025) and at least 5 animal (James et al., 2019) coccidioidomycosis cases due to exposure in Washington state, expanding the known range of *Coccidioides*.

Early events after infection

Although the fungus is endemic in the soil, only 2%–4% of individuals within the endemic area are infected annually (Thompson III GR. Coccidioidomycosis and Valley Fever, 2022), possibly due to arthroconidia being swallowed or removed by mucociliary clearance prior to developing into a spherule. If an arthroconidium reaches the alveolus, the warm, moist environment promotes a switch to the pathogenic yeast phase of the fungus. Initially, the arthroconidium swells becoming an immature spherule, undergoes internal cell division, and develops into a mature spherule, containing several hundred endospores (Fig. 9.2A). Prior to spherule rupture, the spherule is immune masked (Fig. 9.2B). Spherule development does not cause tissue stress or damage, events required to drive recruitment of immune cells and an inflammatory response (Matzinger, 1994). On the pathogen side, *Coccidioides* secretes the metalloproteinase, *Mep1* (Hung et al., 2005), which cleaves an immunogenic spherule outer wall glycoprotein (Hung et al., 2002). After approximately 96–100 hours, the now mature primary spherule ruptures, damaging surrounding cells and releasing the endospores, each of which can develop into a new spherule, establishing a rapid growth of the fungus.

Once the spherule ruptures, localized tissue damage drives a rapid influx of innate immune cells, including resident alveolar macrophages as well as neutrophils and monocytes from circulation. The exposed spherule cell wall, composed primarily of β-glucan and chitin, is then recognized by pattern recognition receptors. The C-type lectin receptor, DECTIN-1, specific for β-glucan, is found on myeloid cells—neutrophils, monocytes, macrophages, and dendritic cells—as well as γδT-cells. Within the lung, additional cells expressing DECTIN-1 include ciliated cells, club cells, Type 2 alveolar epithelial cells, endothelial cells, and smooth muscle cells (Human protein atlas, 2025), indicating recognition and response by both innate immune cells and barrier epithelial cells.

After fungal recognition, the release of cytokines and chemokines recruits additional immune cells. Stimulation of elicited mouse peritoneal macrophages in vitro with formalin-killed spherules resulted in a dose-dependent increase in tumor necrosis factor (TNF)-α, IL-6, and MIP-2, while bone marrow-derived dendritic cells displayed increased TNF-α, IL-6, IL-10, GM-CSF, IL-1α, and IL-1β (Viriyakosol et al., 2013). Fourteen days postinfection, mouse lung lavage fluid showed increases in TNF-α, IL-6, MIP-2, IL-10, IL-4, IL17α, IL-22, IL-23, interferon (IFN)-γ, IL-12p70, IL-1β, and GM-CSF (Viriyakosol et al., 2013). Increased *Tnf*, *Il1a*, *Il17a*, and *Il10* transcripts were observed in mouse lung homogenates 5 days postinfection (Lewis et al., 2015). Among patients, with simple pulmonary coccidioidomycosis shortly after diagnosis, peripheral blood stimulation with *Coccidioides* antigen induced a more than 10-fold increase in IL-1Rα, IL-1β, IFN-γ, GM-CSF, IL-2, IL-13, and TNF-α over unstimulated (Ampel et al., 2018). Comparing previously infected to uninfected individuals, the same cytokines, but not IL-1Rα, were significantly upregulated in infected patients (Ampel et al., 2018). While results are dependent on time since stimulation or infection, cell type assayed, and sample source, specific cytokines, including TNF-α, IL-6, IL-1β, and GM-CSF, are recurrently observed.

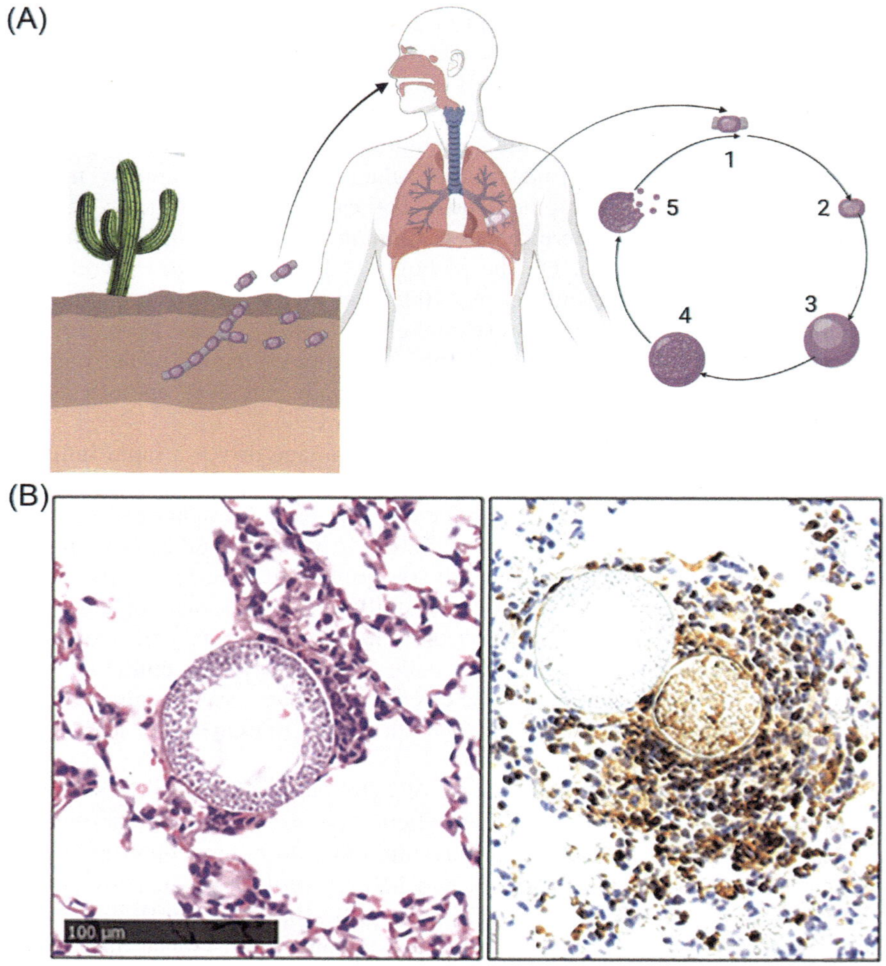

FIGURE 9.2 Inhalation, spherule development, and pulmonary disease progression.

(A) Inhaled arthroconidia, which land in a terminal bronchiole or alveolus allows *Coccidioides* to convert to yeast form, where it will swell, undergo internal cell division, develop endospores, and rupture. (B) Mouse lung showing an immune-masked maturing spherule. Left, hematoxylin and eosin (H&E) stain day 4 post infection. Right, immunohistochemistry for neutrophils (myeloperoxidase, brown), day 5 post infection. Neutrophils surround and invade the lower, ruptured spherule, but the upper, unruptured spherule is not recognized.

From Hsu AP. J Fungi (Basel). 2024;10(4):256.

Known risk factors

Several cohort studies have demonstrated that immunocompromised hosts have an increased risk of severe disease or dissemination. Initial studies of coccidioidomycosis in HIV-infected individuals revealed high rates of dissemination (Bronnimann et al., 1987; Fish et al., 1990; Singh et al., 1996) and mortality (Fish et al., 1990; Singh et al., 1996), leading *Coccidioides* to be considered an opportunistic infection among people living with HIV (Singh et al., 1996; Ampel, 2005). After the introduction of antiretroviral therapy, a significant decrease in newly diagnosed coccidioidomycosis was observed among HIV patients, putting patients with controlled HIV in a similar risk category as the general population (Masannat and Ampel, 2010). Similarly, there is an increased risk of infection among immunosuppressed solid organ transplant recipients (Blair and Logan, 2001). While the majority of cases are diagnosed within the first year posttransplant, recipients continue to face an increased risk in subsequent years (Asbury et al., 2019). Data from lung transplant recipients suggests reactivation of existing disease may occur. Pretransplant surveillance coupled with posttransplant prophylactic antifungals decreases the incidence of severe disease posttransplant (Truong et al., 2022).

Beyond HIV or transplant therapy, direct immunosuppression using corticosteroids or biologics has been shown to increase infection risk. In one study within the endemic region, recipients of TNF-α inhibitors had a more than 10-fold increase in infection rates compared to statewide reported infections (Benedict et al., 2019). A single-center, retrospective study identified 138 patients with diagnoses of both autoimmune disease and coccidioidomycosis. Comparing patients with simple pulmonary disease versus those with disseminated disease revealed a 2.4-fold increased risk of dissemination among those receiving a biologic response modifier, predominantly TNF-α inhibitors (Donovan et al., 2022). Using Medicare claims data for individuals with rheumatic or autoimmune disease, Wilson et al. (2024) observed an increased risk of coccidioidomycosis among those prescribed a biologic response modifier (adjusted hazard ratio 3.94, 95% confidence interval 1.18–13.16), similar to the increased risk reported by Donovan et al. (2022).

Repeatedly in the literature, male sex, pregnancy, and African American ancestry have been documented as risks for severe or disseminated disease (Hsu, 2024; Rosenstein et al., 2001). The risk for severe disease in males diverges from that in females at puberty onset and remains higher through adulthood (McHardy et al., 2022). Male dogs also have increased rates of infection. However, this risk was ameliorated by castration, reducing the risk of neutered male dogs to that of females (McHardy et al., 2022). Unlike transplant-related reactivation, the increased risk of symptomatic disease seen during pregnancy is not affected by prior, resolved disease (Bercovitch et al., 2011). New infections, however, have increased dissemination risk over the course of pregnancy; in one study, 96% of cases in third trimester presented with disseminated disease (Crum and Ballon-Landa, 2006). The underlying causes for this higher dissemination are unknown.

Varying disease presentations have been observed among individuals of different genetic ancestries, the most consistent being a pronounced increase in severity among those with African American ancestry. The annual hospitalization incidence for coccidioidomycosis, which could be used as a marker for disease severity, reveals significantly higher hospitalization rates among African Americans and Asian/Pacific Islanders compared to other ancestries (Kupferwasser and Miller, 2021) (Fig. 9.3A). Comparing disease presentation across ancestries within a California cohort shows that African Americans and East Asians had higher rates of disseminated disease compared to other ancestries (Fig. 9.3B) (Hsu et al., 2022). Together, these findings support a more pronounced infection with increased disease severity among African American individuals. The reasons underlying this increased susceptibility are unknown and require further study. It is noteworthy that increased disease severity among recent African immigrants has not been reported, and the ancestry grouping of "African American" encompasses the diaspora from an entire continent, many of whose ancestors have been in North America for hundreds of years.

Genetic susceptibility

Given the relative rarity of DCM, it is reasonable to consider the possibility that underlying monogenic mutations are causal for the severe phenotype. In 2009 the first monogenic mutation associated with DCM was reported in an adolescent girl with coccidioidal meningitis and a dominant-negative mutation in the transcription factor STAT3 (Powers et al., 2009). Subsequently, patients with mutations in the IFN-γ receptor (IFNγR [*IFNGR1*]) (Vinh et al., 2009) and IL-12 receptor (*IL12RB1*) (Vinh et al., 2011) were reported. These were followed by descriptions of STAT1 gain-of-function (Sampaio et al., 2013), IL12RB2 (Odio et al., 2017), additional STAT3 patients (Odio et al., 2017), and a three-generation family carrying a STAT4 mutation (Powell et al., 2022a,b,c) in DCM patients. With the accessibility of whole-exome sequencing in the early 2010's, it was expected that more causal mutations would be identified. The first cohort collected for whole-exome sequencing was comprised of 67 DCM patients. Using rare variant analysis, only two patients with primary immune deficiency were identified, both carrying *STAT3* point mutations causing premature stop codons (Hsu et al., 2022). Comprehensive literature reviews, however, reveal that monogenic primary immune deficiency mutations are rare among DCM patients, with only 15 disseminated and 3 pulmonary cases reported in the literature (Table 9.1). Review of these mutations indicates a common centrality around the IL-12/IFN-γ signaling pathway with variants observed in *IFNGR1*, *IL12RB1*, *IL12RB2*, *STAT1*, *STAT3*, and *STAT4*, highlighted in Fig. 9.4. While few, these genes provide insights into cellular signaling and transcription events critical to the control of the fungus. Additionally, one patient was homozygous for a *CTPS1* mutation, leading to impaired T-cell proliferation and inability to control *Coccidioides* without antifungal

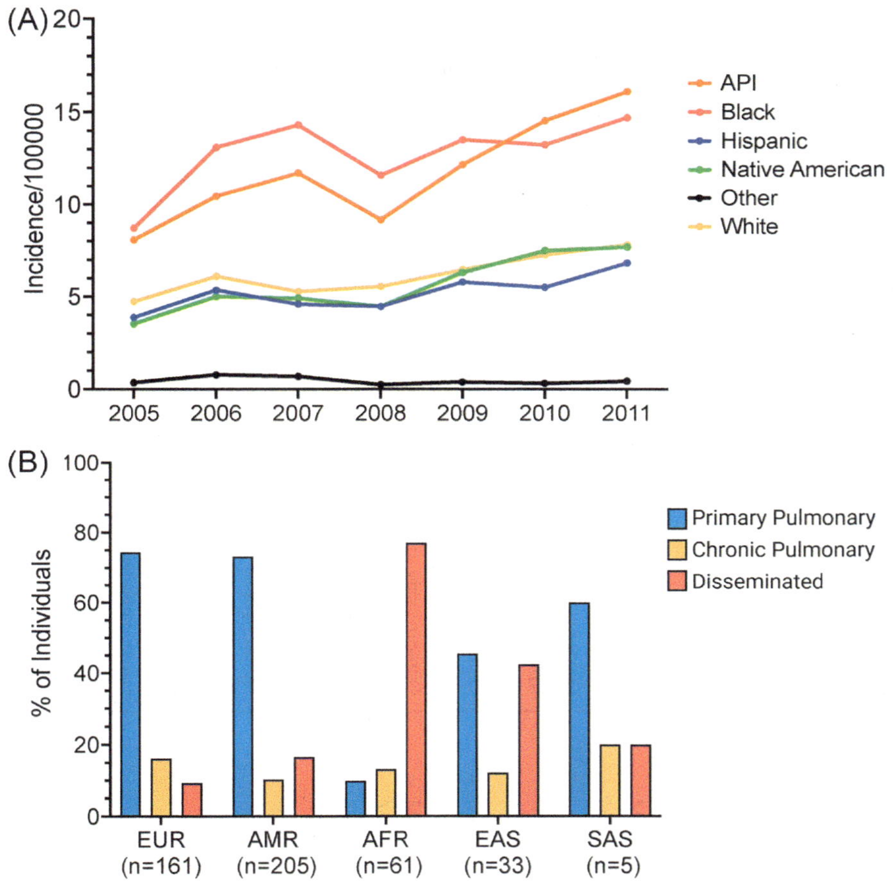

FIGURE 9.3 Impact of genetic ancestry on disease presentation.

(A) Annual coccidioidomycosis hospital incidence rate per 100,000 persons in California and Arizona, separated by self-reported race/ethnicity. API: Asian/Pacific Islander. (B) Disease presentation in a California coccidioidomycosis cohort (n = 468 cases) separated by genetically determined ancestry. EUR: European; AMR: Admixed American; AFR: African American; EAS: East Asian; SAS: South Asian (chronic pulmonary disease is defined as a disease persisting after more than one year of antifungal therapy).

(A) Data adapted from Kupferwasser D, Miller LG. Epidemiol Infect. 2021;149(e127):1–8. (B) Data adapted from Hsu AP et al. JCI Insight. 2022;e159491.

therapy. Individually, primary immune deficiencies are rare genetic events, frequently with increased susceptibility to infection; however, in total, the estimate is approximately 1 in 10,000 affected individuals worldwide (Meyts et al., 2021). Given the rarity

Table 9.1 Coccidioidomycosis in primary immune deficiency patients (DN: dominant negative, AR: autosomal recessive, AD: autosomal dominant, hom: homozygous, GOF: gain of function, NA: not available, DCM: disseminated coccidioidomycosis, PUL: pulmonary coccidioidomycosis).

Case	Gene	Mutation type	Disease	Site of dissemination	Reference
1	*STAT3*	DN	DCM	Meningitis	(Powers et al., 2009)
2	*STAT3*	DN	DCM	Meningitis	(Odio et al., 2017)
3	*STAT3*	DN	DCM	Meningitis	(Stanga and Dajud, 2008)
4	*IFNGR1*	DN	DCM	Osteomyelitis	(Vinh et al., 2009)
5	*IL12RB1*	AR-hom	DCM	Lymphadenitis	(Vinh et al., 2011)
6	*IL12RB1*	AR-hom	DCM	Lymphadenitis; osteomyelitis	(Vinh et al., 2011)
7	*IL12RB2*	AD	DCM	Osteomyelitis, soft tissue, cutaneous	(Odio et al., 2017)
8	*STAT1*	AD-GOF	DCM	Osteomyelitis, soft tissue	(Sampaio et al., 2013)
9	*STAT1*	AD-GOF	DCM	Osteomyelitis, meningitis	(Sampaio et al., 2013)
10	*STAT4*	DN	DCM	Cutaneous	(Powell et al., 2022a,b,c)
11	*STAT4*	DN	DCM	Cutaneous	(Powell et al., 2022a,b,c)
12	*STAT4*	DN	DCM	Osteomyelitis	(Powell et al., 2022a,b,c)
13	*GATA2*	NA	DCM	NA	(Imran and Cui, 2013)
14	*NFKB2*	AD	DCM	Osteomyelitis, skin, joint, soft tissue	(Cavazos et al., 2022)
15	*DOCK8*	AR	DCM	Meningitis	(Krase et al., 2022a,b)
16	*CYBB*	X-linked	PUL		(Krase et al., 2022a,b)
17	*NCF1*	AR	PUL		(Krase et al., 2022a,b)
18	*CTPS1*	AR-hom	PUL	Mediastinal disease	(Krase et al., 2022a,b)

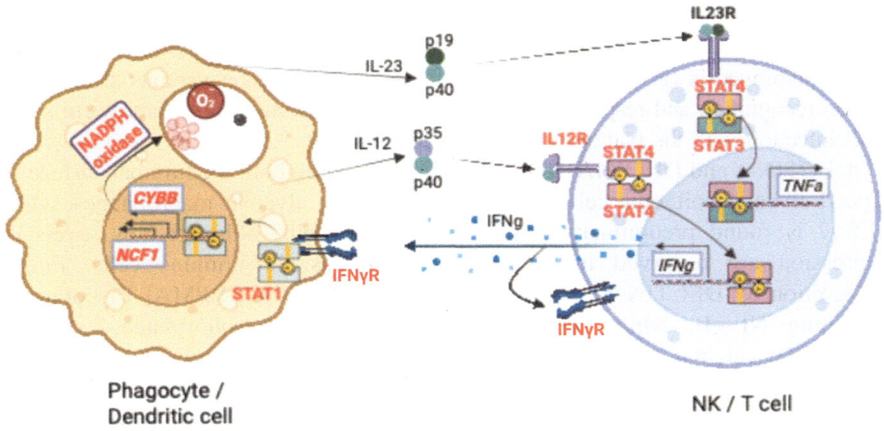

FIGURE 9.4 Primary immune deficiency mutations within the IL-12/IFN-γ pathway.

Phagocytosis of a pathogen such as *Coccidioides* leads to increased NADPH oxidase components gp91phox (CYBB) and p47phox (NCF1) and production of cytokines IL-12 and IL-23. IL-12 binding to the IL12RB1/IL12RB2 heterodimeric receptor on T or natural killer (NK) cells leads to phosphorylation of STAT4 and production of IFN-γ. The heterodimeric IFN-γ receptor (IFNγR), comprised of IFNGR1 and IFNGR2, phosphorylates and activates STAT1. Secreted IL-23 acts through the heterodimeric IL23R comprised of IL23RA and IL12RB1 to activate a STAT3/STAT4 heterodimer. Mutations in proteins shown in red have been identified in primary immune deficiency patients with coccidioidomycosis.

Adapted from Hsu AP. J Fungi (Basel). 2024;10(4):256.

of primary immune deficiencies and the low rate of *Coccidioides* infection within the endemic region, it is less surprising that few patients with primary immune deficiencies have been identified.

Common population variants underlie susceptibility to disseminated disease

Considering the disparity between primary immune deficiency mutations and the incidence of DCM, and understanding a regional, rather than global, *Coccidioides* prevalence provides a "genetics-plus-environment" model in which more common, population-level variants may be driving susceptibility to dissemination. Genetic investigation of DCM patients from Arizona revealed significant overrepresentation of common population variants impairing the function of the fungal β-glucan receptor, DECTIN-1, its downstream signaling partner, PLCγ2, and the pulmonary-epithelial NADPH oxidase, DUOX1/DUOXA1, in more than 50% of one DCM cohort

(Hsu et al., 2022). These findings were validated in a separate California cohort, which included DCM, chronic pulmonary disease, as well as uncomplicated, primary coccidioidomycosis (Hsu et al., 2022). In these cases, common variants affecting β-glucan recognition and response, present within the population in general, were silent until infection with the pathogenic fungus occurred (Fig. 9.5).

DECTIN-1 and DUOX1/DUOXA1 are expressed on both the luminal surface of type II alveolar epithelial cells and on tissue-resident alveolar macrophages, while PLCγ2 is found predominantly in hematopoietic cells, although low levels of expression are observed in pulmonary cell types. In immune cells, fungal recognition by DECTIN-1 signals through the CARD9/BCL10/MALT1 complex, activating NF-κB, while simultaneously PLCγ2 is phosphorylated, releasing intracellular calcium and activating NFAT, together inducing production of TNF-α (Fig. 9.6A). Within the alveolus, intracellular calcium via DECTIN-1 engagement activates the DUOX1/DUOXA1 complex, which produces H_2O_2 in the alveolar space (Fig. 9.6B). Compared to healthy controls, patients carrying DECTIN-1 or PLCγ2 variants showed diminished TNF-α production after β-glucan stimulation (Hsu et al., 2022). Two recurrent DECTIN-1 variants were observed among DCM or chronic pulmonary coccidioidomycosis patients, Y238* and I223S (Hsu et al., 2022). The Y238* mutation has been implicated in susceptibility to other fungal infections, including chronic mucocutaneous candidiasis (Ferwerda et al., 2009) and invasive aspergillosis posthematopoietic stem cell transplant (Cunha et al., 2010), while both

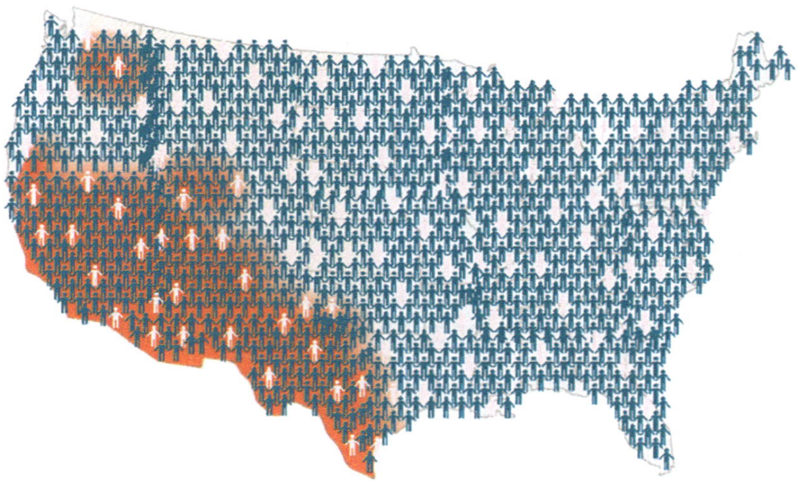

FIGURE 9.5 Overlap of population variants and endemic regions.

Common population variants in fungal recognition and response (pink) are silent unless present within the endemic regions (red shading). Map lines delineate study areas and do not necessarily depict accepted national boundaries.

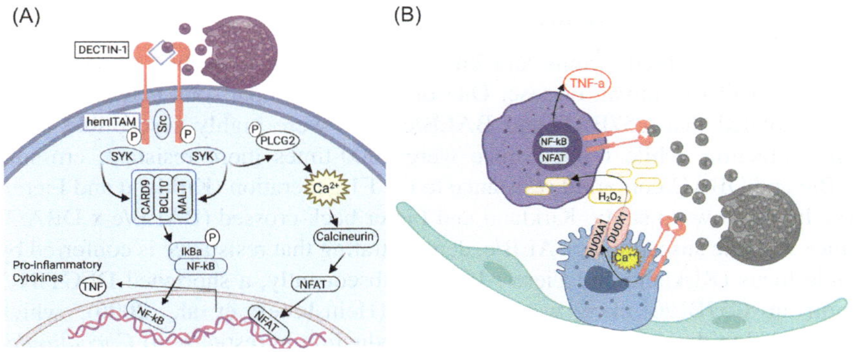

FIGURE 9.6 ***Coccidioides*** **recognition and response.**

(A) *Coccidioides'* β-glucan binding to DECTIN-1 induces phosphorylation of spleen tyrosine kinase (SYK). SYK both activates the CARD9/BCL10/MALT1 complex leading to NF-κB activation, and phosphorylates PLCγ2, causing intracellular calcium release and NFAT activation. Together, NF-κB and NFAT induce pro-inflammatory cytokines, including tumor necrosis factor (TNF)-α. (B) *Coccidioides* recognition by DECTIN-1 on type II alveolar epithelial cells (AEC2) releases intracellular calcium, driving H_2O_2 production by DUOX1/DUOXA1. Alveolar macrophage recognition of *Coccidioides* via DECTIN-1 activates NF-κB and NFAT, as shown in A, potentially amplified by AEC2-produced H_2O_2.

Adapted from Hsu AP, Korzeniowska A, Aguilar CC, et al. JCI Insight. 2022;e159491

variants were found in a cohort of invasive phaeohyphomycosis (Drummond et al., 2022). Severe PLCG2 mutations cause a spectrum of immune disorders ranging from recurrent infections to autoinflammation. In a recent cohort of 76 patients carrying previously uncharacterized *PLCG2* mutations, 11 had fungal infections (14%), including one patient with DCM who was heterozygous for P317L (Baysac et al., 2024). Functional studies demonstrated P317L was hypomorphic with significantly reduced phospho-ERK after B-cell receptor engagement, while both P317L and the DCM-associated R268W variants displayed reduced stimulation-induced calcium flux (Baysac et al., 2024).

Additional DCM-associated variants were identified in the alveolar epithelial NADPH oxidase complex, comprised of DUOX1 and DUOXA1. The DUOX1/DUOXA1 complex is regulated by a DUOX1 intracellular calcium-sensing domain, which, when activated, produces hydrogen peroxide (H_2O_2) in the airway lumen (Forteza et al., 2005). Functionally, β-glucan-activated DECTIN-1 is sufficient to induce H_2O_2 production, and DCM patient variants displayed decreased H_2O_2 after stimulation (Hsu et al., 2022). Cellular models demonstrate H_2O_2 activates NF-κB in a dose- and time-dependent manner (Takada et al., 2003) and amplifies NF-κB response by threefold over H_2O_2 or TNF-α alone (Oliveira-Marques et al., 2013). Identification of this genetic pathway underpinning dissemination susceptibility revealed fungal recognition and response by alveolar epithelial cells as a key initial immune response.

Lessons from mouse models

The presence of inbred strains and known genetic mutations has made mice a common model for human disease. One of the first comparisons between inbred strains revealed that C57BL/6 and BALB/c mice were highly susceptible to *C. immitis* infection, while DBA/2 mice were 1000-times more resistant; crossing BALB/c and DBA/2 conferred resistance to the F1 generation (Kirkland and Fierer, 1983). In a follow-up study, Kirkland and Fierer back-crossed (BALB/c x DBA/2) F1 mice with the susceptible, BALB/c, demonstrating that resistance is conferred by a single locus (Kirkland and Fierer, 1985). Subsequently, a shortened DECTIN-1 isoform in C57BL/6 mice was identified (Heinsbroek et al., 2006), which corresponded to decreased TNF-α and IL-6 production in response to *Coccidioides* spherules (del Pilar Jiménez-A et al., 2008). Similar to the finding of DECTIN-1 variants in human cohorts, comparing C57BL/6 x DBA/2 recombinant inbred lines revealed that *Coccidioides* susceptibility corresponded to the presence of the shortened, C57BL/6 DECTIN-1 isoform (del Pilar Jiménez-A et al., 2008).

While extensive mouse studies have been performed, until recently, they were hampered by the available *Coccidioides* strains. The commonly used *C. posadasii Silveira* or *C. immitis RS* are hypervirulent, with animals succumbing to infection within 2–3 weeks. Despite this limitation, multiple genetically modified mouse models have provided insights to critical immune signaling events and pathways required during *Coccidioides* infection. These have included pattern recognition receptors (*Clec7a*$^{-/-}$ and *Tlr2*$^{-/-}$ (Viriyakosol et al., 2005), cytokine receptors (*Ifngr1*$^{-/-}$ (Shubitz et al., 2021), *Il1r1*$^{-/-}$ (Hung et al., 2014; Viriyakosol et al., 2018), *Il17ra*$^{-/-}$ (Hung et al., 2011), signaling adapter molecules (*Myd88*$^{-/-}$ (Hung et al., 2014; Viriyakosol et al., 2018), *Card9*$^{-/-}$ (Hung et al., 2014)), and transcription factors (mutant-*Stat3* and *Stat4*$^{-/-}$ (Powell et al., 2022a,b,c)). Additionally, genetically modified, avirulent *Coccidioides* strains, such as cts2/ard1/cts3 (Xue et al., 2009) and Δcps1 (Narra et al., 2016), have been demonstrated to protect mice from lethal *Coccidioides* strain challenge. Infection with an avirulent *Coccidioides* strain followed by lethal challenge has been used as a model to examine genes important for the establishment of resistance. Rag1-/-mice, lacking both T and B cells, fail to mount an adaptive response and are not protectable by vaccination (Powell et al., 2022a,b,c). While protection is conferred by vaccination with the avirulent strains, neither strain produces an infection similar to human coccidioidomycosis. More recently, an attenuated, patient-isolate strain, Cp1038, was shown to result in a disease model in which an adaptive immune response occurs, and survival exceeds 8 weeks in C57BL/6 mice (Shubitz et al., 2021). This establishes a more chronic disease model similar to that observed in humans (Shubitz et al., 2021). Lastly, advanced molecular biology and imaging techniques such as single-cell RNA sequencing and spatial transcriptomics are being employed to dissect out specific signaling events and the cell subpopulations contributing to them (Davalos et al., 2025).

Innate immune pathways identified with other pathogens are likely to be mirrored in *Coccidioides* infection. DECTIN-1 defects, observed in DCM, are found in patients with disseminated phaeohyphomycosis (Drummond et al., 2022). Studies using *Legionella* (Liu et al., 2020) and *Aspergillus* (Mills et al., 2025) have revealed IL-1/GM-CSF-mediated crosstalk between the pulmonary epithelium and innate immune cells. Tnf deletion in mice results in a failure of granuloma formation and mortality after *Mycobacterium tuberculosis* infection (Bean et al., 1999), implicating TNF-α in the establishment of the granuloma and control of infection. Similarly, mice infected with *Coccidioides* and treated with TNF-α antibodies display progressive disease and mortality, regardless of whether TNF-α blockade is provided throughout the duration of the infection or only during the first 14 days (Powell et al., 2022a,b,c). Mice given anti-TNF-α 6 weeks after infection, when control has been established, displayed increased lung and splenic fungal burdens and increased mortality (Powell et al., 2022a,b,c).

Moving forward

Although we are solidly in the age of whole genome sequencing and searching for causative mutations, identification of the underlying genetic causes of severe or DCM remains challenging. Two pathways now recognized include the IL-12/IFN-γ pathway identified in rare primary immune-deficient patients, and the DECTIN-1/PLCG2/DUOX1/DUOXA1 pathway involved in fungal recognition and response. One difficulty in searching for genetic risk factors is the inability to reliably identify those previously infected individuals who remained asymptomatic. To date, comparisons have been made using healthy control populations such as 1000 Genomes or population frequency datasets such as gnomAD. These fall short, however, since the exposure risk of any individual within those groups is unknown. Prior studies utilized a coccidioidin skin test to determine infection rate among military service members in the endemic area (Smith and Beard, 1946), although that assay is no longer in widespread use (Benedict et al., 2020). IFN-γ release assays are a promising alternative, currently in development by several laboratories and reported in dogs (Shubitz et al., 2025), which would identify individuals with prior, asymptomatic infections.

A significant number of unanswered questions remain. What is the order of events after spherule rupture? Which cells migrate in, and what are the chemotactic signals used to recruit them? Are all endospores phagocytosed, or do some escape, establishing the ongoing infection? Alternatively, are phagocytosed endospores able to mature within a cell, preventing further immune response until the growing spherule causes rupture? How does dissemination occur—are phagocytosed endospores carried by neutrophils or macrophages into circulation or the lymphatic system? Do dendritic cells phagocytose endospores and carry them to the lymph nodes? What are the key events in granuloma formation, providing a barrier containing the fungus? What cells and signaling pathways maintain the granuloma and keep the fungus quiescent? What events drive the failure of a controlled infection leading to dissemination? Most importantly for patients, what are the underlying genetic drivers that break any one of those pathways leading to susceptibility to severe or disseminated disease?

There are similarities when comparing disseminated or severe coccidioidomycosis to primary immune deficiencies. Primary immune deficiencies are caused by a diverse group of genes, each one relatively rare, impacting a specific aspect of immunity, yet collectively, patients share aberrant infection susceptibility, autoimmunity, or inflammation. It is likely that each individual coccidioidomycosis patient carries one or a few genetic variants impacting specific infection or control processes. Additional genetic underpinnings will continue to be discovered gradually due to the rarity of damaging variants within any given gene or pathway. The continued development of single-cell and spatial analysis, coupled with larger patient cohorts, animal models, and genotype-phenotype databases such as the *All of Us* Research Program, will help address these issues (Bick et al., 2024).

Acknowledgment

This work was supported in part by the Division of Intramural Research, National Institute of Allergy and Infectious Diseases.

References

Ampel, N.M., 2005. Coccidioidomycosis in persons infected with HIV type 1. Clinical Infectious Diseases 41 (8), 1174–1178. Available at https://doi.org/10.1086/444502.

Ampel, N.M., Robey, I., Nguyen, C.T., Roller, B., August, J., Knox, K.S., et al., 2018. Ex vivo cytokine release, determined by a multiplex cytokine assay, in response to coccidioidal antigen stimulation of whole blood among subjects with recently diagnosed primary pulmonary coccidioidomycosis. American Society for Microbiology, United States mSphere 3 (3). Available at https://doi.org/10.1128/mSphere.00065-18, http://msphere.asm.org/content/msph/3/3/e00065-18.full.pdf.

Asbury, K., Blair, J.E., August, J., Beatty, N.L., Mi, L., Carey, E.J., et al., 2019. De novo coccidioidomycosis among solid organ transplant recipients 1 or more years after transplant. American Journal of Transplantation. 19 (9), 2517–2524. Available at https://doi.org/10.1111/ajt.15324, http://onlinelibrary.wiley.com/journal/10.1111/(ISSN)1600-6143.

Baysac, K., Sun, G., Nakano, H., Schmitz, E.G., Cruz, A.C., Fisher, C., et al., 2024. PLCG2-associated immune dysregulation (PLAID) comprises broad and distinct clinical presentations related to functional classes of genetic variants. Journal of Allergy and Clinical Immunology 153 (1), 230–242. Available at https://doi.org/10.1016/j.jaci.2023.08.036.

Bean, A.G.D., Roach, D.R., Briscoe, H., France, M.P., Korner, H., Sedgwick, J.D., et al., 1999. Structural deficiencies in granuloma formation in TNF gene-targeted mice underlie the heightened susceptibility to aerosol Mycobacterium tuberculosis infection, which is not compensated for by lymphotoxin. Journal of Immunology 162 (6), 3504–3511. Available at https://doi.org/10.4049/jimmunol.162.6.3504, http://www.jimmunol.org/.

Benedict, K., McCotter, O.Z., Jackson, B.R., 2020. Coccidioidomycosis skin testing in a commercially insured population, United States, 2014-2017. Emerging Infectious Diseases 26 (3), 619–621. Available at https://doi.org/10.3201/eid2603.190798, https://wwwnc.cdc.gov/eid/article/26/3/19-0798_article.

Benedict, K., McCotter, O.Z., Brady, S., Komatsu, K., Cooksey, G.L.S., Nguyen, A., et al., 2019. Surveillance for Coccidioidomycosis — United States, 2011–2017. MMWR. Surveillance Summaries 68 (7), 1–15. Available at https://doi.org/10.15585/mmwr.ss6807a1.

Bercovitch, R.S., Catanzaro, A., Schwartz, B.S., Pappagianis, D., Heather Watts, D., Ampel, N.M., 2011. Coccidioidomycosis during pregnancy: a review and recommendations for management. Clinical Infectious Diseases 53 (4), 363–368. Available at https://doi.org/10.1093/cid/cir410.

Bick, A.G., Metcalf, G.A., Mayo, K.R., Lichtenstein, L., Rura, S., Carroll, R.J., et al., 2024. Genomic data in the All of Us research program. Nature 627 (8003), 340–346. Available at https://doi.org/10.1038/s41586-023-06957-x.

Blair, J.E., Logan, J.L., 2001. Coccidioidomycosis in solid organ transplantation. Clinical Infectious Diseases 33 (9), 1536–1544. Available at https://doi.org/10.1086/323463.

Bronnimann, D.A., Adam, R.D., Galgiani, J.N., Habib, M.P., Petersen, E.A., Porter, B., et al., 1987. Coccidioidomycosis in the acquired immunodeficiency syndrome. Annals of Internal Medicine 106 (3), 372–379. Available at https://doi.org/10.7326/0003-4819-106-3-372.

Cavazos, S.P., De la Cruz Cruz, R.A., Bejarano, J.I.C., Aparicio, D.N.V., de los Santos, A.H.M., Zárate Hernández, M.del C., 2022. Disseminated coccidioidomycosis as the first presentation of a C-terminal NFKB2 pathogenic variant: a case report and review of the literature. Pediatric Infectious Disease Journal 41 (2), 140–144. Available at https://doi.org/10.1097/INF.0000000000003333, http://journals.lww.com/pidj.

Center for Disease Control. cdc.gov/fungal/php/case-reporting/index.html, accessed 2025.

Centers for Disease Control, 2024. Reportable Fungal Diseases by State. https://www.cdc.gov/fungal/php/case-reporting/index.html.

Crum, N.F., Ballon-Landa, G., 2006. Coccidioidomycosis in pregnancy: case report and review of the literature. American Journal of Medicine 119 (11), 993. Available at https://doi.org/10.1016/j.amjmed.2006.04.022.

Cunha, C., Di Ianni, M., Bozza, S., Giovannini, G., Zagarella, S., Zelante, T., et al., 2010. Dectin-1 Y238X polymorphism associates with susceptibility to invasive aspergillosis in hematopoietic transplantation through impairment of both recipient- and donor-dependent mechanisms of antifungal immunity. Blood 116 (24), 5394–5402. Available at https://doi.org/10.1182/blood-2010-04-279307.

Davalos, O.A., Sebastian, A., Leon, N.F., Rangel, M.V., Miranda, N., Murugesh, D.K., et al., 2025. Spatiotemporal analysis of lung immune dynamics in lethal *Coccidioides posadasii* infection. mBio 16 (5). Available at https://doi.org/10.1128/mbio.02562-24, https://journals.asm.org/doi/10.1128/mbio.02562-24.

del Pilar Jiménez-A, M., Viriyakosol, S., Walls, L., Datta, S.K., Kirkland, T., Heinsbroek, S.E.M., et al., 2008. Susceptibility to *Coccidioides* species in C57BL/6 mice is associated with expression of a truncated splice variant of Dectin-1 (Clec7a). Genes & Immunity 9 (4), 338–348. Available at https://doi.org/10.1038/gene.2008.23.

Donovan, F.M., Ramadan, F.A., Lim, J.R., Buchfuhrer, J.E., Khan, R.N., Dequillfeldt, N.P., et al., 2022. Contribution of biologic response modifiers to the risk of coccidioidomycosis severity. Open Forum Infectious Diseases 9 (3). Available at https://doi.org/10.1093/ofid/ofac032, https://academic.oup.com/ofid.

Drummond, R.A., Desai, J.V., Hsu, A.P., Oikonomou, V., Vinh, D.C., Acklin, J.A., et al., 2022. Human Dectin-1 deficiency impairs macrophage-mediated defense against phaeohyphomycosis. Journal of Clinical Investigation 132 (22). Available at https://doi.org/10.1172/JCI159348, https://www.jci.org/articles/view/159348/pdf.

Ferwerda, B., Ferwerda, G., Plantinga, T.S., Willment, J.A., Van Spriel, A.B., Venselaar, H., et al., 2009. Human dectin-1 deficiency and mucocutaneous fungal infections. Journal of Medicine 361 (18), 1760–1767. Available at https://doi.org/10.1056/NEJMoa0901053, http://content.nejm.org/cgi/reprint/361/18/1760.pdf.

Fish, D.G., Ampel, N.M., Galgiani, J.N., Dols, C.L., Kelly, P.C., Johnson, C.H., et al., 1990. Coccidioidomycosis during human immunodeficiency virus infection: a review of 77 patients. Medicine (United States) 69 (6), 384–391. Available at https://doi.org/10.1097/00005792-199011000-00006.

Forteza, R., Salathe, M., Miot, F., Forteza, R., Conner, G.E., 2005. Regulated hydrogen peroxide production by duox in human airway epithelial cells. American Journal of Respiratory Cell and Molecular Biology 32 (5), 462–469. Available at https://doi.org/10.1165/rcmb.2004-0302OC.

Galgiani, J.N., Hsu, A.P., Powell, D.A., Vyas, J.M., Holland, S.M., 2023. Genetic and other determinants for the severity of coccidioidomycosis: a clinician's perspective. Journal of Fungi 9 (5). Available at https://doi.org/10.3390/jof9050554, www.mdpi.com/journal/jof.

Grizzle, A.J., Wilson, L., Nix, D.E., Galgiani, J.N., 2021. Clinical and economic burden of valley fever in arizona: an incidence-based cost-of-illness analysis. Open Forum Infectious Diseases 8 (2). Available at https://doi.org/10.1093/ofid/ofaa623, https://academic.oup.com/ofid.

Heinsbroek, S.E.M., Taylor, P.R., Rosas, M., Willment, J.A., Williams, D.L., Gordon, S., et al., 2006. Expression of functionally different dectin-1 isoforms by murine macrophages. Journal of Immunology 176 (9), 5513–5518. Available at https://doi.org/10.4049/jimmunol.176.9.5513, http://www.jimmunol.org/.

Hsu, A.P., 2024. The known and unknown "knowns" of human susceptibility to coccidioidomycosis. Journal of Fungi 10 (4). Available at https://doi.org/10.3390/jof10040256.

Hsu, A.P., Korzeniowska, A., Aguilar, C.C., Gu, J., Karlins, E., Oler, A.J., et al., 2022. Immunogenetics associated with severe coccidioidomycosis. JCI Insight 7 (22). Available at https://doi.org/10.1172/jci.insight.159491, https://insight.jci.org/articles/view/159491.

Human protein atlas, 2025. https://www.proteinatlas.org/.

Hung, C.Y., Gonzalez, A., Wüthrich, M., Klein, B.S., Cole, G.T., 2011. Vaccine immunity to coccidioidomycosis occurs by early activation of three signal pathways of T helper cell response (Th1, Th2, and Th17). Infection and Immunity 79 (11), 4511–4522. Available at https://doi.org/10.1128/IAI.05726-11, http://iai.asm.org/content/79/11/4511.full.pdf.

Hung, C.Y., M.d.P. Jiménez-Alzate, A., Gonzalez, M., Wüthrich, B.S., Klein, G.T., Cole, 2014. Interleukin-1 receptor but not toll-like receptor 2 is essential for MyD88-dependent Th17 immunity to *Coccidioides* infection. Infection and Immunity 82 (5), 2106–2114. Available at https://doi.org/10.1128/IAI.01579-13, http://iai.asm.org/content/82/5/2106.full.pdf.

Hung, C.Y., Seshan, K.R., Yu, J.J., Schaller, R., Xue, J., Basrur, V., et al., 2005. A metalloproteinase of *Coccidioides posadasii* contributes to evasion of host detection.

Infection and Immunity 73 (10), 6689–6703. Available at https://doi.org/10.1128/IAI.73.10.6689-6703.2005.

Hung, C.Y., Yu, J.J., Seshan, K.R., Reichard, U., Cole, G.T., 2002. A parasitic phase-specific adhesin of *Coccidioides* immitis contributes to the virulence of this respiratory fungal pathogen. Infection and Immunity 70 (7), 3443–3456. Available at https://doi.org/10.1128/IAI.70.7.3443-3456.2002.

Imran T., Cui, C., 2013. GATA2 transcription factor deficiency predisposing to severe disseminated Coccidioidomycosis. Front. Immunol. Conference Abstract: 15th International Congress of Immunology (ICI). https://doi.org/10.3389/conf.fimmu.2013.02.00408.

James, A.E., Pastenkos, G., Bradway, D., Baszler, T., 2019. Autochthonous transmission of *Coccidioides* in animals, Washington, USA. Emerging Infectious Diseases 25 (1), 123–125. Available at https://doi.org/10.3201/eid2501.180411, https://wwwnc.cdc.gov/eid/article/25/1/pdfs/18-0411.pdf.

Kirkland, T.N., Fierer, J., 1983. Inbred mouse strains differ in resistance to lethal *Coccidioides* immitis infection. Infection and Immunity 40 (3), 912–916. Available at https://doi.org/10.1128/iai.40.3.912-916.1983.

Kirkland, T.N., Fierer, J., 1985. Genetic control of resistance to *Coccidioides* immitis: a single gene that is expressed in spleen cells determines resistance. The Journal of Immunology 135 (1), 548–552. Available at https://doi.org/10.4049/jimmunol.135.1.548.

Krase, I.Z., Garabedian, E., Fuleihan, R., Sacco, K., 2022a. Prevalence of coccidioidomycosis in primary immunodeficiency: data from the USIDNET registry. Clinical Immunology 245, 109135. Available at https://doi.org/10.1016/j.clim.2022.109135.

Krase, I.Z., Woodward, J., Bauer, C.S., Miller, H., Sacco, K., 2022b. Seronegative mediastinal coccidioidomycosis as a novel presentation of CTPS1 combined immunodeficiency. Open Forum Infectious Diseases 9 (8), ofac403. Available at https://doi.org/10.1093/ofid/ofac403, https://academic.oup.com/ofid.

Kupferwasser, D., Miller, L.G., 2021. Sociodemographic factors associated with patients hospitalised for coccidioidomycosis in California and Arizona, State Inpatient Database 2005–2011. Epidemiology and Infection 149. Available at https://doi.org/10.1017/s0950268820002836.

Lewis, E.R.G., David, V.R., Doyle, A.L., Rajabi, K., Kiefer, J.A., Pirrotte, P., et al., 2015. Differences in host innate responses among *Coccidioides* isolates in a murine model of pulmonary coccidioidomycosis. Eukaryotic Cell 14 (10), 1043–1053. Available at https://doi.org/10.1128/EC.00122-15, http://ec.asm.org/content/14/10/1043.full.pdf.

Litvintseva, A.P., Marsden-Haug, N., Hurst, S., Hill, H., Gade, L., Driebe, E.M., et al., 2015. Valley fever: finding new places for an old disease: *Coccidioides* immitis found in Washington state soil associated with recent human infection. Clinical Infectious Diseases 60 (1), e1. Available at https://doi.org/10.1093/cid/ciu681, http://cid.oxfordjournals.org/content/by/year.

Liu, X., Boyer, M.A., Holmgren, A.M., Shin, S., 2020. Legionella-infected macrophages engage the alveolar epithelium to metabolically reprogram myeloid cells and promote antibacterial inflammation. Cell Host and Microbe 28 (5), 683. Available at https://doi.org/10.1016/j.chom.2020.07.019, http://www.elsevier.com.

Masannat, F.Y., Ampel, N.M., 2010. Coccidioidomycosis in patients with HIV-1 infection in the era of potent antiretroviral therapy. Clinical Infectious Diseases 50 (1), 1–7. Available at https://doi.org/10.1086/648719.

Matzinger, P., 1994. Tolerance, danger, and the extended family. Annual Review of Immunology 12 (1), 991–1045. Available at https://doi.org/10.1146/annurev.iy.12.040194.005015.

McHardy, I., Reagan, K.L., Sebastian, J.F., Barker, B., Bays, D.J., Dandekar, S., et al., 2022. Sex differences in susceptibility to coccidioidomycosis. Open Forum Infectious Diseases 9 (3). Available at https://doi.org/10.1093/ofid/ofab543, https://academic.oup.com/ofid.

Meyts, I., Bousfiha, A., Duff, C., Singh, S., Lau, Y.L., Condino-Neto, A., et al., 2021. Primary immunodeficiencies: a decade of progress and a promising future. Frontiers in Immunology 11. Available at https://doi.org/10.3389/fimmu.2020.625753.

Mills, K.A.M., Westermann, F., Espinosa, V., Rosiek, E., Desai, J.V., Aufiero, M.A., et al., 2025. GM-CSF–mediated epithelial-immune cell cross-talk orchestrates pulmonary immunity to *Aspergillus fumigatus*. Science Immunology 10 (105). Available at https://doi.org/10.1126/sciimmunol.adr0547.

Narra, H.P., Shubitz, L.F., Mandel, M.A., Trinh, H.T., Griffin, K., Buntzman, A.S., et al., 2016. A *Coccidioides posadasii* CPS1 deletion mutant is avirulent and protects mice from lethal infection. Infection and Immunity 84 (10), 3007–3016. Available at https://doi.org/10.1128/IAI.00633-16, http://iai.asm.org/content/84/10/3007.full.pdf.

Odio, C.D., Marciano, B.E., Galgiani, J.N., Holland, S.M., 2017. Risk factors for disseminated coccidioidomycosis, United States. Emerging Infectious Diseases 23 (2), 308–311. Available at https://doi.org/10.3201/eid2302.160505, https://wwwnc.cdc.gov/eid/article/23/2/pdfs/16-0505.pdf.

Oliveira-Marques, V., Silva, T., Cunha, F., Covas, G., Marinho, H.S., Antunes, F., et al., 2013. A quantitative study of the cell-type specific modulation of c-Rel by hydrogen peroxide and TNF-α Redox Biology 1 (1), 347–352. Available at https://doi.org/10.1016/j.redox.2013.05.004.

Powell, D.A., Hsu, A.P., Shubitz, L.F., Butkiewicz, C.D., Moale, H., Trinh, H.T., et al., 2022a. Mouse model of a human STAT4 point mutation that predisposes to disseminated coccidiomycosis. ImmunoHorizons 6 (2), 130–143. Available at https://doi.org/10.4049/immunohorizons.2200007, https://www.immunohorizons.org/content/6/2.

Powell, D.A., Hsu, A.P., Butkiewicz, C.D., Trinh, H.T., Frelinger, J.A., Holland, S.M., et al., 2022b. Vaccine protection of mice with primary immunodeficiencies against disseminated coccidioidomycosis. Frontiers in Cellular and Infection Microbiology 11. Available at https://doi.org/10.3389/fcimb.2021.790488, http://www.frontiersin.org/Cellular_and_Infection_Microbiology/archive.

Powell, D.A., Shubitz, L.F., Butkiewicz, C.D., Trinh, H.T., Donovan, F.M., Frelinger, J.A., et al., 2022c. TNFα blockade inhibits both initial and continued control of pulmonary *Coccidioides*. Frontiers in Cellular and Infection Microbiology 11. Available at https://doi.org/10.3389/fcimb.2021.796114.

Powers, A.E., Bender, J.M., Kumánovics, A., Ampofo, K., Augustine, N., Pavia, A.T., et al., 2009. *Coccidioides* immitis meningitis in a patient with hyperimmunoglobulin e syndrome due to a novel mutation in signal transducer and activator of transcription. Pediatric Infectious Disease Journal 28 (7), 664–666. Available at https://doi.org/10.1097/inf.0b013e31819866ec.

Rosenstein, N.E., Emery, K.W., Werner, S.B., Kao, A., Johnson, R., Rogers, D., et al., 2001. Risk factors for severe pulmonary and disseminated coccidioidomycosis: kern County, California, 1995-1996. Clinical Infectious Diseases 32 (5), 708–714. Available at https://doi.org/10.1086/319203.

Sampaio, E.P., Hsu, A.P., Pechacek, J., Bax, H.I., Dias, D.L., Paulson, M.L., et al., 2013. Signal transducer and activator of transcription 1 (STAT1) gain-of-function mutations and disseminated coccidioidomycosis and histoplasmosis. Journal of Allergy and Clinical Immunology 131 (6), 1624. Available at https://doi.org/10.1016/j.jaci.2013.01.052. Available from: http://www.elsevier.com/inca/publications/store/6/2/3/3/6/8/index.htt.

Shubitz, L.F., Powell, D.A., Butkiewicz, C.D., Lewis, M.L., Trinh, H.T., Frelinger, J.A., et al., 2021. A chronic murine disease model of coccidioidomycosis using coccidioides posadasii, strain 1038. Journal of Infectious Diseases 223 (1), 166–173. Available at https://doi.org/10.1093/infdis/jiaa419, http://jid.oxfordjournals.org/content/current.

Shubitz, L.F., Powell, D.A., Butkiewicz, C.D., Frelinger, J.A., Galgiani, J.N., 2025. Recall interferon-γ responses against *Coccidioides* are a surrogate marker for vaccine response in dogs. American Journal of Veterinary Research 86 (9). Available at https://doi.org/10.2460/ajvr.25.04.0119.

Singh, V.R., Smith, D.K., Lawerence, J., Kelly, P.C., Thomas, A.R., Spitz, B., et al., 1996. Coccidioidomycosis in patients infected with human immunodeficiency virus: Review of 91 cases at a single institution. Clinical Infectious Diseases 23 (3), 563–568. Available at https://doi.org/10.1093/clinids/23.3.563, http://cid.oxfordjournals.org/content/by/year.

Smith, C.E., Beard, R.R., 1946. Varieties of coccidioidal infection in relation to the epidemiology and control of the diseases. American journal of public health and the nation's health 36 (12), 1394–1402. Available at https://doi.org/10.2105/ajph.36.12.1394.

Stanga, S.D., Dajud, M.V., 2008. Visual changes in a 4-year-old. Clinical Pediatrics 47 (9), 959–961. Available at https://doi.org/10.1177/0009922808319788.

Takada, Y., Mukhopadhyay, A., Kundu, G.C., Mahabeleshwar, G.H., Singh, S., Aggarwal, B.B., 2003. Hydrogen peroxide activates NF-κB through tyrosine phosphorylation of IκBα and serine phosphorylation of p65. Evidence for the involvement of IκBα kinase and Syk protein-tyrosine kinase. Journal of Biological Chemistry 278 (26), 24233–24241. Available at https://doi.org/10.1074/jbc.M212389200.

Thompson III, G.R., 2022. Coccidioidomycosis and valley fever. https://emedicine.medscape.com/article/215978.

Truong, C.N., Nailor, M.D., Walia, R., Cherrier, L., Nasar, A., Goodlet, K.J., 2022. Universal lifelong fungal prophylaxis and risk of coccidioidomycosis in lung transplant recipients living in an endemic area. Clinical Infectious Diseases 74 (11), 1966–1971. Available at https://doi.org/10.1093/cid/ciab752, http://cid.oxfordjournals.org/content/by/year.

Vinh, D.C., Masannat, F., Dzioba, R.B., Galgiani, J.N., Holland, S.M., 2009. Refractory disseminated coccidioidomycosis and mycobacteriosis in interferon-γ receptor 1 deficiency. Clinical Infectious Diseases 49 (6), e62. Available at https://doi.org/10.1086/6055320.

Vinh, D.C., Schwartz, B., Hsu, A.P., Miranda, D.J., Valdez, P.A., Fink, D., et al., 2011. Interleukin-12 receptor β1 deficiency predisposing to disseminated coccidioidomycosis. linical Infectious Diseases 52 (4), e99. Available at https://doi.org/10.1093/cid/ciq215.

Viriyakosol, S., Fierer, J., Brown, G.D., Kirkland, T.N., 2005. Innate immunity to the pathogenic fungus *Coccidioides posadasii* is dependent on Toll-like receptor 2 and Dectin-1. Infection and Immunity 73 (3), 1553–1560. Available at https://doi.org/10.1128/IAI.73.3.1553-1560.2005.

Viriyakosol, S., Jimenez, Md.P., Gurney, M.A., Ashbaugh, M.E., Fierer, J., 2013. Dectin-1 is required for resistance to coccidioidomycosis in mice. mBio 4 (1). Available at https://doi.org/10.1128/mBio.00597-12, http://mbio.asm.org/content/4/1/e00597-12.full.pdf+html.

Viriyakosol, S., Walls, L., Okamoto, S., Raz, E., Williams, D.L., Fierer, J., et al., 2018. Myeloid differentiation factor 88 and interleukin-1r1 signaling contribute to resistance to *Coccidioides immitis*. Infection and Immunity 86 (6). Available at https://doi.org/10.1128/iai.00028-18.

Washington Department of Health Coccidioidomycosis (Valley Fever), 2025. https://www.doh.wa.gov/public-health-provider-resources/notifiable-conditions/coccidioidomycosis.

Williams, S.L., Benedict, K., Jackson, B.R., Rajeev, M., Cooksey, G., Ruberto, I., et al., 2025. Estimated burden of coccidioidomycosis. JAMA Network Open, e2513572. Available at https://doi.org/10.1001/jamanetworkopen.2025.13572, https://jamanetwork.com/journals/jamanetworkopen.

Wilson, D.L., Zhou, L., Sudano, D.G., Ashbeck, E.L., Kwoh, C.K., Krebs, L., et al., 2024. Risk of coccidioidomycosis infection among individuals using biologic response modifiers, corticosteroids, and oral small molecules. ACR Open Rheumatology 6 (5), 287–293. Available at https://doi.org/10.1002/acr2.11654, https://onlinelibrary.wiley.com/journal/25785745.

Wilson, L., Ting, J., Lin, H., Shah, R., MacLean, M., Peterson, M.W., et al., 2019. The rise of valley fever: prevalence and cost burden of coccidioidomycosis infection in California. International Journal of Environmental Research and Public Health 16 (7), 1113. Available at https://doi.org/10.3390/ijerph16071113.

Xue, J., Chen, X., Selby, D., Hung, C.-Y., Yu, J.-J., Cole, G.T., 2009. A genetically engineered live attenuated vaccine of *Coccidioides posadasii* protects BALB/c Mice against coccidioidomycosis. Infection and Immunity 77 (8), 3196–3208. Available at https://doi.org/10.1128/iai.00459–09.

CHAPTER

10

Immune checkpoint inhibition in the treatment of fungal infections

Sibylle C. Mellinghoff[1,2], Rosanne Sprute[1,2], Michael von Bergwelt-Baildon[3], Oliver A. Cornely[1,2,4] and Sebastian Wurster[5]

[1]University of Cologne, Faculty of Medicine and University Hospital Cologne, Department I of Internal Medicine, Excellence Centre for Medical Mycology (ECMM), Cologne, Germany,
[2]University of Cologne, Faculty of Medicine and University Hospital Cologne, Chair Translational Research, Cologne Excellence Cluster on Cellular Stress Responses in Aging-Associated Diseases (CECAD), Cologne, Germany,
[3]Department of Medicine III, University Hospital, LMU Munich, Munich, Germany,
[4]Faculty of Medicine and University Hospital Cologne, University of Cologne, Cologne, North Rhine-Westphalia, Germany,
[5]Department of Infectious Diseases, Infection Control and Employee Health, The University of Texas MD Anderson Cancer Center, Houston, TX, United States

Introduction

Given the continuous exposure to pathogens, environmental stimuli, and autoantigens, human immune homeostasis requires a finely tuned balance between stimulatory and regulatory signals (Shirafkan et al., 2024). So-called immune checkpoints are an integral part of these immunoregulatory networks and serve as negative feedback loops (comparable to an "off-switch") at critical junctures of innate and adaptive immune interplay (Sharma et al., 2023). While these checkpoints are pivotal for self-tolerance and prevention of overzealous immune responses, they can drive a state of immune paralysis and exhaustion in patients with cancer or infection (Abers et al., 2019; Wherry, 2011). These immunoparalytic mechanisms are best characterized in the context of antitumor immunity and are associated with a progressive loss of T-cell functionality and hyporesponsiveness of other immune cell populations, such as natural killer (NK) cells and phagocytes against cancer cells (Abers et al., 2019; Wherry, 2011; Blank et al., 2019; Wurster and Watowich, 2022) (Fig. 10.1).

Immune checkpoint inhibitors (ICIs) are therapeutic antibodies that block these immunosuppressive feedback loops (Fig. 10.1). Over the past decade, ICIs have led

Immunological Insights and Emerging Therapeutics in Medical Mycology. DOI: https://doi.org/10.1016/B978-0-443-23636-5.00010-1

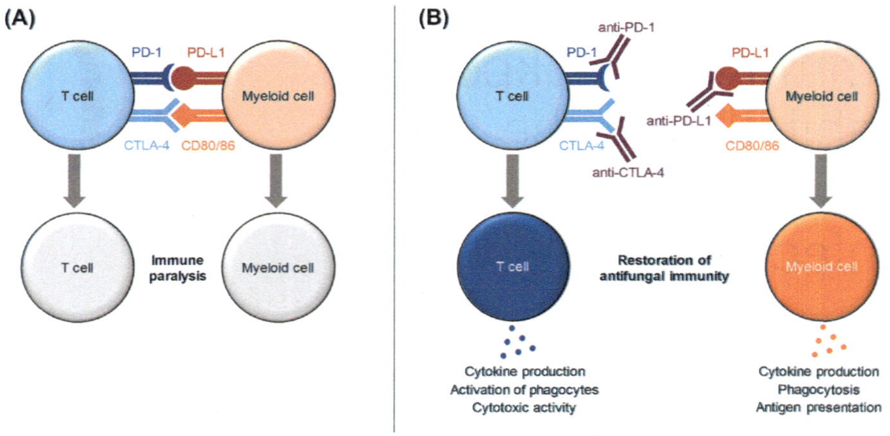

FIGURE 10.1

Role of checkpoint pathways in host defense against malignancies and infections. (A) The interaction of PD-1 and CTLA-4 on T cells with PD-L1 and the CD80/86 complex on myeloid cells serves as a negative (immunoregulatory) feedback loop and can lead to immune paralysis in patients with malignancies or infection. (B) Blockade of the checkpoint targets CTLA-4, PD-1, or PD-L1 with therapeutic antibodies can restore the activation of T cells and myeloid cells and thereby harness host immunity against tumors or pathogens. *CD*, cluster of differentiation; *CTLA-4*, cytotoxic T lymphocyte antigen 4; *PD-1*, programmed cell death protein 1; *PD-L1*, programmed death ligand 1.

to breakthroughs in the treatment of many solid cancers and are also increasingly utilized in the management of hematologic malignancies (Sharma et al., 2023, 2021; Pophali et al., 2024). Although dozens of potentially druggable checkpoint pathways have been identified and new targets are being explored in clinical trials, most ICIs currently approved for cancer immunotherapy either target the programmed cell death protein 1/programmed death ligand 1 (PD-1/PD-L1) pathway or cytotoxic T-lymphocyte antigen 4 (CTLA-4) (Sharma et al., 2023, 2021; Buchbinder and Desai, 2016).

Beyond the success story of ICIs in cancer immunotherapy, a rapidly increasing number of studies have shown an involvement of checkpoint pathways and potential benefit of ICI therapy in infectious diseases, including invasive fungal diseases (IFDs) (Abers et al., 2019; Wurster and Watowich, 2022). In this chapter, we outline the evidence for a role of checkpoint pathways as modulators of antifungal immune defense, summarize preclinical and clinical reports of ICI therapy in medical mycology, discuss critical gaps of knowledge and challenges for clinical translation, and lay out a roadmap to translate the promise of ICIs in IFD management.

The role of checkpoint pathways in regulating antifungal host defense

Several studies found increased expression of checkpoint markers in mouse models and patients with IFDs, often combined with surrogates of functional impairment of antifungal immunity. For instance, increased expression of the exhaustion markers PD-1 and PD-L1 was found in patients with *Candida* sepsis and was associated with suppression of stimulatory signals of T-helper cells (Spec et al., 2016). In another study, expression patterns of checkpoint markers in patients with invasive candidiasis resembled those in tumor-infiltrating lymphocytes (Mellinghoff et al., 2025). Furthermore, the upregulation of PD-1 and other checkpoint markers was associated with poor survival outcomes, and analyses of patient cells revealed PD-1-dependent hypofunctionality of T-cell responses to *Candida albicans* antigens (Mellinghoff et al., 2025). Induction of checkpoint pathways was also demonstrated upon stimulation of mononuclear blood cells from healthy donors with *C. albicans* antigens (Deng et al., 2021) and in mouse models of *C. albicans* (Shindo et al., 2017; Yu et al., 2022) and *C. auris* sepsis (Wurster et al., 2022).

Several recent studies have shed light on the role of checkpoint molecules in *Candida*-induced immune paralysis. PD-L1 induction after β-glucan stimulation or *C. albicans* bloodstream infection was shown to suppress the mobilization of neutrophils from the bone marrow through regulation of chemokine signaling (Yu et al., 2022). Others have identified PD-L1 as a receptor directly binding the ribosomal yeast protein Rpl20b during phagosomal degradation, resulting in enhanced production of both proinflammatory cytokines and IL-10, a cytokine known to induce regulatory T-cell polarization (Li et al., 2024). Similarly, cell-surface glycoproteins of *C. albicans* were shown to bind the checkpoint receptor T cell immunoreceptor with immunoglobulin and ITIM domains (TIGIT), resulting in immune evasion through inhibition of T and NK cells (Charpak-Amikam et al., 2022).

Moreover, several studies have shown robust early upregulation of checkpoint pathways in patients and mice with mold pneumonias. For instance, patients with invasive aspergillosis and mucormycosis displayed an immune phenotype characterized by T-cell exhaustion, with PD-1 being the most significantly upregulated checkpoint marker (Mellinghoff et al., 2025). This observation was partially influenced by underlying malignancies and treatments in these critically ill and multimorbid patients, highlighting the dynamic nature of immune exhaustion in these infections (Mellinghoff et al., 2025). Nuanced differences in immune checkpoint expression suggested that invasive aspergillosis had an overall more profound impact on immune dysregulation than mucormycosis, whereas the latter induced stronger PD-1 upregulation (Mellinghoff et al., 2025).

Induction of exhaustion signals was corroborated by transcriptional profiling of lungs from neutropenic mice with invasive pulmonary aspergillosis, mucormycosis, and fusariosis, indicating the rapid emergence of T-cell exhaustion within seven days after infection, along with paralysis of antifungal effector responses (Wurster et al., 2024). Although the specific contributions of fungal versus host-based drivers of immune exhaustion remain unclear, there is evidence that *Aspergillus* cell wall antigens can stimulate checkpoint pathways and promote T-cell polarization toward a regulatory phenotype (Stephen-Victor et al., 2017). Additionally, quantitative and qualitative changes in cytotoxic T-cell (Wurster et al., 2024) and NK-cell (Mellinghoff et al., 2025; Wurster et al., 2024) responses may contribute to impaired antifungal immunity during mold infections.

Increased expression of checkpoint molecules was also seen in patients and mice with other IFDs. Specifically, elevated PD-1/PD-L1 expression was found on lymphocytes and macrophages of mice with persistent cryptococcal lung infection (Roussey et al., 2017) and on T and B cells of patients with *Pneumocystis* pneumonia (PCP) (Zhang et al., 2020). Expression of these checkpoint markers was associated with impaired phagocytic capacity and T-cell functionality in mice with PCP (Zhang et al., 2020). Furthermore, two studies showed induction of PD-1 and CTLA-4 signaling in patients and mice with paracoccidioidomycosis (Campanelli et al., 2003; Cacere et al., 2008). While the functional relevance of checkpoint induction in paracoccidioidomycosis was debated (Cacere et al., 2008), PD-1 signaling critically compromised host resistance in a histoplasmosis mouse model by attenuating T-cell proliferation and cytokine responses (Lázár-Molnár et al., 2008).

In summary, preclinical models and analyses of specimens from patients with fungal sepsis, invasive yeast infections, mold pneumonias, and endemic mycoses have provided robust evidence for induction of immune checkpoint pathways, especially the PD-1/PD-L1 pathway, by fungal antigen challenge or infection. Moreover, upregulation of these pathways has been associated with attenuated innate immune effector responses, altered immune cell recruitment, and hyporesponsiveness of the T-cell system, suggesting that checkpoint signals contribute to paralyzed immune defense after IFDs (Wurster and Watowich, 2022).

Preclinical studies of immune checkpoint inhibitor therapy in fungal infection models

In addition to the observational immune phenotyping studies discussed above, several groups have explored ICI therapy in murine models of fungal sepsis, mold pneumonias, and other IFDs. Initial proof-of-concept data for the efficacy of antifungal ICI therapy were provided by two landmark studies in the early 2000s: McGaha and Murphy showed that CTLA-4 blockade significantly prolonged survival of mice infected with cryptococcal pneumonia and enhanced responses to immunization with *C. neoformans* antigens (McGaha and Murphy, 2000), while Lázár-Molnár et al. demonstrated that PD-1-deficient mice or those receiving PD-1 inhibitors had improved outcomes after *Histoplasma capsulatum* infection (Lázár-Molnár et al., 2008).

Inspired by the evolving understanding of sepsis-induced immune paralysis (Nakamori et al., 2021; Venet and Monneret, 2018), subsequent work on antifungal ICI therapy focused heavily on fungal sepsis models. Several groups independently showed therapeutic benefits of PD-1/PD-L1 (Shindo et al., 2017; Chang et al., 2013) and CTLA-4 (Chang et al., 2013; Inoue et al., 2011) inhibitors in primary and/or secondary (postperitonitis) *C. albicans* sepsis models. Importantly, adjunct ICI therapy provided an added survival benefit when given along with effective antifungal therapy (fluconazole) (Chang et al., 2013). Similarly, adjunct anti-PD-1 was effective when given along with amphotericin B in a postperitonitis Aspergillus *fumigatus* bloodstream infection model (Vu et al., 2020).

Additionally, several recent studies explored ICI therapy in fungal pneumonia models. For instance, anti-PD-1 therapy significantly improved outcomes and fungal clearance in a neutropenic mouse model of invasive pulmonary aspergillosis, either alone or in synergy with the immunomodulatory antifungal agent caspofungin (Wurster et al., 2020). Likewise, anti-PD-1/PD-L1 monotherapy was effective in neutropenic mice with invasive pulmonary mucormycosis (Preite et al., 2024). A follow-up study corroborated significantly improved outcomes of invasive pulmonary mucormycosis and reversal of infection-induced immune paralysis when anti-PD-L1 was added to first-line antifungal therapy (isavuconazole), especially when anti-PD-L1 was given early (3 days postinfection) (Wurster et al., 2024). Other studies in fungal pneumonia models underscored the promise of PD-1 pathway inhibitors in mice with persistent cryptococcal lung infection (Roussey et al., 2017) and those with PCP (Zhang et al., 2020). Moreover, recent studies demonstrated high efficacy of both anti-PD-1 and anti-CTLA-4 in controlling fungal dissemination and improving outcomes in a mouse model of pulmonary paracoccidioidomycosis (Preite et al., 2024).

Notably, ICI dosing has been highly heterogeneous among these preclinical studies, with most groups using intensive ICI regimens, that is, multidose therapy at oncologic dosing. Although dosing regimens are not immediately transferable between murine and human ICI agents, some preclinical studies in fungal infection models suggested improved tolerability and outcomes with low-dose ICI therapy (Inoue et al., 2011; Wurster et al., 2020).

As extensively reviewed elsewhere (Wurster and Watowich, 2022), surrogates of enhanced antifungal immunity after ICI therapy in preclinical models included a combination of increased T-cell proliferation and activation, more favorable (type-1-prone) polarization of T-cell immunity, increased recruitment of neutrophils to the site of infection due to altered chemokine release, and improved fungicidal activity of mononuclear phagocytes. However, most of these studies relied on narrow and static immunological analyses. Dynamic data on systemic and organ-specific changes in the antifungal immune environment after ICI therapy are scarce, as are detailed data on off-target toxicities and immune-related adverse events (irAEs) in preclinical models.

Clinical exploration of immune checkpoint inhibitor therapy in medical mycology

In addition to emerging evidence from preclinical models, several recent case studies have explored the experimental application of ICI therapy, especially the PD-1 antagonist nivolumab, in patients with refractory IFDs (Grimaldi et al., 2017; Banck et al., 2021; Serris et al., 2022; Lukaszewicz et al., 2022; Khatamzas et al., 2022). These cases frequently involved the concurrent administration of an ICI agent and other immunomodulators like interferon-gamma (IFN-γ) to augment host immune responses against persistent fungal pathogens.

A significant case involved a previously healthy 30-year-old female patient who endured extensive abdominal trauma following a terrorist attack (Grimaldi et al., 2017). She developed peritoneal invasive mucormycosis caused by *Rhizopus* species, which proved refractory to antifungal therapy. The introduction of nivolumab combined with IFN-γ led to substantial clinical improvement and infection control (Banck et al., 2021). In another case, a 51-year-old female with relapsed acute myeloid leukemia following hematopoietic stem cell transplantation presented with coinfections involving sino-orbital mucormycosis (*Lichtheimia ramosa*) and aspergillosis (*A. fumigatus*), both progressive when treated with conventional antifungal regimens (Serris et al., 2022). Administration of nivolumab and IFN-γ resulted in partial clinical response, suggesting that immunotherapy may complement antifungal treatments (Banck et al., 2021). A third case involved a 56-year-old male diabetic patient admitted to the intensive care unit with severe COVID-19 (Serris et al., 2022). He subsequently developed pulmonary aspergillosis and cerebral mucormycosis, both refractory to antifungal agents. The patient was treated with nivolumab in conjunction with IFN-γ, leading initially to a reduction in cerebral abscess size and normalization of fungal biomarkers. However, the patient eventually succumbed to complications from nosocomial infections and multiorgan failure (Serris et al., 2022). Two other patients, one with a polymicrobial soft tissue infection involving *Aspergillus* and various Mucorales species and one with disseminated fusariosis, recovered after ICI therapy (Lukaszewicz et al., 2022; Khatamzas et al., 2022); however, the latter patient developed adrenal insufficiency, possibly due to ICI-induced immunotoxicity (Khatamzas et al., 2022). Moreover, a recent case series from France provided further evidence that combining anti-PD-1 monoclonal antibodies and IFN-γ with standard antifungal treatment can reverse immune paralysis in patients with severe, life-threatening invasive mold diseases. In a cohort of eight patients with refractory infections—primarily mucormycosis—who exhibited high T-cell PD-1 expression, six survived following adjunctive immunotherapy (Serris et al., 2026).

These clinical observations underscore the potential utility of ICIs, especially as part of multimodal therapy, for managing refractory IFD by potentiating host immune defense. The varied outcomes highlight the complexity of these infections and emphasize the need for comprehensive research to elucidate optimal patient selection criteria, therapeutic timing, and safety considerations. Robust clinical trials are now imperative to further evaluate the efficacy and safety of this approach, identify patient subgroups most likely to benefit, and assess the balance between therapeutic gains and potential adverse effects.

Gaps of knowledge

Despite the apparent parallels between the microenvironment of tumors and infectious diseases (Abers et al., 2019), numerous questions remain regarding pathogen-specific and organ-specific changes during IFDs. Systematic preclinical and, prospectively, clinical studies on synergies with antifungal agents and other immunomodulators are necessary to further assess the clinical application of antifungal immune checkpoint therapy. This should include detailed analyses of synergies with immunopharmacological effects of existing (Wurster and Watowich, 2022; Wurster et al., 2020; Ben-Ami et al., 2008) and new antifungal agents (Matsuo et al., 2024). Omics-driven analyses (Eisfeld et al., 2024) of tissues from advanced preclinical models and sequentially collected patient specimens would provide multidimensional data to characterize systemic and site-specific immune dynamics after antifungal ICI therapy.

Although it has been hypothesized that oncologic ICI therapy may provide an added "double hit" benefit by boosting host defense against opportunistic pathogens (Daver and Kontoyiannis, 2017), this hypothesis remains to be confirmed by epidemiologic or experimental data. While firm epidemiologic studies with robust denominators are lacking, reports of IFDs have been exceedingly rare in cancer patients receiving ICIs and have been partially associated with immunosuppressive therapies to mitigate ICI-induced irAEs (Bernardes and Hohl, 2020). However, ICIs have historically been used predominantly in cancer entities associated with a relatively low underlying IFD risk (e.g., melanoma, lung cancer) (Sharma et al., 2023), precluding firm conclusions regarding their "double hit" benefit in strengthening antifungal immunity.

Thus far, all preclinical studies in fungal infection models have focused on the PD-1/PD-L1 and CTLA-4 pathways, and all published clinical reports involved anti-PD-1. However, numerous other checkpoint targets, such as T-cell immunoglobulin and mucin-domain containing-3, LAG-3, and TIGIT, are being explored in investigational cancer immunology studies (Pant et al., 2020; Cai et al., 2023), and the LAG3 antibody relatlimab has obtained FDA approval for combination therapy of advanced melanomas (FDA approves Opdualag for unresectable or metastatic melanoma, 2022). Systematic exploration of these targets, some of which were shown to be upregulated in patients with IFDs (Mellinghoff et al., 2025), might provide new avenues to boost antifungal immunity. Notably, some of the newer ICI agents targeting these "alternative" checkpoint pathways have highly favorable toxicity profiles (Cai et al., 2023) and might therefore provide advantages in the inflammatory environment of an acute infection.

Furthermore, the optimal timing of ICI administration in patients with IFDs remains elusive. Based on the more advanced experience with ICIs in the management of JC virus-associated encephalitis in severely immunocompromised patients, effective reinvigoration of host defense tends to rely on both the antigenic burden and the degree of immune exhaustion (Beck and Cortese, 2020). This optimal "window of opportunity" will need to be elucidated in experimental and clinical mycology studies. Although the importance of timely initiation of salvage immunotherapy was acknowledged in a clinical case report (Serris et al., 2022), only one preliminary preclinical study has explored timing-dependent benefits of antifungal ICI therapy, finding that early adjunct ICI therapy combined with first-line antifungals was the most promising strategy to alleviate immune paralysis and improve outcomes in mice with invasive pulmonary mucormycosis (Wurster et al., 2024). However, many additional variables, such as underlying malignancies, novel molecularly targeted anticancer agents, and coinfections, can significantly alter the immune dynamics and responses to antifungal immunotherapy. Thus far, these variables are largely unexplored in preclinical models.

As discussed above, optimal dosing of ICI agents in patients with IFDs will also need to be defined and may depend on the time of administration (i.e., preemptive therapy vs salvage settings), degree of inflammation, antigen burden, and severity of immune exhaustion. Establishing an optimal dosing strategy that balances efficacy and safety remains a key hurdle in advancing ICI therapy towards routine clinical use for infectious diseases.

How to advance immune checkpoint inhibitor therapy toward clinical translation

To advance ICI therapy towards clinical translation in patients with IFDs, well-designed clinical trials will be essential. This section will discuss key considerations for such clinical trials (Fig. 10.2).

Patient selection and trial designs

Defining criteria for patient eligibility is crucial. This includes assessing immune status, comorbidities, fungal pathogen characteristics, and previous antifungal treatment responses. Adaptive trial designs may provide flexibility to adjust treatment protocols based on interim results. Dose optimization studies will be critical to balance therapeutic benefits with toxicity risks. Phase II studies can then expand to assess efficacy and immunological responses in specific patient subgroups and explore combinations of ICIs with existing antifungal agents and immunomodulators like IFN-γ. Eventually, randomized controlled trials comparing

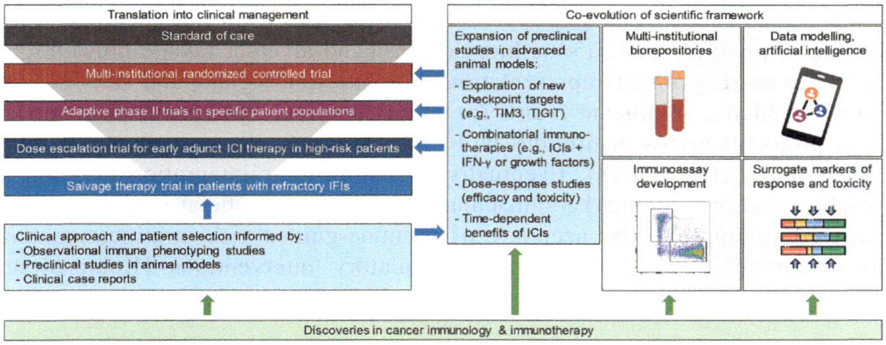

FIGURE 10.2

Roadmap toward clinical translation of ICI therapy in medical mycology. *ICIs*, immune checkpoint inhibitors; *IFIs*, invasive fungal infections; *IFN-γ*, interferon gamma; *TIGIT*, T cell immunoreceptor with immunoglobulin and ITIM domains; *TIM-3*, T-cell immunoglobulin and mucin-domain containing-3.

standard antifungal therapy with and without ICI adjuncts are necessary for rigorous evaluation of safety and efficacy.

Endpoints and longitudinal follow-up

To allow for comparability, primary endpoints should be informed by established outcome parameters for antifungal trials (Segal et al., 2008). This includes time to resolution of clinical symptoms, microbiological infection clearance, radiological improvement, and survival outcomes. Secondary endpoints should assess immune reconstitution, fungal load reduction, and quality-of-life improvements. Posttrial surveillance will be necessary to monitor for late-onset irAEs (Keam et al., 2024; Johnson et al., 2022), recurrence of fungal infections, and long-term changes to adaptive immunity, providing insights into long-term safety and durability of the immune response.

Biomarker integration

Biomarkers for immune exhaustion, such as PD-L1 expression, maturation and activity of antigen-presenting cells, cytokine profiles, and fungal-specific immune markers, should be tracked to correlate with clinical outcomes. Such biomarkers would then guide study designs and patient selection to identify those most likely to benefit from ICI therapy. To do so, immunoassay protocols that are predominantly designed for research settings need to be tailored to clinical needs, for example, by developing robust whole blood-based assay systems (Lauruschkat et al., 2021). Additionally, analysis of biospecimens from the site of infection (e.g., tissue biopsies, broncho-alveolar lavage fluid) might provide a more granular representation of exhaustion signals and site-specific immune deficits. Significant efforts for quality assurance and standardization of assay protocols across institutions will be needed to facilitate multicenter trials (Albert-Vega et al., 2018). Eventually, algorithms for integration of clinical variables and immune markers, machine learning, and artificial intelligence are expected to improve the accuracy of immune-guided risk stratification and inform timely personalized immunomodulatory interventions (Komorowski et al., 2022).

Conclusion

A continuously growing body of experimental studies using a combination of in vitro experiments, murine infection models, and immune profiling of patient specimens have revealed upregulation of immune checkpoint markers such as PD-1/PD-L1 and CTLA-4 in response to many IFDs. Although the functional consequences of checkpoint induction in patients and mice with IFDs are not fully understood, several studies have shown that upregulation of these exhaustion signals was associated with paralyzed antifungal immune defense (Wurster and Watowich, 2022). Consequently, initial clinical evidence suggests that immune checkpoint upregulation might have prognostic implications in patients with IFDs (Mellinghoff et al., 2025). Moreover, several preclinical proof-of-concept studies in fungal sepsis and pneumonia models have demonstrated the safety and efficacy of ICI immunotherapy, either alone or combined with antifungal therapy, and provided initial mechanistic insights into therapeutic immunomodulation. Likewise, anecdotal clinical reports suggested potential utility of ICIs as salvage therapy for recalcitrant mold infections; however, heterogeneity of outcomes, potential reporting bias, limited immunologic data, and lack of systematic clinical studies preclude firm conclusions.

Given the complexities surrounding immune modulation in immunocompromised patients, a cautious and stepwise approach is required to mitigate risks while maximizing therapeutic benefits. Thus innovative trial designs will be pivotal for translating preclinical findings into clinical practice. A combination of more advanced preclinical models, multiinstitutional biorepositories of patient specimens, high-dimensional immune profiling studies, and evolving data science capabilities is expected to inform clinical translation and drive new discoveries to intercept paralyzed antifungal immunity. Ultimately, thorough biomarker integration and immune-guided risk models might pave the way toward personalized precision medicine in antifungal immunotherapy.

References

Abers, M.S., Lionakis, M.S., Kontoyiannis, D.P., 2019. Checkpoint inhibition and infectious diseases: a good thing? Trends in Molecular Medicine 25 (12), 1080–1093. Available at https://doi.org/10.1016/j.molmed.2019.08.004, www.elsevier.com/locate/molmed.

Albert-Vega, C., Tawfik, D.M., Trouillet-Assant, S., Vachot, L., Mallet, F., Textoris, J., 2018. Immune functional assays, from custom to standardized tests for precision medicine. Frontiers in Immunology 9. Available at https://doi.org/10.3389/fimmu.2018.02367, https://www.frontiersin.org/journals/immunology#.

Banck, J.C., Mueller, N., Mellinghoff, S.C., Thelen, M., Fraccaroli, A., Blumenberg, V., et al., 2021. Immune checkpoint blockade for aspergillosis and mucormycosis coinfection. HemaSphere 5 (3), E530. Available at https://doi.org/10.1097/HS9.0000000000000530, https://journals.lww.com/hemasphere/pages/default.aspx.

Beck, E.S., Cortese, I., 2020. Checkpoint inhibitors for the treatment of JC virus-related progressive multifocal leukoencephalopathy. Current Opinion in Virology 40, 19–27. Available at https://doi.org/10.1016/j.coviro.2020.02.005, http://www.elsevier.com/wps/find/journaldescription.cws_home/724700/description#description.

Ben-Ami, R., Lewis, R.E., Kontoyiannis, D.P., 2008. Immunocompromised hosts: immunopharmacology of modern antifungals. Clinical Infectious Diseases 47 (2), 226–235. Available at https://doi.org/10.1086/589290.

Bernardes, M., Hohl, T.M., 2020. Fungal infections associated with the use of novel immunotherapeutic agents. Current Clinical Microbiology Reports 7 (4), 142–149. Available at https://doi.org/10.1007/s40588-020-00154-4, springer.com/biomed/medical+microbiology/journal/40588.

Blank, C.U., Haining, W.N., Held, W., Hogan, P.G., Kallies, A., Lugli, E., et al., 2019. Defining 'T cell exhaustion' Nature Reviews. Immunology 19 (11), 665–674. Available at https://doi.org/10.1038/s41577-019-0221-9, http://www.nature.com/nri/index.html.

Buchbinder, E.I., Desai, A., 2016. CTLA-4 and PD-1 pathways similarities, differences, and implications of their inhibition. American Journal of Clinical Oncology: Cancer Clinical Trials 39 (1), 98–106. Available at https://doi.org/10.1097/COC.0000000000000239, http://journals.lww.com/amjclinicaloncology/pages/default.aspx.

Cacere, C.R., Mendes-Giannini, M.J.S., Fontes, C.J., Kono, A., Duarte, A.J.S., Benard, G., 2008. Altered expression of the costimulatory molecules CD80, CD86, CD152, PD-1 and ICOS on T-cells from paracoccidioidomycosis patients: lack of correlation with T-cell hyporesponsiveness. Clinical Immunology 129 (2), 341–349. Available at https://doi.org/10.1016/j.clim.2008.07.008.

Cai, L., Li, Y., Tan, J., Xu, L., Li, Y., 2023. Targeting LAG-3, TIM-3, and TIGIT for cancer immunotherapy. Journal of Hematology & Oncology 16 (1). Available at https://doi.org/10.1186/s13045-023-01499-1.

Campanelli, A.P., Martins, G.A., Souto, J.T., Pereira, M.S.F., Livonesi, M.C., Martinez, R., et al., 2003. Fas-Fas ligand (CD95-CD95L) and cytotoxic T lymphocyte antigen-4 engagement mediate T cell unresponsiveness in patients with paracoccidioidomycosis. Journal of Infectious Diseases 187 (9), 1496–1505. Available at https://doi.org/10.1086/374646.

Chang, Burnham, Compton, et al., 2013. Blockade of the negative co-stimulatory molecules PD-1 and CTLA-4 improves survival in primary and secondary fungal sepsis. Critical Care (London, England) 17 (3).

Charpak-Amikam, Y., Lapidus, T., Isaacson, B., Duev-Cohen, A., Levinson, T., Elbaz, A., et al., 2022. Candida albicans evades NK cell elimination via binding of agglutinin-like sequence proteins to the checkpoint receptor TIGIT. Nature Communications 13 (1). Available at https://doi.org/10.1038/s41467-022-30087-z.

Daver, N., Kontoyiannis, D.P., 2017. Checkpoint inhibitors and aspergillosis in AML: the double hit hypothesis. The Lancet Oncology 18 (12), 1571–1573. Available at https://doi.org/10.1016/S1470–2045(17)30852-5, http://www.journals.elsevier.com/the-lancet-oncology/.

Deng, W., Su, Z., Liang, P., Ma, Y., Liu, Y., Zhang, K., et al., 2021. Single-cell immune checkpoint landscape of PBMCs stimulated with *Candida albicans*. Emerging Microbes & Infections 10 (1), 1272–1283. Available at https://doi.org/10.1080/22221751.2021.1942228.

Eisfeld, A.J., Anderson, L.N., Fan, S., Walters, K.B., Halfmann, P.J., Westhoff Smith, D., et al., 2024. A compendium of multi-omics data illuminating host responses to lethal human virus infections. Scientific Data 11 (1). Available at https://doi.org/10.1038/s41597-024-03124-3, https://www.nature.com/sdata/.

FDA approves Opdualag for unresectable or metastatic melanoma. 2022 3 21 https://www.fda.gov/drugs/resources-information-approved-drugs/fda-approves-opdualag-unresectable-or-metastatic-melanoma.

Grimaldi, D., Pradier, O., Hotchkiss, R.S., Vincent, J.L., 2017. Nivolumab plus interferon-γ in the treatment of intractable mucormycosis. The Lancet Infectious Diseases 17 (1), 18. Available at https://doi.org/10.1016/S1473–3099(16)30541-2, http://www.journals.elsevier.com/the-lancet-infectious-diseases.

Inoue, S., Bo, L., Bian, J., Unsinger, J., Chang, K., Hotchkiss, R.S., 2011. Dose-dependent effect of anti-CTLA-4 on survival in sepsis. Shock (Augusta, Ga.) 36 (1), 38–44. Available at https://doi.org/10.1097/shk.0b013e3182168cce.

Johnson, D.B., Nebhan, C.A., Moslehi, J.J., Balko, J.M., 2022. Immune-checkpoint inhibitors: long-term implications of toxicity. Nature Reviews Clinical Oncology 19 (4), 254–267. Available at https://doi.org/10.1038/s41571-022-00600-w, http://www.nature.com/nrclinonc/archive/index.html.

Keam, S., Turner, N., Kugeratski, F.G., Rico, R., Colunga-Minutti, J., Poojary, R., et al., 2024. Toxicity in the era of immune checkpoint inhibitor therapy. Frontiers in Immunology 15. Available at https://doi.org/10.3389/fimmu.2024.1447021, https://www.frontiersin.org/journals/immunology#.

Khatamzas, E., Mellinghoff, S.C., Thelen, M., Schlößer, H.A., Kunz, W., Buerkle, C., et al., 2022. Nivolumab induces long-term remission in a patient with fusariosis. European Journal of Cancer 173, 91–94. Available at https://doi.org/10.1016/j.ejca.2022.06.035, http://www.journals.elsevier.com/european-journal-of-cancer/.

Komorowski, M., Green, A., Tatham, K.C., Seymour, C., Antcliffe, D., 2022. Sepsis biomarkers and diagnostic tools with a focus on machine learning. eBioMedicine 86, 104394. Available at https://doi.org/10.1016/j.ebiom.2022.104394.

Lauruschkat, C.D., Page, L., White, P.L., Etter, S., Davies, H.E., Duckers, J., et al., 2021. Development of a simple and robust whole blood assay with dual co-stimulation to quantify the release of T-cellular signature cytokines in response to *Aspergillus fumigatus* antigens. Journal of Fungi 7 (6), 462. Available at https://doi.org/10.3390/jof7060462.

Lázár-Molnár, E., Gácser, A., Freeman, G.J., Almo, S.C., Nathenson, S.G., Nosanchuk, J.D., 2008. The PD-1/PD-L costimulatory pathway critically affects host resistance to the pathogenic fungus *Histoplasma capsulatum*. Proceedings of the National Academy of

Sciences of the United States of America 105 (7), 2658–2663. Available at https://doi.org/10.1073/pnas.0711918105, http://www.pnas.org/cgi/reprint/105/7/2658.

Li, K., Chatterjee, A., Qian, C., Lagree, K., Wang, Y., Becker, C.A., et al., 2024. Profiling phagosome proteins identifies PD-L1 as a fungal-binding receptor. Nature 630 (8017), 736–743. Available at https://doi.org/10.1038/s41586-024-07499-6.

Lukaszewicz, A.C., Venet, F., Boibieux, A., Lherm, M., Devigne, B., Monneret, G., 2022. Nivolumab and interferon-γ rescue therapy to control mixed mould and bacterial superinfection after necrotizing fasciitis and septic shock. Medical Mycology Case Reports 37, 19–22. Available at https://doi.org/10.1016/j.mmcr.2022.06.003, http://www.journals.elsevier.com/medical-mycology-case-reports/.

Matsuo, T., Wurster, S., Kontoyiannis, D.P., 2024. Good outcomes in salvage therapy of fusariosis in patients with leukemia: is it the host or the drug? Clinical Infectious Diseases 79 (2), 571–572. Available at https://doi.org/10.1093/cid/ciad768, http://cid.oxfordjournals.org/content/by/year.

McGaha, T., Murphy, J.W., 2000. CTLA-4 down-regulates the protective anticryptococcal cell-mediated immune response. Infection and Immunity 68 (8), 4624–4630. Available at https://doi.org/10.1128/IAI.68.8.4624-4630.2000.

Mellinghoff, S.C., Thelen, M., von Bergwelt-Baildon, M., Schlößer, H.A., Cornely, O.A., Sprute, R., et al., 2025. Immune phenotypes in patients with invasive mould infection support the use of PD-1 inhibition as potential treatment option. Mycoses 68 (3). Available at https://doi.org/10.1111/myc.70044, http://onlinelibrary.wiley.com/journal/10.1111/(ISSN)1439-0507.

Nakamori, Y., Park, E.J., Shimaoka, M., 2021. Immune deregulation in sepsis and septic shock: reversing immune paralysis by targeting PD-1/PD-L1 pathway. Frontiers in Immunology 11. Available at https://doi.org/10.3389/fimmu.2020.624279, https://www.frontiersin.org/journals/immunology#.

Pant, A., Medikonda, R., Lim, M., 2020. Alternative checkpoints as targets for immunotherapy. Current Oncology Reports 22 (12). Available at https://doi.org/10.1007/s11912-020-00983-y.

Pophali, P., Varela, J.C., Rosenblatt, J., 2024. Immune checkpoint blockade in hematological malignancies: current state and future potential. Frontiers in Oncology 14. Available at https://doi.org/10.3389/fonc.2024.1323914, http://www.frontiersin.org/Oncology/about.

Preite, N.W., Borges, B.M., Kaminski, Vd.L., Ayupe, M.C., Gonçalves, L.M., dos Santos, B.V., et al., 2024. Blocking the CTLA-4 and PD-1 pathways during pulmonary paracoccidioidomycosis improves immunity, reduces disease severity, and increases the survival of infected mice. Frontiers in Immunology 15. Available at https://doi.org/10.3389/fimmu.2024.1347318, https://www.frontiersin.org/journals/immunology#.

Roussey, J.A., Viglianti, S.P., Teitz-Tennenbaum, S., Olszewski, M.A., Osterholzer, J.J., 2017. Anti-PD-1 antibody treatment promotes clearance of persistent cryptococcal lung infection in mice. Journal of Immunology 199 (10), 3535–3546. Available at https://doi.org/10.4049/jimmunol.1700840, http://www.jimmunol.org/content/jimmunol/199/10/3535.full.pdf.

Segal, B.H., Herbrecht, R., Stevens, D.A., Ostrosky-Zeichner, L., Sobel, J., Viscoli, C., et al., 2008. Defining responses to therapy and study outcomes in clinical trials of invasive fungal diseases: mycoses study group and European Organization for Research and Treatment of Cancer Consensus Criteria. Clinical Infectious Diseases 47 (5), 674–683. Available at https://doi.org/10.1086/590566.

Serris, A., Guihot, A., Joffre, J., Dessajan, J., Dahuron, L., Bosch, A., et al., 2026. Emerging evidence for anti-PD-1 and IFN-γ as adjunctive immunotherapy in invasive mold infections. mBio 17, e00230–26. Available at https://doi.org/10.1128/mbio.00230-26.

Serris, A., Ouedrani, A., Uhel, F., Gazzano, M., Bedarida, V., Rouzaud, C., et al., 2022. Case report: immune checkpoint blockade plus interferon-Γ add-on antifungal therapy in the treatment of refractory Covid-associated pulmonary aspergillosis and cerebral mucormycosis. Frontiers in Immunology 13. Available at https://doi.org/10.3389/fimmu.2022.900522.

Sharma, P., Siddiqui, B.A., Anandhan, S., Yadav, S.S., Subudhi, S.K., Gao, J., et al., 2021. The next decade of immune checkpoint therapy. Cancer Discovery 11 (4), 838–857. Available at https://doi.org/10.1158/2159-8290.CD-20-1680, https://cancerdiscovery.aacrjournals.org/content/11/4/838.full.pdf.

Sharma, P., Goswami, S., Raychaudhuri, D., Siddiqui, B.A., Singh, P., Nagarajan, A., et al., 2023. Immune checkpoint therapy—current perspectives and future directions. Cell 186 (8), 1652–1669. Available at https://doi.org/10.1016/j.cell.2023.03.006.

Shindo, Y., McDonough, J.S., Chang, K.C., Ramachandra, M., Sasikumar, P.G., Hotchkiss, R.S., 2017. Anti-PD-L1 peptide improves survival in sepsis. Journal of Surgical Research 208, 33–39. Available at https://doi.org/10.1016/j.jss.2016.08.099, http://www.elsevier.com/inca/publications/store/6/2/2/9/0/1/index.htt.

Shirafkan, F., Hensel, L., Rattay, K., 2024. Immune tolerance and the prevention of autoimmune diseases essentially depend on thymic tissue homeostasis. Frontiers in Immunology 15. Available at https://doi.org/10.3389/fimmu.2024.1339714.

Spec, A., Shindo, Y., Burnham, C.-A.D., Wilson, S., Ablordeppey, E.A., Beiter, E.R., et al., 2016. T cells from patients with *Candida sepsis* display a suppressive immunophenotype. Critical Care 20 (1). Available at https://doi.org/10.1186/s13054-016-1182-z.

Stephen-Victor, E., Karnam, A., Fontaine, T., Beauvais, A., Das, M., Hegde, P., et al., 2017. *Aspergillus fumigatus* cell Wall α-(1,3)-glucan stimulates regulatory T-cell polarization by inducing PD-L1 expression on human dendritic cells. The Journal of Infectious Diseases 216 (10), 1281–1294. Available at https://doi.org/10.1093/infdis/jix469.

Venet, F., Monneret, G., 2018. Advances in the understanding and treatment of sepsis-induced immunosuppression. Nature Reviews Nephrology 14 (2), 121–137. Available at https://doi.org/10.1038/nrneph.2017.165.

Vu, C.T.B., Thammahong, A., Yagita, H., Azuma, M., Hirankarn, N., Ritprajak, P., et al., 2020. Blockade of PD-1 attenuated postsepsis aspergillosis via the activation of IFN-γ and the dampening of IL-10. Shock (Augusta, Ga.) 53 (4), 514–524. Available at https://doi.org/10.1097/SHK.0000000000001392, http://journals.lww.com/shockjournal.

Wherry, E.J., 2011. T cell exhaustion. Nature Immunology 12 (6), 492–499. Available at https://doi.org/10.1038/ni.2035.

Wurster, S., Robinson, P., Albert, N.D., Tarrand, J.J., Goff, M., Swamydas, M., et al., 2020. Protective activity of programmed cell death protein 1 blockade and synergy with caspofungin in a murine invasive pulmonary aspergillosis model. Journal of Infectious Diseases 222 (6), 989–994. Available at https://doi.org/10.1093/infdis/jiaa264, http://jid.oxfordjournals.org/content/current.

Wurster, S., Albert, N.D., Kontoyiannis, D.P., 2022. Candida auris bloodstream infection induces upregulation of the PD-1/PD-L1 immune checkpoint pathway in an immunocompetent mouse model. mSphere 7 (2). Available at https://doi.org/10.1128/msphere.00817-21, https://journals.asm.org/doi/10.1128/msphere.00817-21.

Wurster, S., Watowich, S., Kontoyiannis, D.P., 2022. Checkpoint inhibitors as immunotherapy for fungal infections: promises, challenges, and unanswered questions. Frontiers in Immunology 13.

Wurster, Albert, N.D., Kontoyiannis, 2024. Early combination therapy with isavuconazole and immune checkpoint inhibitors improves infection outcomes and alleviates paralyzed antifungal host immunity in neutropenic mice with invasive pulmonary mucormycosis. Open Forum Infect Dis 12 (S1).

Yu, Y., Wang, R.R., Miao, N.J., Tang, J.J., Zhang, Y.W., Lu, X.R., et al., 2022. PD-L1 negatively regulates antifungal immunity by inhibiting neutrophil release from bone marrow. Nature Communications 13 (1). Available at https://doi.org/10.1038/s41467-022-34722-7, https://www.nature.com/ncomms/.

Zhang, C., Rong, H.M., Li, T., Zhai, K., Tong, Z.H., 2020. PD-1 Deficiency promotes macrophage activation and T-helper cell type 1/T-helper cell type 17 response in pneumocystis pneumonia. American Journal of Respiratory Cell and Molecular Biology 62 (6), 767–782. Available at https://doi.org/10.1165/rcmb.2019-0234oc, https://www.atsjournals.org/doi/10.1165/rcmb.2019-0234OC.

CHAPTER

Bioengineering T cells for the treatment of invasive aspergillosis

11

Beeke Tappe and Juergen Loeffler

Department of Internal Medicine II, University Hospital of Wuerzburg, Wuerzburg, Germany

Introduction

Conidia from the saprophytic pathogen *Aspergillus fumigatus* are ubiquitously present in the environment, exposing humans constantly to the airborne fungal spores (Latgé, 2001). In immunocompetent individuals, conidia are killed and cleared by a variety of immune cells. In some individuals, nevertheless, the pulmonary system fails to eliminate the conidia, resulting in their germination and subsequent formation of hyphae into the lung tissue, a disease called invasive pulmonary aspergillosis (IPA). An inflammatory reaction of the immune system subsequently strengthens the alveolar damage, even leading to angio-invasion and hematogenous dissemination of *A. fumigatus* (Van De Veerdonk et al., 2017). Factors contributing to the development of IPA include neutropenia, treatments that compromise the immune system, such as those for stem cell or solid organ transplantation, and underlying viral infections, including those caused by the influenza virus, SARS-CoV-2, or HIV (Hoenigl et al., 2022; Latge and Chamilos, 2019; Salazar et al., 2022; Tappe et al., 2022).

The treatment of invasive aspergillosis (IA) remains complicated, especially for immunocompromised patients. Their weakened immune systems impair their ability to fight infections and may result in complications with conventional treatments. The Infectious Diseases Society of America guidelines on aspergillosis, for example, highlight the complexity of managing fungal infections in such patients, stressing the need for tailored therapeutic approaches and the challenges in achieving effective treatment outcomes (Patterson et al., 2016).

The efficacy of antifungal therapies, including polyenes, triazoles, and echinocandins, is limited by late diagnosis, drug toxicity, and emerging resistance. Improved diagnostic methods and real-time monitoring biomarkers are essential for advancing IA treatment, but novel therapeutics are also needed (Denning and Hope, 2010). The idea of utilizing immunomodulating therapeutic agents that specifically target the host's immune response, aiming to enhance the effectiveness of conventional antifungal therapy, was introduced (Gellin et al., 2001). Immunomodulation involves leveraging the patient's immune system to control, stabilize, and potentially eradicate the disease, a

Immunological Insights and Emerging Therapeutics in Medical Mycology. DOI: https://doi.org/10.1016/B978-0-443-23636-5.00009-5

strategy further advocated by Sam and colleagues for its potential to directly address the causes of treatment failure (Sam et al., 2018).

Genetic engineering of immune cells holds great potential to improve and complement the conventional treatment of invasive fungal diseases (IFD). Chimeric antigen receptor (CAR) engineered T cells are already used in the treatment of cancer, but due to their important role in the immune response against *A. fumigatus*, engineered T cells might be an attractive alternative to standard treatments for IPA.

Immune responses to *Aspergillus fumigatus*

Several immune cell populations are involved in the host response to *A. fumigatus*. Conidia that are not removed mechanically by the physical barrier of the respiratory tract and the antimicrobial peptides produced by the respiratory epithelial cells escape into the alveoli, where they are most often phagocytosed by alveolar macrophages (Brakhage et al., 2010; Papadopoulou et al., 2016). Neutrophils are recruited to the local infection site by chemokines and anaphylatoxins, subsequently release reactive oxygen species, and form extracellular traps (Brakhage et al., 2010; Bruns et al., 2010). Additionally, natural killer (NK) cells are recruited to the infection site and are the most significant contributors to interferon-gamma (IFN-γ) secretion (Park et al., 2009; Wang et al., 2017). Furthermore, the cross-reaction of immune cells is detrimental to the effective host response against *A. fumigatus*. NK cells can, for example, directly interact with dendritic cells (DCs) (Weiss et al., 2018). DCs not only recruit immune cells by secreting several chemokines, such as interleukin-8 (IL-8), CCL-20, and CXCL-10 and further pro-inflammatory cytokines, such as tumor necrosis factor-alpha (TNF-α) and IL-1, but also engage the adaptive immune system by presenting fungal antigens (Thammasit et al., 2021). T cells are crucial in providing protective and therapeutic responses against *A. fumigatus*. In individuals suffering from IPA, a positive correlation between the presence of *A. fumigatus*-specific T cells producing IFN-γ and improved clinical outcomes was detected (Hebart et al., 2002; Jolink et al., 2014). Consequently, research is exploring the adoptive transfer of these specific T cells, sourced from the patient's own T-cell repertoire, as an adjunct therapy for IPA, as reviewed in Ademe (2020); Papadopoulou et al. (2016).

Adoptive transfer of T cells to treat invasive pulmonary aspergillosis

There are several reasons why classical antimycotic treatments might fail, especially in immunocompromised patients. On the one hand, antifungal resistances are rising, clinically relevant strains carrying antimycotic resistance were detected

(Vitiello et al., 2023). Furthermore, the therapeutics need to reach effective concentrations at the site of infection, which has to happen in a passive manner (Zhao et al., 2019). Not only can specific interactions with other drugs affect the efficacy of antifungals, but individual patient factors, such as immune status and organ function, can impact the effectiveness of treatment (Lin et al., 2001).

Adoptive T-cell therapy, typically employed following allogeneic stem cell transplantation, leverages the adaptive immune system and the targeted increase of specific T cells to eliminate fungal infections, as demonstrated in research by Bacher and colleagues in 2015 (Bacher et al., 2015). This approach has been validated through both murine and human clinical studies, in which in vitro expanded fungus-specific T cells have shown significant clinical efficacy, as reviewed by Deo and Gottlieb (2015). Specifically, the use of *Aspergillus*-specific $CD4^+$ T cells, isolated from the spleens of immunized mice and restimulated in vitro, not only offered protection but also prolonged the survival of mice (Deo and Gottlieb, 2015).

The challenge of IPA postneutrophil recovery in up to two-thirds of alloSCT patients—during a period when adaptive immune responses are still compromised—raises a critical concern. Adoptive T-cell transfer presents a promising solution to this problem, with T cells playing a pivotal role in managing infectious diseases. The efficiency of the adoptive transfer of *Aspergillus*-specific T cells has been proven in mouse models (Bozza et al., 2003; Maldini et al., 2018). These protective T cells can be expanded ex vivo from peripheral blood, presenting a viable option for adoptive therapy. Moreover, a clinical trial by Perruccio et al. (2005) showed that recipients of haploidentical stem cell transplants suffering from IA who received a single infusion of expanded donor-derived anti-*Aspergillus* T-cell clones experienced clearance of the infection in 90% of cases within an average of approximately 8 weeks.

However, *A. fumigatus*-specific T cells are usually scarce and exhibit considerable variation in the efficacy of their T-cell receptor (TCR) concerning specificity and responsiveness. This variation poses a substantial challenge for the production and distribution of these cells for therapeutic applications (Ademe, 2020; Papadopoulou et al., 2016).

The approval of CAR T-cell therapies by the U.S. FDA in 2017 for use in cancer treatments, alongside the success of CAR T cells in B-cell malignancies, has prompted research into the application of CARs for treating infections, including fungal diseases (Seif et al., 2019). A previous study showed promising results for CAR T-cell treatment against *A. fumigatus* (Kumaresan et al., 2014). In this study, T cells were engineered with a Dectin-1 (D-) CAR that recognizes carbohydrate antigens through Dectin-1. This method effectively redirects T-cell specificity, enabling them to produce cytokines and proliferate in response to fungi. Clinically relevant numbers of D-CAR T cells could be expanded for adoptive transfer, and their ability to lyse *Aspergillus* germlings and their T_{CM} phenotype, enabling self-renewal and differentiation into effector T cells in vivo, was shown (Kumaresan et al., 2014). The research confirms D-CAR T-cells' capacity to directly target and manage *Aspergillus* infection, providing a promising basis for further studies. Beta-glucans, nevertheless, are not restricted to one species or even fungi, and therefore Dectin-1-mediated T-cell activation might interfere with a broad range of commensal and pathogenic microorganisms. Consequently, it would be advantageous to redirect the T cells to antigens derived from fungal species.

Basics of chimeric antigen receptor T cells

CARs are artificial receptors that combine antigen-binding and T-cell activating functions. These recombinant receptors consist of an antigen-recognizing extracellular targeting element, mostly a single-chain variable fragment (scFv), and an intracellular signaling domain (Wu et al., 2020). The CAR molecule is guided by a transmembrane domain through the cellular membrane. The extracellular domain is linked by a hinge region, or spacer, to a transmembrane domain, which is commonly derived from IgG, CD8, or CD28, as reviewed in Guedan et al., (2019). The biological activity of CARs, and therefore their design, has evolved over the past decades. A first improvement, inventing the so-called second-generation CAR, brought the introduction of a costimulatory domain, which is a necessity for full activation of T cells (van der Stegen et al., 2015). The most common costimulatory domains are CD28 or 4-1BB. They act through different pathways and might therefore have complementary functions. In a third generation of CARs, consequently, two signaling domains were merged, leading to better expansion and longer persistence (Ramos et al., 2018; Roselli et al., 2021). Another common modification of the CAR design is the integration of a cytokine, mainly IL-12, which enhances the CAR T-cell activity by autocrine stimulation, a construct called "T cells redirected for universal cytokine killing" (Chmielewski and Abken, 2012). Further innovations in the CAR field are the generation of universal CARs. This technique involves the disruption of genes for TCR or major histocompatibility complex (MHC) with subsequent abrogated expression (Zhao et al., 2018). The trafficking of CAR T cells can be enhanced using self-driving CARs, enabling cells to carry chemokine receptors for mediators released by target cells (Liu et al., 2020). Armored CARs can maintain efficiency in immunosuppressive microenvironments created by malignant cells by secreting cytokines or expressing soluble tethered ligands (Yeku and Brentjens, 2016; Yeku et al., 2017). Cells expressing self-destruct CARs comprise a safety switch with which apoptosis can be induced by administration of external signals (Straathof et al., 2005). On the contrary, conditional CARs require the administration of external signals to initiate their activity (Park et al., 2021).

CAR T-cell products approved by the FDA and most clinical trials consist of second generation CARs, whereas a lot of research is focusing on new-generation CARs. Their advantages lie in increasing the efficacy by modulating immune checkpoint pathways, the induction of cytokine secretion, or implementing safety-switch mechanism to control cytokine release syndrome (Tomasik et al., 2022).

Research findings

A study by Seif and colleagues in 2022 introduced a CAR engineered to recognize and redirect T cells against an epitope on the cell wall of *A. fumigatus* hyphae (Seif et al., 2022). The CAR utilizes a scFv from the AB90-E8 monoclonal antibody (mAb). Unlike CARs based on Dectin-1, the Af-CAR's design aims for specificity to *A. fumigatus* by targeting a conserved protein absent in other species. Af-CAR T cells have shown specific efficacy in identifying strains and clinical isolates of *A. fumigatus*, without targeting other *Aspergillus* species. The modified T cells demonstrate essential effector and helper T-cell functions, effectively combating fungal infections both in vitro and in vivo by releasing the cytotoxic mediators perforin and granzyme B. Upon encountering *A. fumigatus*, Af-CAR T cells release a range of cytokines indicative of a Th1 immune response, including GM-CSF, TNF-α, IFN-γ, and IL-2. The secretion of these cytokines leads to the recruitment and activation of macrophages, which play a crucial role in the immune response against fungal infections, as previously described. Moreover, the secreted cytokines are necessary to properly induce a pro-inflammatory state in macrophages. In an in vivo model of IPA in immunodeficient mice, Af-CAR T cells localized to the lungs, released perforin and various cytokines that enhance T-cell proliferation and cytolytic activity, and reduced fungal burden. Unlike antimycotics, which need to reach the lungs in a passive way and might therefore not reach suitable concentrations at the site of infection, Af-CAR T cells are recruited and actively migrate to the lungs (Denning and Hope, 2010; Zhao et al., 2019). Additionally, human chemokines secreted by Af-CAR T cells were detected, indicating the recruitment of mononuclear cells and neutrophils to the infection site, a key aspect of the protective immune response. Moreover, Seif and colleagues explored spacer design within the CAR structure, finding that a longer spacer enhances target recognition, essential for effective epitope binding. Furthermore, the transgenic T cells of the subgroups of $CD8^+$ and $CD4^+$ cells were investigated separately. $CD8^+$ Af-CAR T cells secreted perforin and granzyme B and damaged *A. fumigatus* hyphae. $CD8^+$ and $CD4^+$ Af-CAR T cells secreted cytokines in concentrations sufficient to activate other immune cells and potentiate their antifungal effect. In vivo, $CD8^+$ Af-CAR T cells were detected in the lungs at the site of infection; they engaged immune cells and reduced fungal burden in the lung. $CD4^+$ and $CD8^+$ T-cell treatment resulted in an improved overall survival.

In conclusion, in this study, an *A. fumigatus*-specific CAR was invented, successfully brought into T cells, redirecting them to recognize *A. fumigatus* hyphae and confer an antifungal effect. Additionally, Af-CAR T cells activated macrophages, which play an essential role in the clearance of fungus. These data show the potential of gene-engineered T cells for an adoptive add-on therapy for IPA (Seif et al., 2022).

Evaluation of literature

The study group that invented the first fungus-specific CAR T cell using a Dectin-1 targeting CAR recently published a new study, in which they used an mAb (AF-

269-5) as an scFv, comparable to the study of Seif and colleagues. In contrast, instead of using a nonviral system, they employed a lentiviral expression system for generating Af-CAR T cells. Nevertheless, these cells were also engineered to specifically target mature *A. fumigatus* hyphae. AF-CAR T cells enhanced persistence in the bloodstream and reduced immunotoxicity. The choice of the CD137/4-1BB costimulatory domain and the use of a lentiviral vector are highlighted as improvements over previous designs, aimed at boosting clinical-grade production efficiency and cell performance. Furthermore, the CAR triggers nuclear factor of activated T cells signaling in response to hyphal lysate, and cells subsequently produce functional cytokines, showcasing their potential to attack the fungus directly and stimulate a host immune response. Different cytokine expansion regimens were tested, all showing a type 1-prone polarization, minimizing the release of regulatory and type-2 T-cell cytokines. This indicates a strong antifungal effector response leading to combating fungal infections. In vivo experiments in an IPA model in immunocompromised mice, AF-CAR T cells demonstrated significant protection against *A. fumigatus*, even under severe immunosuppression and chemotherapy-induced neutropenia. In in vitro assays to study the hyphal length of *A. fumigatus*, it was shown that the CAR T cells reduced the mycelial growth. Furthermore, it was observed that the presence of caspofungin enhances the antifungal activity of AF-CAR T cells in vitro by delaying fungal growth and possibly increasing the antigen's accessibility. This suggests a synergistic potential between antifungal drugs and CAR T-cell therapy, offering a strategic advantage in treating fungal infections (Kumaresan et al., 2024).

Alternative bioengineering strategies

Besides engineering T cells to express CARs on their surface, T cells can be equipped with TCRs that recognize *A. fumigatus* antigens. This approach involves identifying and targeting peptides derived from fungal proteins that are presented on the surface of antigen-presenting cells. T-cell activation mediated through the TCR is dependent on the peptide presentation by human leukocyte antigen (HLA) molecules. TCRs can recognize a high number of fungal antigens, whereas CARs are limited to their scFv. Unlike TCRs that can recognize both surface and intracellular proteins, CARs are designed to identify cell-surface antigens exclusively (Chmielewski and Abken, 2012). The specific activation by a CAR, nevertheless, is not HLA restricted. The independence from the need for antigen processing and presentation by the HLA system makes CARs a more universally applicable option across diverse HLA patient groups (Sadelain et al., 2013). Another technique, successful in oncology, was translated into the field of IFD. Immune checkpoint inhibitors (ICIs) have been shown to enhance antifungal immunity by restoring T-cell responses (Daver and Kontoyiannis, 2017). There have been preclinical studies and clinical case reports that show that blockade of programmed cell death protein 1 (PD-1) immune checkpoint pathways works promisingly in adjunct immune enhancement in the treatment strategies for opportunistic fungal infections (Wurster et al., 2022). In an in vivo study exploring ICIs as immunotherapy for neutropenic IPA, anti-PD-1 checkpoint blockade significantly improved survival, reduced fungal burden, and enhanced secretion of pro-inflammatory cytokines and chemokines required for neutrophil recruitment in the lungs. Nevertheless, there remain concerns about potential hyperinflammatory toxicity, highlighting the importance of balancing immune activation and damage (Wurster et al., 2020). As reviewed in Wurster et al. (2022), PD-L1 inhibitors may provide more consistent protection than PD-1 inhibitors due to differences in immune modulation and the risk of inflammatory responses.

Moreover, Cenci and colleagues concluded over two decades ago that there might be *Aspergillus* antigens suitable for vaccination against IPA. The Th1-mediated resistance to IPA was proven in a mouse model (Cenci et al., 2000).

Challenges, limitations, and future perspectives

Several studies have shown that fungus-specific CAR T cells are a promising tool for the treatment of opportunistic fungal infections. Nevertheless, until now, most CAR T-cell products need to be generated autologously because of the risk of graft-versus-host disease (GvHD) when using allogeneic T cells. This process is time-consuming, and cells from severely ill patients might be compromised in function (Depil et al., 2020; Thommen and Schumacher, 2018). Since patients with rapidly progressing diseases, including IPA, need effective treatments urgently, the interest in allogeneic cell sources as off-the-shelf products is rising. This would potentially reduce costs and provide treatments readily available to a broader patient base without the need for individualized production (Depil et al., 2020).

New approaches, addressing these challenges in allogeneic CAR T-cell therapy, involve genome editing to eliminate T-cell alloreactivity by suppressing the expression of TCRs and/or MHC class I complexes (Zhao et al., 2018). This strategy aims to create "universal" CAR T cells, enabling large-scale manufacturing from healthy donors. UCART19, one such off-the-shelf CAR T-cell product, is currently in clinical trials for treating B-cell acute lymphoblastic leukemia (Benjamin et al., 2022).

Still, CAR T cells have already shown substantial protection in short-term mouse models, but clinically relevant questions remain, such as the optimal dosing, the integration with conventional antifungal treatments, and potential synergies with other underlying immunotherapies (Kumaresan et al., 2014, 2024; Seif et al., 2022).

Another alternative to T-cell therapies includes using other immune effector cells, such as NK cells, which possess high cytotoxic potential and a lower risk of GvHD in allogeneic settings (Albinger et al., 2021).

Conclusion

The rising number of patients at risk of developing IPA, caused by factors such as underlying viral infections as seen during the SARS-CoV-2 pandemic, or neutropenia after intensive chemotherapeutic treatment or immunotherapy, underlines the urgency for novel therapeutic strategies (Hoenigl et al., 2022; Latge and Chamilos, 2019). The effectiveness of standard antimycotic treatments is diminished by resistance, side effects, or insufficient immune response in certain groups (Denning and Hope, 2010). Immunomodulation emerges as a promising option, through the use of ICIs that enhance anti-*Aspergillus* responses (Daver and Kontoyiannis, 2017). However, diminished immune cell counts, as in severe lymphopenia after alloSCT, limit the efficacy of these approaches. Furthermore, adoptive T-cell transfer was already shown to have great potential to treat patients with IA (Bacher et al., 2015). The effective activation of antigen-specific adaptive immune responses is dependent on the activation of pathogen-detection mechanisms of the innate immune system. This PRR activation, on the other hand, might cause tissue damage because of severe inflammation and therefore promote infection or might not be present in patients that have illnesses, such as neutropenia and granulomatous (Romani, 2011). Therefore we suggest the adoptive transfer of CAR T cells, which are activated by fungal recognition without the need for other immune cells, as highly beneficial. CARs can redirect T-cell activity to a specific target. Previously, it was shown that Dectin-1 CAR T cells are effective against *A. fumigatus* in an IPA mouse model. But this CAR might also target commensal fungi (Kumaresan et al., 2014). Therefore our group designed a CAR whose scFv consists of a mAb derived from a conserved cell wall antigen on *A. fumigatus*, which was shown to be highly specific. In animal models, this CAR T-cell product showed very promising results and shows an opportunity to improve the treatment for patients suffering from IA (Seif et al., 2022). However, obstacles such as the production times under good manufacturing practice conditions remain significant challenges, particularly for an acute infection requiring rapid treatment. A potential solution lies in allogeneic, off-the-shelf CAR products, such as universal T cells or other efficacious immune cell types, such as NK cells, which have demonstrated potential in cancer treatment and are already being explored in clinical trials (Albinger et al., 2021). In conclusion, combining innovative therapies such as CAR-T or NK-cell therapies with existing antifungal treatments could offer a synergistic approach, potentially overcoming the limitations of current strategies and markedly enhancing patient outcomes in IPA.

AI disclosure

During the preparation of this work, the author(s) used ChatGPT 4 in order to improve readability and language edits. After using this tool/service, the author(s) reviewed and edited the content as needed and take(s) full responsibility for the content of the publication.

References

Ademe, M., 2020. Immunomodulation for the treatment of fungal infections: opportunities and challenges. Frontiers in Cellular and Infection Microbiology 10. Available at https://doi.org/10.3389/fcimb.2020.00469.

Albinger, N., Hartmann, J., Ullrich, E., 2021. Current status and perspective of CAR-T and CAR-NK cell therapy trials in Germany. Gene Therapy 28 (9), 513–527. Available at https://doi.org/10.1038/s41434-021-00246-w.

Bacher, P., Jochheim-Richter, A., Mockel-Tenbrink, N., Kniemeyer, O., Wingenfeld, E., Alex, R., et al., 2015. Clinical-scale isolation of the total *Aspergillus fumigatus*-reactive T-helper cell repertoire for adoptive transfer. Cytotherapy 17 (10), 1396–1405. Available at https://doi.org/10.1016/j.jcyt.2015.05.011, http://www.journals.elsevier.com/cytotherapy.

Benjamin, R., Jain, N., Maus, M.V., Boissel, N., Graham, C., Jozwik, A., et al., 2022. UCART19, a first-in-class allogeneic anti-CD19 chimeric antigen receptor T-cell therapy for adults with relapsed or refractory B-cell acute lymphoblastic leukaemia (CALM): a phase 1, dose-escalation trial. The Lancet Haematology 9 (11), e833. Available at https://doi.org/10.1016/S2352-3026(22)00245-9, http://www.journals.elsevier.com/the-lancet-haematology/.

Bozza, S., Perruccio, K., Montagnoli, C., Gaziano, R., Bellocchio, S., Burchielli, E., et al., 2003. A dendritic cell vaccine against invasive aspergillosis in allogeneic hematopoietic transplantation. Blood 102 (10), 3807–3814. Available at https://doi.org/10.1182/blood-2003-03-0748.

Brakhage, A.A., Bruns, S., Thywissen, A., Zipfel, P.F., Behnsen, J., 2010. Interaction of phagocytes with filamentous fungi. Current Opinion in Microbiology 13 (4), 409–415. Available at https://doi.org/10.1016/j.mib.2010.04.009.

Bruns, S., Kniemeyer, O., Hasenberg, M., Aimanianda, V., Nietzsche, S., Thywien, A., et al., 2010. Production of extracellular traps against *Aspergillus fumigatus* in vitro and in infected lung tissue is dependent on invading neutrophils and influenced by hydrophobin roda. PLoS Pathogens 6 (4), 1–18. Available at https://doi.org/10.1371/journal.ppat.1000873, http://www.plospathogens.org/article/fetchObjectAttachment.action?uri=info%3Adoi%2F10.1371%2Fjournal.ppat.1000873&representation=PDF.

Cenci, E., Mencacci, A., Bacci, A., Bistoni, F., Kurup, V.P., Romani, L., 2000. T cell vaccination in mice with invasive pulmonary aspergillosis. Journal of Immunology 165 (1), 381–388. Available at https://doi.org/10.4049/jimmunol.165.1.381, http://www.jimmunol.org/.

Chmielewski, M., Abken, H., 2012. CAR T cells transform to trucks: chimeric antigen receptor–redirected T cells engineered to deliver inducible IL-12 modulate the tumour stroma to combat cancer. Cancer Immunology, Immunotherapy 61 (8), 1269–1277. Available at https://doi.org/10.1007/s00262-012-1202-z.

Daver, N., Kontoyiannis, D.P., 2017. Checkpoint inhibitors and aspergillosis in AML: the double hit hypothesis. The Lancet Oncology 18 (12), 1571–1573. Available at https://doi.org/10.1016/S1470-2045(17)30852-5, http://www.journals.elsevier.com/the-lancet-oncology/.

Denning, D.W., Hope, W.W., 2010. Therapy for fungal diseases: opportunities and priorities. Trends in Microbiology 18 (5), 195–204. Available at https://doi.org/10.1016/j.tim.2010.02.004.

Deo, S.S., Gottlieb, D.J., 2015. Adoptive T-cell therapy for fungal infections in haematology patients. Clinical and Translational Immunology 4 (8). Available at https://doi.org/10.1038/cti.2015.16, https://onlinelibrary.wiley.com/loi/20500068.

Depil, S., Duchateau, P., Grupp, S.A., Mufti, G., Poirot, L., 2020. Off-the-shelf' allogeneic CAR T cells: development and challenges. Nature Reviews. Drug Discovery 19 (3), 185–199. Available at https://doi.org/10.1038/s41573-019-0051-2.

Gellin, B., Modlin, J.F., Casadevall, A., Pirofski, L.A., 2001. Adjunctive immune therapy for fungal infections. Clinical Infectious Diseases 33 (7), 1048–1056.

Guedan, S., Calderon, H., Posey, A.D., Maus, M.V., 2019. Engineering and design of chimeric antigen receptors. Molecular Therapy Methods and Clinical Development 12, 145–156. Available at https://doi.org/10.1016/j.omtm.2018.12.009, https://www.journals.elsevier.com/molecular-therapy-methods-and-clinical-development/.

Hebart, H., Bollinger, C., Fisch, P., Sarfati, J., Meisner, C., Baur, M., et al., 2002. Analysis of T-cell responses to *Aspergillus fumigatus* antigens in healthy individuals and patients with hematologic malignancies. Blood 100 (13), 4521–4528. Available at https://doi.org/10.1182/blood-2002-01-0265, https://www.journals.elsevier.com/blood.

Hoenigl, M., Seidel, D., Sprute, R., Cunha, C., Oliverio, M., Goldman, G.H., et al., 2022. COVID-19-associated fungal infections. Nature Microbiology 7 (8), 1127–1140. Available at https://doi.org/10.1038/s41564-022-01172-2, www.nature.com/nmicrobiol/.

Jolink, H., Hagedoorn, R.S., Lagendijk, E.L., Drijfhout, J.W., van Dissel, J.T., Falkenburg, J.H.F., et al., 2014. Induction of A. fumigatus-specific CD4-positive T cells in patients recovering from invasive aspergillosis. Haematologica 99 (7), 1255–1263. Available at https://doi.org/10.3324/haematol.2013.098830.

Kumaresan, P.R., Manuri, P.R., Albert, N.D., Maiti, S., Singh, H., Mi, T., et al., 2014. Bioengineering T cells to target carbohydrate to treat opportunistic fungal infection. Proceedings of the National Academy of Sciences of the United States of America 111 (29), 10660–10665. Available at https://doi.org/10.1073/pnas.1312789111, http://www.pnas.org/content/111/29/10660.full.pdf+html.

Kumaresan, P.R., Wurster, S., Bavisi, K., da Silva, T.A., Hauser, P., Kinnitt, J., et al., 2024. A novel lentiviral vector-based approach to generate chimeric antigen receptor T cells targeting *Aspergillus fumigatus*. mBio 15 (4). Available at https://doi.org/10.1128/mbio.03413-23, https://journals.asm.org/toc/mbio/current.

Latge, J.P., Chamilos, G., 2019. *Aspergillus fumigatus* and aspergillosis in 2019. Clinical Microbiology Reviews 33 (1). Available at https://doi.org/10.1128/CMR.00140-18.

Latgé, J.-P., 2001. The pathobiology of *Aspergillus fumigatus*. Trends in Microbiology 9 (8), 382–389. Available at https://doi.org/10.1016/s0966-842x(01)02104-7.

Lin, S.-J., Schranz, J., Teutsch, S.M., 2001. Aspergillosis case-fatality rate: systematic review of the literature. Clinical Infectious Diseases 32 (3), 358–366. Available at https://doi.org/10.1086/318483.

Liu, G., Rui, W., Zheng, H., Huang, D., Yu, F., Zhang, Y., et al., 2020. CXCR2-modified CAR-T cells have enhanced trafficking ability that improves treatment of hepatocellular carcinoma. European Journal of Immunology 50 (5), 712–724. Available at https://doi.org/10.1002/eji.201948457.

Maldini, C.R., Ellis, G.I., Riley, J.L., 2018. CAR T cells for infection, autoimmunity and allotransplantation. Nature Reviews. Immunology 18 (10), 605–616. Available at https://doi.org/10.1038/s41577-018-0042-2, http://www.nature.com/nri/index.html.

Papadopoulou, A., Kaloyannidis, P., Yannaki, E., Cruz, C.R., 2016. Adoptive transfer of *Aspergillus*-specific T cells as a novel anti-fungal therapy for hematopoietic stem cell transplant recipients: progress and challenges. Critical Reviews in Oncology/Hematology 98, 62–72. Available at https://doi.org/10.1016/j.critrevonc.2015.10.005, www.elsevier.com/locate/critrevonc.

Park, S., Pascua, E., Lindquist, K.C., Kimberlin, C., Deng, X., Mak, Y.S.L., et al., 2021. Direct control of CAR T cells through small molecule-regulated antibodies. Nature Communications 12 (1). Available at https://doi.org/10.1038/s41467-020-20671-6, http://www.nature.com/ncomms/index.html.

Park, S.J., Hughes, M.A., Burdick, M., Strieter, R.M., Mehrad, B., 2009. Early NK cell-derived IFN-γ is essential to host defense in neutropenic invasive aspergillosis. Journal of Immunology 182 (7), 4306–4312. Available at https://doi.org/10.4049/jimmunol.0803462, http://www.jimmunol.org/cgi/reprint/182/7/4306.

Patterson, T.F., Thompson, G.R., Denning, D.W., Fishman, J.A., Hadley, S., Herbrecht, R., et al., 2016. Practice guidelines for the diagnosis and management of aspergillosis: 2016 update by the infectious diseases society of America. Clinical Infectious Diseases 63 (4), e1. Available at https://doi.org/10.1093/cid/ciw326, http://cid.oxfordjournals.org/content/by/year.

Perruccio, K., Tosti, A., Burchielli, E., Topini, F., Ruggeri, L., Carotti, A., et al., 2005. Transferring functional immune responses to pathogens after haploidentical hematopoietic transplantation. Blood 106 (13), 4397–4406. Available at https://doi.org/10.1182/blood-2005-05-1775, http://www.bloodjournal.org/cgi/reprint/106/13/4397.

Ramos, C.A., Rouce, R., Robertson, C.S., Reyna, A., Narala, N., Vyas, G., et al., 2018. In vivo fate and activity of second- versus third-generation CD19-specific CAR-T cells in B cell non-hodgkin's lymphomas. Molecular Therapy 26 (12), 2727–2737. Available at https://doi.org/10.1016/j.ymthe.2018.09.009, https://www.journals.elsevier.com/molecular-therapy.

Romani, L., 2011. Immunity to fungal infections. Nature Reviews. Immunology 11 (4), 275–288. Available at https://doi.org/10.1038/nri2939.

Roselli, E., Boucher, J.C., Li, G., Kotani, H., Spitler, K., Reid, K., et al., 2021. 4-1BB and optimized CD28 co-stimulation enhances function of human mono-specific and bi-specific third-generation CAR T cells. Journal for ImmunoTherapy of Cancer 9 (10). Available at https://doi.org/10.1136/jitc-2021-003354, http://www.immunotherapyofcancer.org/.

Sadelain, M., Brentjens, R., Rivière, I., 2013. The basic principles of chimeric antigen receptor design. Cancer Discovery 3 (4), 388–398. Available at https://doi.org/10.1158/2159-8290.CD-12-0548, http://cancerdiscovery.aacrjournals.org/content/3/4/388.full.pdf+html.

Salazar, F., Bignell, E., Brown, G.D., Cook, P.C., Warris, A., 2022. Pathogenesis of respiratory viral and fungal coinfections. Clinical Microbiology Reviews 35 (1). Available at https://doi.org/10.1128/CMR.00094-21, https://journals.asm.org/doi/10.1128/CMR.00094-21.

Sam, Q.H., Yew, W.S., Seneviratne, C.J., Chang, M.W., Chai, L.Y.A., 2018. Immunomodulation as therapy for fungal infection: are we closer? Frontiers in Microbiology 9. Available at https://doi.org/10.3389/fmicb.2018.01612, https://www.frontiersin.org/articles/10.3389/fmicb.2018.01612/full.

Seif, M., Einsele, H., Löffler, J., 2019. CAR T cells beyond cancer: hope for immunomodulatory therapy of infectious diseases. Frontiers in Immunology 10. Available at https://doi.org/10.3389/fimmu.2019.02711, https://www.frontiersin.org/journals/immunology#.

Seif, M., Kakoschke, T.K., Ebel, F., Bellet, M.M., Trinks, N., Renga, G., et al., 2022. CAR T cells targeting *Aspergillus fumigatus* are effective at treating invasive pulmonary aspergillosis in preclinical models. Science Translational Medicine 14 (664). Available at https://doi.org/10.1126/scitranslmed.abh1209, https://www.science.org/doi/10.1126/scitranslmed.abh1209.

Straathof, K.C., Pulè, M.A., Yotnda, P., Dotti, G., Vanin, E.F., Brenner, M.K., et al., 2005. An inducible caspase 9 safety switch for T-cell therapy. Blood 105 (11), 4247–4254. Available at https://doi.org/10.1182/blood-2004-11-4564, https://www.journals.elsevier.com/blood.

Tappe, B., Lauruschkat, C.D., Strobel, L., Pantaleón García, J., Kurzai, O., Rebhan, S., et al., 2022. COVID-19 patients share common, corticosteroid-independent features of impaired host immunity to pathogenic molds. Frontiers in Immunology 13. Available at https://doi.org/10.3389/fimmu.2022.954985, https://www.frontiersin.org/journals/immunology#.

Thammasit, P., Sripetchwandee, J., Nosanchuk, J.D., Chattipakorn, S.C., Chattipakorn, N., Youngchim, S., 2021. Cytokine and chemokine responses in invasive aspergillosis following hematopoietic stem cell transplantation: past evidence for future therapy of aspergillosis. Journal of Fungi 7 (9). Available at https://doi.org/10.3390/jof7090753, https://www.mdpi.com/2309-608X/7/9/753/pdf.

Thommen, D.S., Schumacher, T.N., 2018. T cell dysfunction in cancer. Cancer Cell 33 (4), 547–562. Available at https://doi.org/10.1016/j.ccell.2018.03.012, https://www.journals.elsevier.com/cancer-cell.

Tomasik, J., Jasiński, M., Basak, G.W., 2022. Next generations of CAR-T cells - new therapeutic opportunities in hematology? Frontiers in Immunology 13. Available at https://doi.org/10.3389/fimmu.2022.1034707, https://www.frontiersin.org/journals/immunology#.

van der Stegen, S.J.C., Hamieh, M., Sadelain, M., 2015. The pharmacology of second-generation chimeric antigen receptors. Nature Reviews. Drug Discovery 14 (7), 499–509. Available at https://doi.org/10.1038/nrd4597.

Van De Veerdonk, F.L., Gresnigt, M.S., Romani, L., Netea, M.G., Latgé, J.P., 2017. *Aspergillus fumigatus* morphology and dynamic host interactions. Nature Reviews. Microbiology 15 (11), 661–674. Available at https://doi.org/10.1038/nrmicro.2017.90, http://www.nature.com/nrmicro/index.html.

Vitiello, A., Ferrara, F., Boccellino, M., Ponzo, A., Cimmino, C., Comberiati, E., et al., 2023. Antifungal drug resistance: an emergent health threat. Biomedicines 11 (4), 1063. Available at https://doi.org/10.3390/biomedicines11041063.

Wang, C., Sun, W., Ye, Y., Bomba, H.N., Gu, Z., 2017. Bioengineering of artificial antigen presenting cells and lymphoid organs. Theranostics 7 (14), 3504–3516. Available at https://doi.org/10.7150/thno.19017, http://www.thno.org/v07p3504.pdf.

Weiss, E., Ziegler, S., Fliesser, M., Schmitt, A.L., Hünniger, K., Kurzai, O., et al., 2018. First insights in NK-DC cross-talk and the importance of soluble factors during infection with *Aspergillus fumigatus*. Frontiers in Cellular and Infection Microbiology 8. Available at https://doi.org/10.3389/fcimb.2018.00288, https://www.frontiersin.org/articles/10.3389/fcimb.2018.00288/full.

Wu, L., Wei, Q., Brzostek, J., Gascoigne, N.R.J., 2020. Signaling from T cell receptors (TCRs) and chimeric antigen receptors (CARs) on T cells. Cellular and Molecular Immunology 17 (6), 600–612. Available at https://doi.org/10.1038/s41423-020-0470-3, http://www.nature.com/cmi/archive/index.html.

Wurster, S., Robinson, P., Albert, N.D., Tarrand, J.J., Goff, M., Swamydas, M., et al., 2020. Protective activity of programmed cell death protein 1 blockade and synergy with caspofungin in a murine invasive pulmonary aspergillosis model. Journal of Infectious Diseases 222 (6), 989–994. Available at https://doi.org/10.1093/infdis/jiaa264, http://jid.oxfordjournals.org/content/current.

Wurster, S., Watowich, S.S., Kontoyiannis, D.P., 2022. Checkpoint inhibitors as immunotherapy for fungal infections: promises, challenges, and unanswered questions. Frontiers in Immunology 13. Available at https://doi.org/10.3389/fimmu.2022.1018202, https://www.frontiersin.org/journals/immunology#.

Yeku, O.O., Purdon, T.J., Koneru, M., Spriggs, D., Brentjens, R.J., 2017. Armored CAR T cells enhance antitumor efficacy and overcome the tumor microenvironment. Scientific Reports 7 (1). Available at https://doi.org/10.1038/s41598-017-10940-8, www.nature.com/srep/index.html.

Yeku, O.O., Brentjens, R.J., 2016. Armored CAR T-cells: utilizing cytokines and pro-inflammatory ligands to enhance CAR T-cell anti-tumour efficacy. Biochemical Society Transactions 44 (2), 412–418. Available at https://doi.org/10.1042/bst20150291.

Zhao, J., Lin, Q., Song, Y., Liu, D., 2018. Universal CARs, universal T cells, and universal CAR T cells. Journal of Hematology & Oncology 11 (1). Available at https://doi.org/10.1186/s13045-018-0677-2.

Zhao, Y., Prideaux, B., Baistrocchi, S., Sheppard, D.C., Perlin, D.S., 2019. Beyond tissue concentrations: antifungal penetration at the site of infection. Medical Mycology 57, S161. Available at https://doi.org/10.1093/mmy/myy067, https://mmy.oxfordjournals.org/.

Index

Note: Page numbers followed by "*f*" and "*t*" refer to figures and tables, respectively.

K

L

M

N

9780443236365